Safeguarding

The Critically Ill

ISCCM
INDIAN SOCIETY OF
CRITICAL CARE MEDICINE

Safeguarding

The Critically Ill

Editors

Pradip Kumar Bhattacharya
MD ACME FICCM FCCCM FCCM
Professor and Head
Department of Critical Care Medicine
In-Charge (Trauma and Emergency)
Dean Research and PhD Coordinator
Rajendra Institute of Medical Sciences (RIMS)
Ranchi, Jharkhand, India
Immediate Past President, ISCCM National (2025–2026)

Bharat G Jagiasi
MD FICCM IDCCM
Director
Department of Critical Care
Kokilaben Dhirubhai Ambani Hospital
Navi Mumbai, Maharashtra, India
General Secretary, ISCCM (2024–2025)

JAYPEE BROTHERS MEDICAL PUBLISHERS
The Health Sciences Publisher
New Delhi | London

JAYPEE **Jaypee Brothers Medical Publishers (P) Ltd.**

Headquarters
EMCA House, 23/23-B
Ansari Road, Daryaganj
New Delhi 110 002, India
Landline: +91-11-23272143, +91-11-23272703
+91-11-23282021, +91-11-23245672
e-mail: jaypee@jaypeebrothers.com

Corporate Office
4838/24, Ansari Road, Daryaganj
New Delhi 110 002, India
Phone: +91-11-43574357
Fax: +91-11-43574314
e-mail: jaypee@jaypeebrothers.com

Overseas Office
JP Medical Ltd
83 Victoria Street, London
SW1H 0HW (UK)
Phone: +44-20 3170 8910
e-mail: info@jpmedpub.com

EU GPSR Authorised Representative
Logos Europe, 9 rue Nicolas Poussin
17000, La Rochelle, France
Phone: +33 (0) 6 67 93 73 78
e-mail: contact@logoseurope.eu

Website: www.jaypeebrothers.com
Website: www.jaypeedigital.com

Inquiries for bulk sales may be solicited at: jaypee@jaypeebrothers.com

Safeguarding: The Critically Ill

First Edition: **2026**

ISBN: 978-93-6616-874-6

Printed at: Samrat Offset Pvt. Ltd.

Dedication

I dedicate this book to the esteemed authors whose expertise and dedication have illuminated the complexities of critical care for infectious diseases. Your contributions have transformed this project into a comprehensive and invaluable resource.

I sincerely appreciate Dr Bharat G Jagiasi's tireless dedication and unwavering commitment to bringing this book to fruition.

I am deeply grateful to my inspiring teachers who instilled in me the foundations of medical knowledge and ignited my passion for learning. Your guidance continues to shape my practice and inspire my pursuit of excellence.

To my loving family, whose unwavering support, patience, and understanding have been my constant source of strength. Your sacrifices and encouragement have allowed me to pursue my professional aspirations.

I am deeply grateful to my dedicated colleagues and peers, whose collaborative spirit and shared commitment to patient care have enriched my professional life. Your insights and support have been invaluable in navigating the challenges of critical care.

Most importantly, the patients are the true heroes of this story. Your resilience in the face of adversity and your trust in our care have been the driving forces behind this work. Because of you, we strive to advance our knowledge and improve the outcomes of critical illness.

May this book serve as a testament to the collective effort and unwavering dedication of all those who strive to safeguard the critically ill.

Pradip Kumar Bhattacharya

To the Supreme Power, whose grace and guidance have illuminated my path;

To my parents and sisters, who have been my guiding light;

To my wife, Anaya, and my son, Atiksh, for their love, patience, and sacrifices;

To all those striving to make ICUs safer for patients worldwide;

And to the many kind souls whose unseen support has been a source of strength during this journey.

Bharat G Jagiasi

Section Editors

Aruna Poojary
MD DNB (Micro) D (ABMM) DipHIC (UK)
CIC (USA) DipRCpath
Lab Director
Department of Pathology and
Microbiology
Breach Candy Hospital Trust
Mumbai, Maharashtra, India

Binila Chacko
MBBS MD DNB DM (Critical Care) FICCM FCICM
Professor and Head
Department of Critical Care Medicine
Christian Medical College
Vellore, Tamil Nadu, India

Nishant Kumar
DA DNB MNAMS
Professor of Anesthesiology
Department of Anesthesiology and
Critical Care
Lady Hardinge Medical College and
SSK and KSC Hospitals
New Delhi, India

Contributors

Afreen Kidwai Abdul Razak
MBBS DNB DrNB
Associate Consultant
Department of Critical Care
Sindhu Hospital
Hyderabad, Telangana, India

Amarja Ashok Havaldar MBBS MD
PDF (Neuroanesthesia) DNB DM FNB EDIC
PGDMLE (NLSIU)
Associate Professor
Department of Critical Care Medicine
St John's Medical College
Bengaluru, Karnataka, India

Anu Prasad MBBS MD FNB
Consultant
Department of Critical Care Medicine
Tata Main Hospital
Jamshedpur, Jharkhand, India

Archana Srivastava
MBBS DA IDCCM IFCCM EDICM
Head
Department of Critical Care and
Emergency
MGM New Bombay Hospital
Navi Mumbai, Maharashtra, India

Asif Ahmed MBBS DNB (Gold Medal)
IDCCM FICCM
Consultant and Head
Department of Critical Care Medicine
Tata Main Hospital
Jamshedpur, Jharkhand, India

Bhavna Sunil Ghewari
Basic BSc Nursing
Staff Nurse
Department of Infection Control Team
Breach Candy Hospital Trust
Mumbai, Maharashtra, India

Bhuvna Ahuja MBBS MD
Assistant Professor
Neuroanesthesia and Neurocritical
Care Unit
Department of Neurosurgery
Lok Nayak Hospital
New Delhi, India

Biswabikash Mohanty
MBBS MD DrNB (Critical Care Medicine)
Associate Consultant
Department of Critical Care Medicine
Apollo Multispeciality Hospital
Kolkata, West Bengal, India

Debottam Gangopadhyay
MBBS MD DrNB (Critical Care Medicine)
Associate Consultant
Department of Critical Care Medicine
Apollo Multispeciality Hospital
Kolkata, West Bengal, India

Dipanjan Hojai MBBS (IPGMER, Kolkata)
DA (KEM, Mumbai) DNB DrNB Critical Care
Medicine Academic Registrar
Department of Critical Care Medicine
Apollo Multispecialty Hospital
Kolkata, West Bengal, India

Gyanendra Agarwal
MBBS MD (Internal Medicine)
DM (Pulmonary and Critical Care Medicine)
Director
Department of Pulmonary and Critical
Care Medicine
Max Superspecialty Hospital
Noida, Uttar Pradesh, India

Kamal P Bhutada
MBBS MD DNB (Med) MNAMS IDCCM EDIC
Senior Physician and Critical Care
Consultant
Director of ICU
Department of Critical Care
CARE Hospital
Nagpur, Maharashtra, India

Krishna K Chaitanya
MBBS MD (Anesthesia)
DrNB (Critical Care Medicine)
Associate Consultant
Department of Critical Care
Sindhu Hospitals
Hyderabad, Telangana, India

Kuldeep Singh MBBS MD DrNB CCM
Associate Consultant
Department of Critical Care Medical
Max Hospital
Ghaziabad, Uttar Pradesh, India

Mahajyoti Chakravorty MBBS DNB
Consultant
Department of Critical Care Medicine
Tata Main Hospital
Jamshedpur, Jharkhand, India

Monalisa Mishra
MBBS MD FNB (Critical Care Medicine)
Consultant Critical Care
Department of Critical Care Medicine
Apollo Multispecialty Hospital
Kolkata, West Bengal, India

Naseema Shaik
MBBS MD (Microbiology)
Associate Professor
Department of Microbiology
NRI Medical College
Guntur, Andhra Pradesh, India

Nishant Sahay MBBS DNB
Professor
Department of Anesthesia and
Critical Care
All India Institute of Medical Sciences
Patna, Bihar, India

Poonam Gupta
MBBS MD (Microbiology) PGDHCM
Lab Head and Lead Consultant
(Microbiology and Infection Prevention)
Kokilaben Dhirubhai Ambani Hospital
Navi Mumbai, Maharashtra, India

Pradeep Kumar Bhatia
MBBS MD FICCM FICA
Professor and Head
Department of Anesthesiology
and Critical Care
All India Institute of Medical Sciences
Jodhpur, Rajasthan, India

Prashant Narayan Walse MBBS MD
DNB (Medicine) IDCCM IFCCM EDIC
Consultant Physician and Intensive
Department of Medicine and
Critical Care
Asian Citicare Superspeciality Hospital
Chhatrapati Sambhaji Nagar
Maharashtra, India

Priyanka H Chhabra MBBS MD DNB
Associate Professor
Department of Anesthesia and
Intensive Care
Vardhman Mahavir Medical College
and Safdarjung Hospital
New Delhi, India

Priyanka Patil BHMS MBA (HCA) CIC
Senior Infection Control Officer
Department of Pathology and
Microbiology
Breach Candy Hospital Trust
Mumbai, Maharashtra, India

Rachana Ambarkar MBBS MD
Senior Resident
Department of Microbiology
Lokmanya Tilak Municipal Medical
College and General Hospital
Mumbai, Maharashtra, India

Rajesh Kumar
MBBS DA MD (Anesthesiology)
Assistant Professor
Department of Anesthesia and
Critical Care
All India Institute of Medical Sciences
Patna, Bihar, India

Sadik Mohammed MBBS MD
Additional Professor
Department of Anesthesiology and Critical Care
All India Institute of Medical Sciences
Jodhpur, Rajasthan, India

Sahil Diwan MBBS MD DNB
Professor, Department of Anesthesia and Intensive Care
Vardhman Mahavir Medical College and Safdarjung Hospital
New Delhi, India

Samvveda Shirish Samel
MBBS MD DNB (General Medicine)
Consultant
Department of General Medicine
Samveda Clinic
Mumbai, Maharashtra, India

Saswati Sinha
MBBS MD (Medicine) IDCCM EDIC
Senior Consultant
Department of Critical Care
Manipal Hospitals
Kolkata, West Bengal, India

Shaik Arif Pasha MBBS MD IDCCM FICCM (NIMS) FCCM (ICCCM) EDIC
Professor and Head
Department of Critical Care Medicine
NRI Medical College
Guntur, Andhra Pradesh, India

Shailesh Kumar Sahu
MBBS MD PDCC DrNB (Critical Care Medicine)
Consultant
Department of Critical Care Medicine
Jaiprakash Hospital and Research Centre
Rourkela, Odisha, India

(Lt Col) Shibu Sasidharan
MBBS MD DNB EDIC MRCA (UK) MRCEM (UK) MNAMS
Consultant in Anesthesiology, Critical Care Medicine, and Emergency Medicine
Department of Anesthesiology and Critical Care
Base Hospital, Delhi Cantt
New Delhi, India

Shripad Taklikar MBBS MD
Professor Additional
Department of Microbiology
Lokmanya Tilak Municipal Medical College and General Hospital
Mumbai, Maharashtra, India

Siva Prabodh Vuddandi
MBBS MD (Biochemistry)
Professor and Head
Department of Biochemistry
NRI Medical College
Guntur, Andhra Pradesh, India

Smita Sharma MBBS MD IDCCM
Senior Consultant, Department of Pulmonary and Critical Care Medicine
Max Superspecialty Hospital
Noida, Uttar Pradesh, India

Sneha Johnson BSc Nursing
International Infection Prevention and Control Certificate Course (IIPCC)
Senior Staff Nurse
(Infection Control Nurse)
Department of Infection Control Team
Breach Candy Hospital Trust
Mumbai, Maharashtra, India

Srikant Behera
MBBS MD PDCC DM (Critical Care Medicine)
Assistant Professor
Department of Medicine
All India Institute of Medical Sciences
Bhubaneswar, Odisha, India

Srinivas Samavedam MBBS MD DNB FRCP FNB EDIC FICCM MBA
Chief Intensivist
Department of Critical Care
Ramdev Rao Hospital
Hyderabad, Telangana, India

Subhash Todi MBBS MD (Medicine) MRCP
Director, Department of Critical Care
Manipal Hospitals
Kolkata, West Bengal, India
Head, Department of Academics and Research
Manipal Hospital
Past Research Chairperson, ISCCM Research Committee

Suresh Ramasubbaman
AB-Internal-Medicine/Pulmonary/CCM
Senior Consultant
Department of Pulmonary and CCM
Apollo Multispecialty Hospitals
Kolkata, West Bengal, India

Suryasnata Das MBBS MD (Microbiology)
Director
Department of Laboratory Medicine
Max Superspecialty Hospital
Noida, Uttar Pradesh, India

Susovan Mitra
MBBS MD MRCP (London) FCCM SCE-RCP-Geriatric Medicine (Cal)
Consultant
Intensive Care Unit/Critical Care Medicine
Gericare Hospital
Chennai, Tamil Nadu, India

Swapna Khanzode MBBS DNB (Internal Medicine) IDCC FIDM
Consultant Medicine and Critical Care
Department of Internal Medicine and Critical Care
Ketki Research Institute of Medical Sciences
Nagpur, Maharashtra, India
American Oncology Institute
Nagpur, Maharashtra, India

Swati Singh MBBS MD
Senior Resident (Neuroanesthesia and Neurocritical Care Unit)
Department of Neurosurgery
Lok Nayak Hospital
New Delhi, India

Vrunda Vijay Agre MBBS CCTM
Associate Consultant
Department of Critical Care
Kokilaben Dhirubhai Ambani Hospital
Navi Mumbai, Maharashtra, India

Yasmin Muhammed
MBBS MD (Microbiology)
Junior Consultant
Department of Microbiology
Base Hospital, Delhi Cantt
New Delhi, India

Preface

Life-threatening challenges confront the most vulnerable patients in the Critical Care Unit. Infections, particularly those caused by resistant organisms and those affecting immunocompromised individuals, pose a formidable threat. *Safeguarding: The Critically Ill* is born from the urgent need to equip clinicians with the most current and effective strategies to combat and control these complex infections.

This book is not merely a compilation of information but a collaborative effort, a synthesis of expertise from some of our country's brightest minds. Recognizing the multifaceted nature of infectious diseases in the Critical Care Unit, I have carefully selected authors who are leaders in their respective fields, ensuring that each chapter reflects the most up-to-date knowledge and best practices.

Our goal is to create a complete guide covering all types of infections seen in the critical care unit, from common bacterial infections to the most challenging cases involving organisms resistant to multiple drugs and infections in people with weak immune systems. We delve into the intricacies of diagnosis, treatment, and prevention, offering practical guidance that can be readily applied at the bedside.

The challenges of managing critically ill patients with infections are ever-evolving. New pathogens emerge, resistance patterns shift, and the landscape of critical care continues to transform. I sincerely hope that *Safeguarding: The Critically Ill* will serve as a valuable tool for intensivists, infectious disease specialists, nurses, and all healthcare professionals dedicated to improving the outcomes of these vulnerable patients.

I extend my deepest gratitude to the esteemed authors who have contributed their expertise to this project. Their dedication and commitment to advancing the field of critical care infectious diseases have made this book possible.

This work is dedicated to the patients we serve and to the tireless efforts of all those who strive to protect them from the devastating impact of infection.

Pradip Kumar Bhattacharya

Preface

Acknowledgments

I extend my deepest gratitude to my teachers, whose knowledge and mentorship have been instrumental in shaping my understanding of infection prevention in critical care. Their guidance has been invaluable throughout my journey.

I am sincerely grateful to Professor Pradip Kumar Bhattacharya, President of ISCCM (2024–2025), for giving me this opportunity and for his leadership in advancing critical care in India. His support has been instrumental in bringing this book to life.

A heartfelt thanks to Dr Aruna Poojary, whose unwavering support and encouragement during the formulation of this book played a crucial role in its development.

Above all, I am profoundly thankful to my parents, my sisters, my family, and my wife, Anaya, and son, Atiksh, for their patience and understanding. Their support allowed me to dedicate time to this book, often at the cost of family moments.

To all my colleagues and mentors who contributed in ways big and small—thank you. This book is a reflection of your influence, and I hope it serves as a valuable resource in advancing infection prevention in the ICU.

I would also like to acknowledge the countless acts of kindness and encouragement I received along the way. Each of them, often unnoticed, played a part in bringing this book to completion.

Bharat G Jagiasi

Contents

SECTION 4: Multidrug-resistant Organisms and Antibiotic Stewardship

Section Editor: *Nishant Kumar*

SECTION 5: Special Considerations in Infection Control

Section Editor: *Nishant Kumar*

SECTION 6: Innovations and Future Directions

Section Editor: *Binila Chacko*

SECTION 7: Practical Tools and Appendices

Section Editor: *Aruna Poojary*

Plate 1

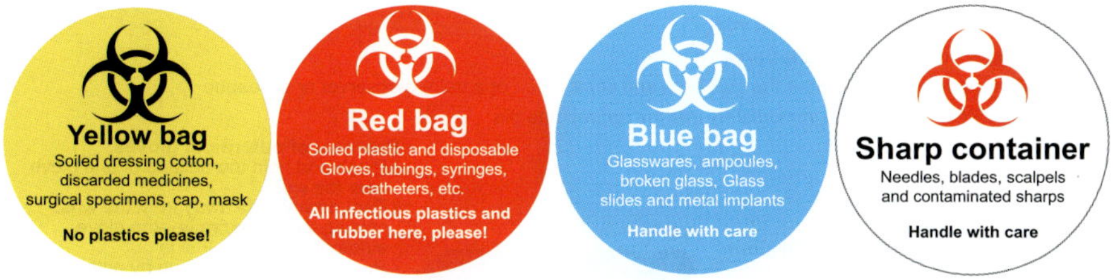
Yellow bag
Soiled dressing cotton, discarded medicines, surgical specimens, cap, mask
No plastics please!
Red bag
Soiled plastic and disposable Gloves, tubings, syringes, catheters, etc.
All infectious plastics and rubber here, please!
Blue bag
Glasswares, ampoules, broken glass, Glass slides and metal implants
Handle with care
Sharp container
Needles, blades, scalpels and contaminated sharps
Handle with care

Fig. 2: Biomedical waste segregation color-coded ***(Chapter 3)***.

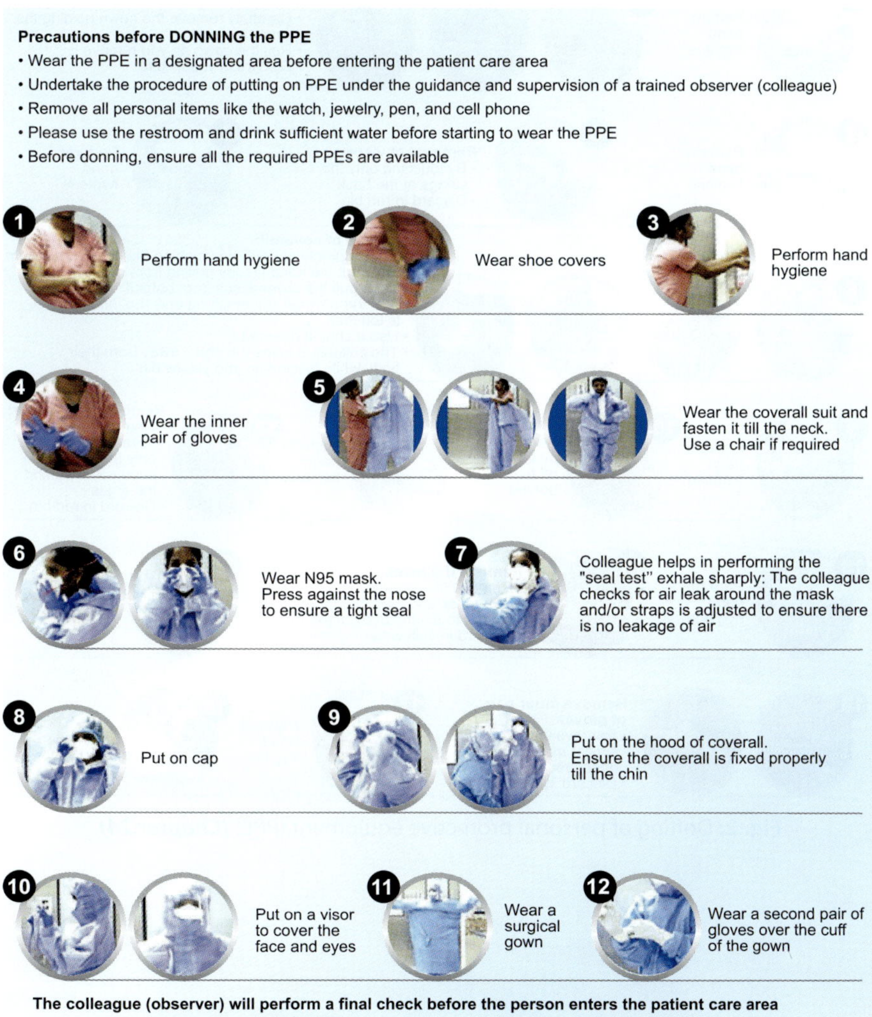

Fig. 1: Donning of personal protective equipment (PPE) ***(Chapter 24)***.

Plate 2

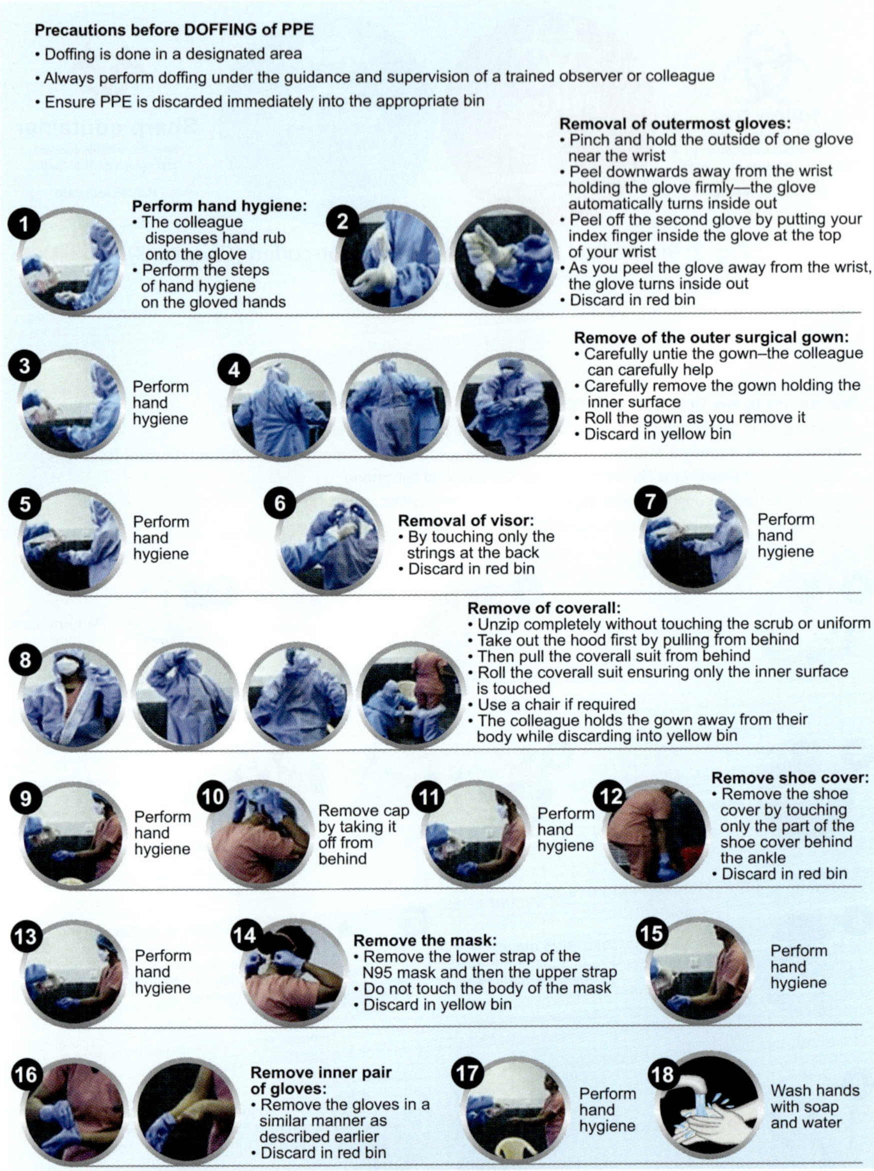

Fig. 2: Doffing of personal protective equipment (PPE) ***(Chapter 24)***.

SECTION 1

Fundamentals of Intensive Care Unit Infections

Section Editor: *Aruna Poojary*

1 CHAPTER

Introduction to Intensive Care Unit Infections

Amarja Ashok Havaldar

LEARNING OBJECTIVES

- Epidemiological triad.
- Community vs Hospital acquired infections.
- Global burden of infection.
- Importance of infection prevention.
- Cost of treating infection.
- Global action plan.

INTRODUCTION

Intensive care unit infections are associated with prolonged hospitalization and adverse outcomes. Understanding the epidemiology of infections is necessary to find out strategies to control infections. The global burden of infections is huge and associated with higher cost of treatment. Global action plan is one of the steps that can help in mitigating the problem of infections.

EPIDEMIOLOGY OF INTENSIVE CARE UNIT INFECTIONS

Epidemiology

Epidemiology is the study of the distribution and determinants of diseases in a specified population. Host factors, agents, and the environment form the epidemiological triad **(Fig. 1)**. This helps in understanding factors contributing to infection and helps in planning solutions.[1] The development of infections is due to the interaction between these factors. For instance,

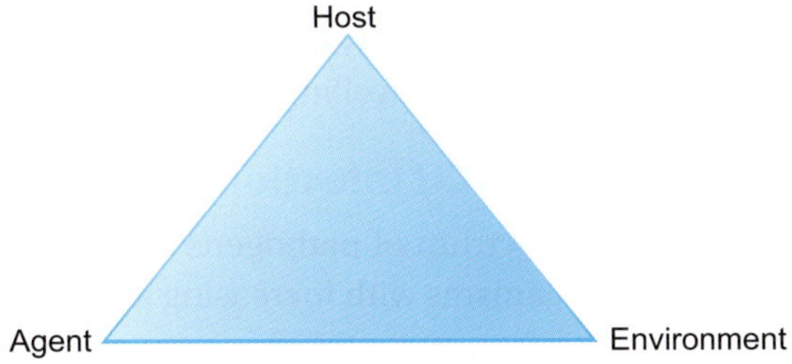

Fig. 1: Epidemiological triad.

ventilator-associated pneumonia (VAP) results from the interaction of patient factors (associated comorbidities and immunity), causative agents (*Acinetobacter baumannii* and *Klebsiella pneumoniae*) and the environment (presence of endotracheal tube and impaired mucociliary secretions).

Community-acquired Infections

Patients are admitted to intensive care unit (ICU) with various community-acquired infections such as pneumonia, urinary tract infection, meningitis, and abdominal infections. Tropical infections constitute a large number of cases admitted to ICU. The reason for ICU admission in such cases is severe infections requiring ventilator support, hemodynamic monitoring, or extracorporeal therapies. Virk, et al. in the study on community-acquired infections showed higher burden of tropical illness and also highlighted rising resistance of gram-negative bacteria to third-generation cephalosporins and carbapenems.[2]

Healthcare-associated Infections

Similarly, infections developed after 48 hours of hospitalization are called healthcare-associated infections (HAIs), e.g., VAP, central line-associated bloodstream infection (CLABSI), catheter-associated urinary tract infection (CAUTI), and surgical site infections (SSI).[3,4] Among these, VAP is the most common HAI infection with the incidence ranging from 5 to 40%.[4]

Risk Factors for Development of Healthcare-associated Infections[5]

- *Extremes of age*: Congenital disorders associated with impaired immune function or premature neonates and elderly with impaired immune function
- *Immunocompromised status*: Retroviral disease or acquired immune deficiencies. Patients on immunomodulators such as steroids and postchemotherapy
- *Comorbidities*: Diabetes mellitus, chronic kidney disease, and terminal illness
- *Prolonged hospitalization*: It can lead to development of infection with resistant bacteria, and immune paralysis.
- Use of intravascular devices or indwelling catheters

Types of Bacteria Causing ICU Infections

As per the published data, spectrum of pathogens has changed from gram-positive to gram-negative organisms with increasing antibiotic resistance.[6]

ESKAPE[7] pathogens are resistant bacteria which include:
- *Enterococcus faecium*
- *Staphylococcus aureus*

- *Klebsiella pneumoniae*
- *Acinetobacter baumannii* complex
- *Pseudomonas aeruginosa*
- *Enterobacter* species

With increasing antimicrobial resistance (AMR), very few effective antibiotics remain available.[7] Hence, infection prevention is paramount and underscores any other intervention.

Pathogens like *Elizabethkingia meningoseptica, Stenotrophomonas maltophilia,* and *Burkholderia cepacia* complex are isolated in patients with prolonged hospitalization. An Indian study showed a 28-day mortality rate of around 34.1% with these pathogens.[8] Mortality was higher in patients with hemodynamic instability and those who were on steroids. The antibiotic choices, cotrimoxazole, minocycline, and levofloxacin demonstrated variable sensitivity across different bacteria. Implementing strict infection control practices is therefore crucial to minimize these infections.

A study on the global burden of AMR, published in 2019 indicated highest burden of AMR in low-resource settings. This study highlighted limitations in data collection systems and laboratory capacity in low-income countries.[9]

Burden and Impact of ICU-acquired Infections: Key Learnings from Important Global and Indian Studies

A point prevalence multicentric study from Europe by Vincent et al. in 1995, comprising 10,038 patients, showed a total of 44.8% of patients in the ICU were infected, and 20.6% of patients had ICU-acquired infections.[10] Respiratory infection was the most common followed by urinary and bloodstream infections. Predominant organisms responsible for the infections were *Enterobacterales, S. aureus, P. aeruginosa,* coagulase negative staphylococci, and fungi. Among gram-positive infections, 60% were *Methicillin-resistant S. aureus (MRSA)* **(Table 1)**.

Risk factors for developing infection included an ICU stay over 48 hours, mechanical ventilation, trauma, venous catheters, urinary catheter, and stress ulcer prophylaxis. The study confirmed that VAP was linked to the duration of exposure, illness severity, and use of invasive ventilator support. Notably, the APACHE score was not a significant factor in the multiple logistic regression model.

Another European study called Sepsis Occurrence in Acutely Ill Patients (SOAP), published in 2006 showed age, comorbidities, septic shock, positive fluid balance, cancer, and medical admissions were associated with higher mortality. Respiratory infections were the most common followed by abdominal sepsis. The predominant isolated bacteria were *S. aureus, Pseudomonas,* and *Escherichia coli.*[11]

TABLE1: Global studies on infection and resistance patterns.

Name of study and year	*Primary objective*	*Sample size*	*Outcome*	*Bacteria isolated*	*Most common site of infection*
EPIC I (1995)	Prevalence of nosocomial infections	10,038	• 44.8% patients were infected • 20.6% had ICU-acquired infections	*Enterobacterales, Staphylococcus aureus, Pseudomonas aeruginosa,* coagulase negative staphylococci, and fungi. Among gram-positive infections ,60% *Methicillin-resistant S. aureus (MRSA)*	Respiratory
SOAP (2006)	Incidence of sepsis and characteristics of critically ill patients	3,147	37.4% had sepsis, 24.7% sepsis on admission. Cultures positive in 60% of sepsis cases	*S. aureus* was the common organism	Respiratory
EPIC II (2009)	Prevalence of nosocomial infections	13,796	• 51% were infected • 71% were receiving antibiotics	Gram-negative followed by gram-positive and fungal infections	Respiratory
EUROBACT-1 International Cohort Study (2012)	HA-BSI epidemiology and drug resistance and it is impact on patient outcomes	1,156	76% of infections were ICU-acquired, with a median diagnosis time of 14 days postadmission; 12% were polymicrobial	Gram-negative, followed by gram-positive, fungal and anaerobes. Overall, 47.8% of isolates were MDR, including 20.5% XDR and 0.4% PDR	
INDICAPS I (2016)	Organizational aspects, case mix and practices in Indian ICU		Infection rate was 12.2%, 60.7% of patients received antibiotics without infection	Gram-negative followed by gram-positive and fungi	

Contd...

Contd...

Name of study and year	*Primary objective*	*Sample size*	*Outcome*	*Bacteria isolated*	*Most common site of infection*
INDICAPS II (2021)	Organizational aspects, case mix and practices in Indian ICU		25.6% of patients were infected and 29.3% had sepsis during their ICU stay	Gram-negative infection was more prevalent, followed by gram-positive and fungal infection	
EUROBACT-2 International Cohort Study (2023)	To update the epidemiology and main factors associated with day-28 mortality in ICU patients with HA-BSI	2,600	• 78% were ICU-acquired infections. Gram-negative bacteria (59.0%) were the primary pathogens. Overall, 23.5% exhibited DTR, with 1.5% PDR • Overall mortality—37.1%	• Gram-negative (*Klebsiella, Acinetobacter*, • *Escherichia coli,* • *Pseudomonas)* • Gram-positive • *Enterococcus* species • Coagulase-negative staphylococci and • *Staphylococcus aureus* • Anaerobes *Bacteroides* species • Fungi—*Candida albicans* • *Candida* non-*albicans*, and other	Pneumonia and intravascular catheters

(DTR: difficult-to-treat resistance; HA-BSI: healthcare-associated bloodstream infection; ICU: intensive care unit; MDR: multidrug-resistant; PDR: pan-drug resistant; XDR: extensively drug resistant)

The Extended Prevalence of Infection in Intensive Care study published in 2009 was also a point prevalence study which included 13,796 patients, showing 51% were infected and 71% were receiving antibiotics.[12] Respiratory infections were predominant, and culture positivity was around 70%. Most pathogens were gram-negative followed by gram-positive bacteria and fungal pathogens. Infection rates were higher in patients with comorbidities and severe illness as shown by the Simplified Acute Physiology Score (SAPS II) and Sequential Organ Failure Assessment (SOFA) score. A limitation of the study was differences in the prevalence rate due to lead time bias.

Another key observation was that expenditure on gross domestic product (GDP) was inversely proportional to the rate of infections. However, evaluating the amount of GDP allocated specifically for ICU would have helped study this relationship further. Other factors that can influence infection rates were national antibiotic policy, infection control practices, and public awareness.[12]

When we compare Indian data, the first INDICAPS study of around 4,000 patients, infection rate was 12.2%.[13] Severe sepsis or septic shock was seen in 28.3% of patients. Around 60.7% of patients received antibiotics without infection. The identified pathogens were gram-negative (68.9%), gram-positive (15.9%), and fungi (7.5%). Mycobacteria, viruses, and parasites were uncommon.

The subsequent INDICAPS II study of 4,669 patients showed 25.6% of patients were infected and 29.3% had sepsis during their ICU stay. Gram-negative infection was more prevalent, followed by gram-positive and fungal infection.[14]

Characteristics and determinants of hospital-acquired infection evaluated in the EUROBACT I study showed that the isolation of multidrug resistant bacteria was associated with higher odds of 28-day mortality with odds ratio (OR), 1.49; 95 % confidence interval (CI), 1.07–2.06.[15]

The Epidemiology and Determinants of the Outcomes of Hospital Acquired Blood stream Infections in the intensive care, EUROBACT II study describes hospital-acquired blood stream infection as predominantly caused by gram-negative bacteria and associated with carbapenem-resistant and difficult-to-treat pathogens.[16] Difficult-to-treat resistance pathogens (DTR) are defined as gram-negative blood stream infections resistant to carbapenem, beta-lactam, and fluoroquinolones.[17]

Infection and Patient Outcomes

As per the literature, it is clear that the isolation of the resistant bacteria is associated with higher mortality, increased length of ICU stay, cost of care, and associated with the higher mortality.[9,18,19] The multinational study by Rosenthal et al. showed CLABSI and VAP were associated with mortality. Age, female gender, and length of ICU stay were the risk factors associated with development of HAI.[18] The global burden of the sepsis study with data from 1990 to 2017 showed 48.9 million cases of sepsis were reported and 11 million were sepsis-related deaths. AMR is a serious concern in low-resource settings. The pathogens associated with death include ESKAPE pathogens with *Streptococcus pneumoniae*. Hence improving laboratory facilities and data collection facilities is necessary. The lower sociodemographic index group had higher burden of the disease.[9,20]

An Indian study evaluating healthcare-associated blood stream and urinary tract infections in network hospitals resulted in the implementation of locally adapted protocols.[21] A surveillance study on VAP including 13 hospitals showed a VAP rate of 6.4 per 1,000 ventilator days, and *Acinetobacter* was the most common species followed by *Klebsiella*.[22] A study by Lakbar et al., on patients admitted with highly antibiotic resistant bacteria and patients without resistant bacteria showed infections with *S. aureus, P. aeruginosa*, Enterobacterales such as *E. coli, Klebsiella pneumoniae, Enterobacter cloacae*, or *Acinetobacter baumannii* complex. Patients infected with multidrug-resistant bacteria had significantly higher mortality 40.3% versus 30% ($p < 0.001$).[19] A study by Gandra et al., observed distinct types of bacteria and the resistant patterns in low-income countries as compared to high-income countries. The gram-negative bacteria with MDR or XDR resistance pattern had higher odds of mortality. Among gram-positive infections, MRSA with aminoglycosides resistance also associated with higher mortality.[6]

The largest study on antimicrobial resistance from 1990 to 2021 and forecasting about 2050, showed reduced incidence of infections in patients <5 years of age. A higher incidence of infection was observed in elderly compared to younger patients. It also emphasized the importance of infection prevention, vaccination, minimizing inappropriate use of antibiotics in agriculture and humans, and identifying newer antibiotic molecules.[23]

Cost of Treating Nosocomial Infection

A study of 499 patients admitted to a tertiary care hospital from India evaluated attributable cost of nosocomial infections in the ICU. In this cohort of patients who developed infection had higher treatment cost [median (interquartile range—IQR) Indian National Rupee INR 92,893 (United States USD 1,523) (IQR 57,168–140,286) vs. INR 180469 (USD 2958) (IQR 140,030–237,525); $p < 0.001$. The development of infection was also associated with increased length of ICU and hospital stay.[24] Similar results were observed by Iranian study suggesting higher cost in patients who developed infection [3,264 ± 6,078 (USD)] as compared to those without infection [2,451 ± 3,098 USD].[25]

An ongoing systematic review on economic evaluation of healthcare infection prevention can help in designing cost-effective interventions for infection control.[26]

IMPORTANCE OF INFECTION PREVENTION

- *ICU layout*: Infrastructure—recommended bed space is 150–200 sq feet, and distance between the two beds should be at least 6 feet. Availability of positive and negative pressure rooms for high-risk patients is preferable.[27]
- *Human resources—adequate nurse to patient ratio, housekeeping, and trained doctors:* Nurse to patient ratio—a cross-sectional survey showed nurse to patient allocation ratio-based staffing was associated with improvement in infection control practices. Minimum staffing ratio was 1:4. However, there is no clarity about which settings nurses were working, ICU, or ward.[28] Another survey done in eight ICUs showed mean patient-to-nurse ratio was 1.95. Increased missed care and higher workload were associated with higher hospital-acquired infections.[29]
- *Availability of other resources:* Hand rubs, hand wash solution, cleaning materials, disinfectants, safety devices, etc.
- *Training all healthcare workers (HCWs):* Induction and in service for all including doctors
- Surveillance for HCAIs especially device-associated infections
- Audits for various processes

To prevent hospital-acquired infections, single intervention has not proven effective. Hence the use of prevention bundles, such as those for VAP or CLABSI, where multiple interventions are implemented, is crucial.

A study on CLABSI prevention by Rosenthal et al., conducted in 30 different ICUs showed that the implementation of care bundle comprising of 11 elements was feasible and that resulted in a reduction in CLABSI rates postintervention. The intervention led to steady decline in the CLABSI rate from 15.34 at the baseline to 2.23 per 1,000 central line days over 29 months. ICU all-cause mortality also dropped from 16.17% to 13.68%. The findings also suggested the generalizability of these results, indicating that these interventions could be implemented in other ICUs.[30]

Antimicrobial Use and Misuse

Antimicrobial resistance is multifactorial and antibiotic stewardship is necessary to combat this global threat. The WHO's initiative in response to this issue is antibiotic stewardship.

An antibiotic stewardship program is an effort to improve and measure antibiotic prescription practices across the hospital. Such programs involve various components **(Fig. 2)**.[31]

The access, watch, and reserve (AWaRe) classification of antibiotics by World Health Organization (WHO) released in 2017, is updated every 2 years. The aim is that 60% of the antibiotic use should be from the Access group of antibiotics **(Fig. 3)**.[32,33]

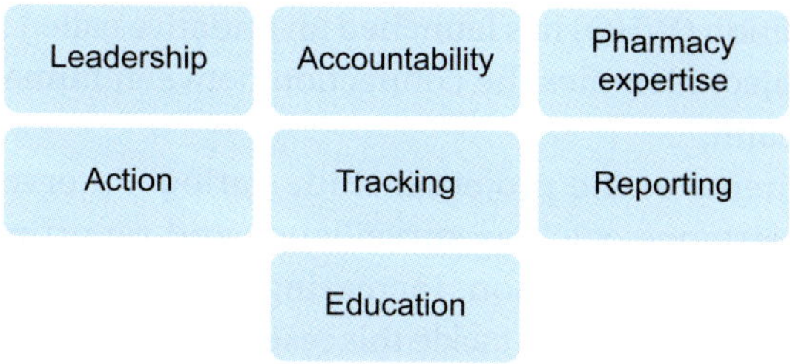

Fig. 2: Elements of hospital antibiotic stewardship program.

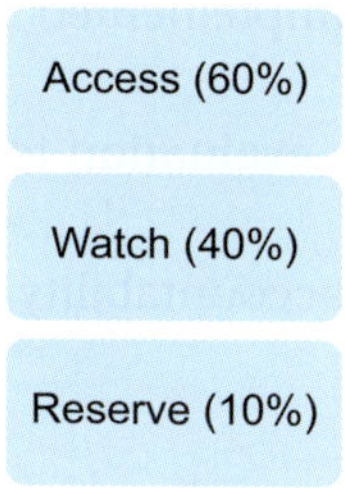

Fig. 3: Aware classification of antibiotics by WHO.

- *Access:* This group of antibiotics is recommended as essential first- or second-choice empiric treatment options for infectious syndromes (e.g., clindamycin and doxycycline).
- *Watch:* This group includes antibiotic classes that have higher resistance potential and form the key targets for stewardship program. (e.g., piperacillin + tazobactam and meropenem). This constitutes around 40% of the antibiotics.
- *Reserve:* This is the group of antibiotics reserved for the treatment of confirmed or suspected infections due to multidrug-resistant organisms (e.g., colistin and tigecycline). This group constitutes approximately 10% of total antibiotic use.

Difficulties in implementing WHO classification of antibiotics:[32]

- Lack of public awareness
- Lack of awareness among HCWs
- Nonavailability of access antibiotics
- Limited resources for implementing this framework
- Lack of political support

GLOBAL ACTION PLAN (WHO) AGAINST RESISTANT INFECTION

One Health Project

Antibiotic resistance is considered as a global emergency. With the increasing AMR and the nonavailability of effective antibiotics in the pipeline, the World

Health Organization (WHO) has launched an initiative called the One Health Project. The project identifies the connection between human, animal, and environment health.

Key components of the project include various interventions related to antibiotic resistance, such as surveillance and reporting of antibiotic resistance, tracking transmission, increasing awareness, policy decisions, and preparing the workforce to tackle this resistance.

Implementing surveillance systems and rationalized and regulated use of antibiotics can help in reducing AMR.

Many countries have already implemented national surveillance system and stewardship programs.

Global antibiotic stewardship evaluation tool (G-ASET): There are five domains included:[34]

1. Leadership commitment and accountability
2. Resources
3. Education and training
4. Antibiotic stewardship actions
5. Antibiotic use tracking, monitoring, and reporting

Regarding the use of antibiotics in farming and animal husbandry, the use of antimicrobials in farming and the administration of antibiotics to animals need to be regulated. Infection in animals can affect food quality and transmit diseases to humans.

The Ministry of Health and Family Welfare has released the national guidelines for antimicrobial use in infectious diseases. The guidelines are extensive and include various infectious diseases, treatment options, and preventive aspects. This is a useful resource for managing infectious diseases with guidelines based on local epidemiology.[35]

Diagnostic Tests

Rapid diagnostic tests, polymerase chain reaction (PCR), and whole genome sequencing can help identify pathogens early and know the resistance gene responsible for the resistance.

CONCLUSION

Understanding the epidemiology of ICU infections is vital. The ICU-acquired infections are associated with prolonged hospitalization, increased treatment cost, and also associated with the higher mortality. National surveillance system and public awareness and increasing allocation of GDP toward healthcare are the possible options to tackle this menace and improve the ecosystem. Implementing infection prevention and control (IPC) practices, and antibiotic stewardship programs, and regular audits on antibiotic usage is the need of the hour.

REFERENCES

1. Bonita R, Beaglehole R, Kjellström T, World Health Organization. Basic epidemiology, 2nd edition. [online] Available from https://iris.who.int/handle/10665/43541 [Last accessed August, 2025].
2. Virk HS, Biemond JJ, Earny VA, Chowdhury S, Frölke RI, Khanna SM, et al. Unraveling Sepsis Epidemiology in a Low- and Middle-Income Intensive Care Setting Reveals the Alarming Burden of Tropical Infections and Antimicrobial Resistance: A Prospective Observational Study (MARS-India). Clin Infect Dis. 2025;80(1):101-7.
3. Kollef MH, Torres A, Shorr AF, Martin-Loeches I, Micek ST. Nosocomial Infection. Crit Care Med. 2021;49:169-87.
4. Teng J, Imani S, Zhou A, Zhao Y, Du L, Deng S, et al. Combatting resistance: Understanding multi-drug resistant pathogens in intensive care units. Biomed Pharmacother. 2023;167:115564.
5. Liu X, Long Y, Greenhalgh C, Steeg S, Wilkinson J, Li H, et al. A systematic review and meta-analysis of risk factors associated with healthcare-associated infections among hospitalized patients in Chinese general hospitals from 2001 to2022. J Hospital Infect. 2023;135:37-49.
6. Gandra S, Tseng KK, Arora A, Bhowmik B, Robinson ML, Panigrahi B, et al. The Mortality Burden of Multidrug-resistant Pathogens in India: A Retrospective, Observational Study. Clin Infect Dis. 2019;69:563-70.
7. Daruka L, Czikkely MS, Szili P, Farkas Z, Balogh D, Grézal G, et al. ESKAPE pathogens rapidly develop resistance against antibiotics in development in vitro. Nat Microbiol. 2025;10:313-31.
8. Prayag PS, Rajhans P, Mahale N, Patwardhan SA, Dhekane PN, Soman RN, et al. Bacteremia Caused by Rare NFGNB in the ICU: A Single-center Experience. Indian J Crit Care Med. 2025;29:345-51.
9. Antimicrobial Resistance Collaborators. Global burden of bacterial antimicrobial resistance in 2019: a systematic analysis. The Lancet. 2022;399:629-55.
10. Vincent JL. The Prevalence of Nosocomial Infection in Intensive Care Units in Europe: Results of the European Prevalence of Infection in Intensive Care (EPIC) Study. JAMA. 1995;274:639.
11. Vincent JL, Sakr Y, Sprung CL, Ranieri VM, Reinhart K, Gerlach H, et al. Sepsis in European intensive care units: Results of the SOAP study*: Crit Care Med. 2006;34:344-53.
12. Vincent JL. International Study of the Prevalence and Outcomes of Infection in Intensive Care Units. JAMA. 2009;302:2323.
13. Divatia JV, Amin PR, Ramakrishnan N, Kapadia FN, Todi S, Sahu S, et al. Intensive Care in India: The Indian Intensive Care Case Mix and Practice Patterns Study. Indian J Crit Care Med. 2016;20:216-25.
14. Divatia JV, Mehta Y, Govil D, Zirpe K, Amin PR, Ramakrishnan N, et al. Intensive Care in India in 2018–2019: The Second Indian Intensive Care Case Mix and Practice Patterns Study. Indian J Crit Care Med. 2021;25:1093-107.
15. Tabah A, Koulenti D, Laupland K, Misset B, Valles J, Bruzzi de Carvalho F, et al. Characteristics and determinants of outcome of hospital-acquired bloodstream infections in intensive care units: the EUROBACT International Cohort Study. Intensive Care Med. 2012;38:1930-45.

16. Tabah A, Buetti N, Staiquly Q, Ruckly S, Akova M, Aslan AT, et al. Epidemiology and outcomes of hospital-acquired bloodstream infections in intensive care unit patients: the EUROBACT-2 international cohort study. Intensive Care Med. 2023;49:178-90.
17. Dettori S, Portunato F, Vena A, Giacobbe DR, Bassetti M. Severe infections caused by difficult-to-treat Gram-negative bacteria. Curr Opin Crit Care. 2023;29:438-45.
18. Rosenthal VD, Yin R, Lu Y, Rodrigues C, Myatra SN, Kharbanda M, et al. The impact of healthcare-associated infections on mortality in ICU: A prospective study in Asia, Africa, Eastern Europe, Latin America, and the Middle East. Am J Infect Control. 2023;51:675-82.
19. Lakbar I, Medam S, Ronflé R, Cassir N, Delamarre L, Hammad E, et al. Association between mortality and highly antimicrobial-resistant bacteria in intensive care unit-acquired pneumonia. Sci Rep. 2021;11:16497.
20. Rudd KE, Johnson SC, Agesa KM, Shackelford KA, Tsoi D, Kievlan DR, et al. Global, regional, and national sepsis incidence and mortality, 1990–2017: analysis for the Global Burden of Disease Study. Lancet. 2020;395:200-11.
21. Mathur P, Malpiedi P, Walia K, Srikantiah P, Gupta S, Lohiya A, et al. Health-care-associated bloodstream and urinary tract infections in a network of hospitals in India: a multicentre, hospital-based, prospective surveillance study. Lancet Glob Health. 2022;10:e1317-25.
22. Mathur P, Ningombam A, Soni KD, Aggrawal R, Singh KV, Samanta P, et al. Surveillance of ventilator associated pneumonia in a network of Indian hospitals using modified definitions: a pilot study. Lancet Reg Health-Southeast Asia. 2024;28:100450.
23. GBD 2021 Antimicrobial Resistance Collaborators. Global burden of bacterial antimicrobial resistance 1990–2021: A systematic analysis with forecasts to 2050. Lancet. 2024;404:1199-226.
24. Chacko B, Thomas K, David T, Paul H, Jeyaseelan L, Peter JV. Attributable cost of a nosocomial infection in the intensive care unit: A prospective cohort study. World J Crit Care Med. 2017;6:79-84.
25. Soleymani F, Safari Palangi H, Sarabi Asiabar A, Keshtkar A, Mohammadi M, Akbari Sari A, et al. Costs of hospital-acquired infection for patients hospitalized in intensive care unit of an Iranian referral hospital. Med J Islam Repub Iran. 2018;32:67.
26. Tchouaket EN, Kruglova K, Beogo I, Sia D, Robins S, Bélanger E, et al. Economic evaluation of healthcare-associated infection prevention and control in long-term care: a systematic review protocol. Syst Rev. 2022;11:261.
27. Rungta N, Zirpe KG, Dixit SB, Mehta Y, Chaudhry D, Govil D, et al. Indian Society of Critical Care Medicine Experts Committee Consensus Statement on ICU Planning and Designing, 2020. Indian J Crit Care Med. 2020;24:S43-60.
28. Tencic M, Roche MA. Nurse–patient ratios and infection control practices: A cross-sectional study. Collegian. 2023;30:828-34.
29. Alanazi FK, Lapkin S, Molloy L, Sim J. Healthcare-associated infections in adult intensive care units: A multisource study examining nurses' safety attitudes, quality of care, missed care, and nurse staffing. Intensive Crit Care Nurs. 2023;78:103480.
30. Rosenthal VD, Jin Z, Brown EC, Dongol R, De Moros DA, Alarcon-Rua J, et al. Decreasing central line-associated bloodstream infections rates in intensive

care units in 30 low- and middle-income countries: An INICC approach. Am J Infect Control. 2024;52:580-87.

31. CDC. (2024). Core Elements of Antibiotic Stewardship for Health Departments. [online] Available from https://www.cdc.gov/antibiotic-use/hcp/core-elements/index.html [Last accessed August, 2025].
32. Mudenda S, Daka V, Matafwali SK. World Health Organization AWaRe framework for antibiotic stewardship: Where are we now and where do we need to go? An expert viewpoint. Antimicrob Steward Healthc Epidemiol. 2023;3:e84.
33. Zanichelli V, Sharland M, Cappello B, Moja L, Getahun H, Pessoa-Silva C, et al. The WHO AWaRe (Access, Watch, Reserve) antibiotic book and prevention of antimicrobial resistance. Bull World Health Organ. 2023;101:290-6.
34. CDC. (2025). Global Antibiotic Stewardship Evaluation Tool (G-ASET) for Inpatient Healthcare Facilities. [online] Available from https://www.cdc.gov/international-infection-control/hcp/communications-resources/g-aset.html#:~:text=G%2DASET%20for%20Inpatient%20Healthcare,related%20to%20antibiotic%20stewardship%20practices [Last accessed August, 2025].
35. Ministry of Health and Family Welfare. Government of India. (2016). National Treatment Guidelines for Antimicrobial Use in Infectious Diseases. [online] Available from https://ncdc.mohfw.gov.in/wp-content/uploads/2024/04/File622.pdf [Last accessed August, 2025].

2

CHAPTER

Pathophysiology of Infections in the Intensive Care Unit

Asif Ahmed, Mahajyoti Chakravorty, Anu Prasad

LEARNING OBJECTIVES

- Causes and mechanism of infection in an intensive care unit.
- Specific type of infections acquired in the intensive care unit and the culprit pathogen that cause these infections and their virulence.
- Host immune response to infection.
- Molecular mechanisms of immune response in the form of pathogen associated molecular patterns (PAMPs) and damage associated molecular patterns (DAMPs) and their influence on tissue damage and disease progression.
- Risk of increased coagulation and thrombosis due to endothelial injury and release of tissue factor as a result of cytokine response.
- Immune imbalance due to overexpression of proinflammatory (systemic inflammatory response syndrome) and anti-inflammatory (compensatory anti-inflammatory response syndrome) response, leading to multiorgan failure, complications of sepsis, and even death.
- Predilection of certain pathogens for specific organ systems.

INTRODUCTION

Patients in intensive care units (ICUs) are always at high risk of developing healthcare-associated infections (HAIs) due to the high prevalence of invasive procedures and devices, in the background of immunosuppression, comorbidities, frailty, and increased age. HAIs are infections acquired in an acute care setting which were not present or incubating at the time of admission and arise after 48 hours of admission.[1]

The incidence of HAIs in ICUs in India, according to a retrospective study, ranges between 9.6% and 17.7%.[2] The high incidence highlights the concern as these are associated with increased ICU stay and mortality. It is therefore important to have a detailed understanding of the pathophysiology of infections in the ICU to have a better insight into management and care of the patients. The common infection-causing agents in the ICUs are *Klebsiella, Acinetobacter, Escherichia coli, Pseudomonas, Staphylococcus aureus,* and *Candida.*[3,4]

MECHANISM OF INFECTION IN THE INTENSIVE CARE UNIT

Infection in a critically ill patient involves the colonization of bacteria, followed by adhesion, invasion, and multiplication inside the host, and ultimately leading to the development of a disease. The pathogen can be transmitted by various routes including contact, air, and droplet as well as through various devices inserted in the patient. The risk of developing a HAI is linked to the prevalence and virulence of the pathogens, the immunocompromised state of host, advanced age, presence of multiple comorbidities, indwelling devices, mechanical ventilation support, invasive procedures, and prolonged length of stay in the ICU or hospital. Certain specific infections that are most common in ICUs are catheter-associated urinary tract infection (CAUTI), hospital-acquired pneumonia (HAP), central line-associated bloodstream infection (CLABSI), surgical site infection (SSI) and *Clostridium difficile* infection (CDI). The mechanism of infection can be unique to each of these entities.

SPECIFIC INFECTIONS AND THEIR MECHANISM

Catheter-associated Urinary Tract Infection

The most significant risk factor for CAUTI is an indwelling urinary catheter, followed by other factors such as female gender, diabetes mellitus, chronic bedridden state, cerebrovascular disease, poor maintenance and care of the catheter, and long duration of catheterization. Invasion of microorganisms can be through intra- or extraluminal colonization, retrograde ascent, periurethral entry, or biofilm formation on the indwelling catheter. Common culprits are the skin and fecal microflora, which include gram-negative bacteria, *Enterococci*, *Staphylococci*, and *Candida* species. Fibrinogen protein plays a specific role in CAUTI, where urinary catheterization causes an inflammatory reaction that can cause the host to release fibrinogen in the urethra and the bladder. This fibrinogen acts as a binding protein for the pathogens and is a source of nutrition. The most common pathogens are *E. coli* and *Klebsiella*. The mechanism of virulence of *Pseudomonas aeruginosa* is via the production of rhamnolipids which promotes catheter adherence and migration along with production of elastase/lectins and other toxins. *Enterococci* are protease-producing organisms that split fibrinogen and use it as a scaffold to adhere to the catheter surface. *Enterococci* also cause endocarditis and biofilm-associated pili for adherence and colonization of the urinary catheter. Staphylococci produce clumping factor B that binds to fibrinogen. *Proteus mirabilis* produces mannose-resistant *Proteus*-like fimbria to attach to the luminal surface of urinary bladder and flagella to cause ascending urinary tract infection. *Proteus* also produces ureases that can split urea and increase the pH of urine that can produce a crystalline biofilm on the inner surface of the urinary catheter and cause blockage to urine flow. *Candida* has a predilection for colonizing latex catheter more than silicone and binds to urinary catheter via fibrinogen.[5]

Hospital-acquired Pneumonia

Hospital-acquired pneumonia is defined as pneumonia that develops in a patient after >48 hours of hospitalization. Ventilator-associated pneumonia (VAP) is a type of HAP which occurs in patients on mechanical ventilation for >48 hours. The risk factors include malnutrition, antibiotic use, aspiration (overt and covert), sedation or muscle relaxant when on mechanical ventilation, major surgery, advanced age, and renal failure on hemodialysis. Most of the factors involved are related to impaired swallowing, presence of an enteral feeding tube, and colonization of the oropharynx with pathogenic microorganisms. Common organisms causing infection are *Acinetobacter baumannii, Klebsiella pneumoniae*, and *P. aeruginosa*. Contamination during procedures such as tracheal suctioning, fiber-optic bronchoscopy, humidification, and frequent disconnection of ventilator circuits are some additional exogenous factors for developing VAP. The endotracheal tube plays a noticeable role in the mechanism of VAP by acting as a surface for biofilm formation apart from lowering the cough reflex and mucociliary clearance. Endotracheal tube insertion can also cause airway trauma which can cause bacteria to bind the tracheal surface apart from causing a direct inoculation of the lower airway with oral flora during the procedure. The biofilm formed on the endotracheal tube acts as a reservoir for VAP pathogens, especially the ESKAPE organisms (*Enterococcus faecalis, Staphylococcus aureus, Klebsiella pneumoniae, Acinetobacter baumannii, Pseudomonas aeruginosa, and Enterobacter),* which can stay under the cover of the biofilm and develop resistance to antimicrobial therapy.[6]

Central Line-associated Bloodstream Infection

Risk factors for CLABSI are prolonged hospitalization, chronic illness, parenteral nutrition, neutropenia, multilumen central vein cannula (CVC), and break in antiseptic technique during insertion. Bacteria can migrate from the skin exit site of catheter toward the intravenous space. The most common mechanism is due to contamination of catheter hub, when handled with unsterile hands during drug administration, and less commonly by hematogenous spread and contaminated infusions. Catheter site selection (femoral vs. internal-jugular), catheter type (nontunneled vs. tunneled), insertion condition (emergency vs. elective), and operator skills are other factors which can influence the risk of CLABSI. Organisms which commonly cause infection are *Staphylococcus, Enterococcus, Bacteroides,* and *Candida* species. Biofilm formation is a phenomenon which is common to both gram-positive and gram-negative bacteria. Broad-spectrum antibiotics, parenteral nutrition, malignancy, diabetes mellitus, and femoral catheterization add the risk for *Candida* infection.[7]

Surgical Site Infections

Surgical site infection can manifest anytime within 30 days of surgery to 90 days of device implantation. The patient's own healthy microflora of the skin or genitourinary tract can be the cause of SSI if the surgical wound lies in the vicinity of the contaminated area. Risk factors include tobacco addiction, hyperglycemia, obesity, malnutrition, immunosuppressed conditions, wound drains, prolonged length of stay, and poor local hygiene. Endogenous routes such as skin flora and opened viscus and exogenous routes such as from healthcare providers or operation theater environment can contribute to the development of SSI. The intraoperative phase can seed the pathogen in the wound if it is an urgent procedure, requires prolonged time, or the patient was hypovolemic or hypoxemic during the surgery. Additional factors include blood transfusion, the anatomical site operated upon, or the type of implant placed. The risk is higher with a dirty, contaminated wound rather than a clean wound. The common pathogens involved are *E. coli*, *Staphylococcus*, coagulase-negative Staphylococci, *Enterobacter*, *Enterococcus*, and *Klebsiella*. Pathogens vary according to the surgical location like *S. aureus* and *Streptococcus* species are more common for skin or superficial site infections, whereas *E. coli* and *Enterococcus* species are commonly found after gastrointestinal (GI) procedures. Surgical instrument or environmental contamination can lead to clusters of cases in a post-surgery unit or ICU.[1]

Clostridium Difficile Infection

Clostridium difficile is a gram-positive, anaerobic, spore-forming, and toxin-producing bacterium that can colonize the gut of healthy individuals without causing infections. The bacteria are mainly transmitted by the fecal–oral route or through the aerosol spread of spores. CDI is characterized by pseudomembranous colitis and diarrhea. The single-most important risk factor for CDI is the use of broad-spectrum antibiotics, especially cephalosporins, clindamycin, fluoroquinolones, and penicillins. Other risk factors are advanced age, prolonged hospitalization, gastric acid suppressants, comorbidities, and immunosuppression. *Clostridium difficile* produces two toxins: (1) Toxin A (enterotoxin) and (2) toxin B (cytotoxin), which cause injury to enterocytes, disruption of tight junctions, and release of fluid in the lumen of the gut along with an inflammation of the submucosa and the lamina propria (neutrophilic chemotaxis). Severe CDI can lead to fulminant colitis, sepsis, and even death.[8]

PATHOPHYSIOLOGY OF INFECTIONS IN CRITICALLY ILL PATIENTS

In critically ill patients, infections can occur due to pathogen invasion, host response, immune dysregulation, and organ dysfunction. All these mechanisms contribute to sepsis, multiorgan failure, and increased mortality.[9]

Immune Response and Host Factors

Nonspecific innate immune response is the primary line of defense against an infection. The innate immune response has three components: (1) Physical barrier, (2) cellular component, and (3) humoral response. An invading pathogen first encounters natural barriers, such as skin and mucous membranes of respiratory, GI, and urogenital tracts, that block the entry of microbes. The acidic pH of stomach, immunoglobulin A (IgA) in mucosal secretions, presence of lysozymes in tears and saliva, and commensal bacteria in the GI tract are some natural physiochemical barriers that block the entry of pathogens. Once these barriers are crossed, the host body is systemically exposed to microbes and activates the cellular component consisting of macrophages, dendritic cells, mast cells, neutrophils, eosinophils, and natural killer (NK) cells. The humoral component of innate immunity consists of complement proteins, C-reactive proteins, and components of the coagulation system.[10]

The pathophysiology of infection primarily depends on the complex interaction of pathogens with the host immune response. Microbes such as bacteria, viruses, and fungi differ in structure, ability to cause infection, and infection mechanism, but they all have PAMPs. Bacterial lipopolysaccharide (LPS) of gram-negative bacteria, lipoteichoic acid of gram-positive bacteria, and viral ribonucleic acid (RNA) and deoxyribonucleic acid (DNA) are few examples of PAMPs.[11-13] PAMPs help to identify the pathogens. The neutrophils, monocytes, and macrophages detect the pathogens' PAMPs through specialized pattern recognition receptors (PRRs). Toll-like receptors (TLRs), nucleotide-binding oligomerization domain (NOD)-like receptors (NLRs), and C-type leptin receptors (CLRs) are some prominent PRRs. Cytokines are small polypeptides that act as messenger molecules which activate the systemic inflammatory response with resultant endothelial activation.

In sepsis, the pathogen load is very high and PRRs are persistently stimulated, causing hyperinflammation and tissue injury. This causes release of various intracellular materials known as damage-associated molecular patterns.[14] They can be proteins such as heat shock proteins, high mobility group box 1 (HMGB1), and nonprotein metabolites such as adenosine triphosphate (ATP). Apart from recognizing the exogeneous PAMPs, the PRRs also interact with these endogenous DAMPs, and both PAMPs and DAMPs initiate activation of neutrophils and a series of inflammatory pathways, cellular metabolism, and adaptive immunity, leading to cell injury and hyperinflammation.[15,16] The activated neutrophils release various mediators such as reactive oxygen species (ROS), prostaglandins, etc., that constantly disrupt the endothelial glycocalyx and endothelium. This loss of barrier function leads to increase in permeability and capillary leak. The resultant redistribution of fluids from vascular to extravascular space leads to interstitial edema and hypovolemia, a hallmark feature of the initial part of sepsis.[17]

The endothelial injury also causes release of tissue factor (TF) that initiates the extrinsic clotting system. In addition, cytokines amplify the procoagulant response by releasing a large quantity of TF from macrophages. The uncontrolled systemic coagulation is kept in check by several anticoagulants including activated protein C (APC) and tissue plasminogen activators. However, during inflammatory surge, depressed levels of APC and downregulation of the fibrinolytic system tilt the balance toward an intense procoagulant response. Excessive thrombin formation in microvessels leads to local ischemia that contributes to multiorgan dysfunction.[18] The inflammatory process and coagulation disorder are closely interlinked in sepsis. Thrombocytopenia, elevated D-dimer and fibrinogen degradation products, and low levels of APC, which are suggestive of low-grade disseminated intravascular coagulation (DIC), are seen in patients with sepsis. However, most of these subtle abnormalities are not detected in a routine laboratory test.[19]

The cytokine response is bimodal with the initial release of pro-inflammatory mediators such as interleukin 1, interleukin 6, tumor necrosis factor α (TNF-α), and later anti-inflammatory response that includes interleukin 10, interleukin 4, and tumor growth factor β(TGF-β). Overexpression of inflammatory response leads to systemic inflammatory response syndrome (SIRS) and organ dysfunction, whereas excessive release of anti-inflammatory response leads to compensatory anti-inflammatory response syndrome (CARS) and immune paralysis.[20]

Anti-inflammatory response is a protective mechanism to limit collateral damage caused by hyperinflammatory response and to restore homeostasis. However, in sepsis, overexpression and sustained inflammatory response lead to over-exhaustion of compensatory mechanisms and immune paralytic state. During this immune-paralytic phase, the possibility of secondary and opportunistic infections increases.[21] Cellular apoptosis, reprogramming of antigen-presenting cells, immune cell depletion, and T-cell exhaustion, combined together, result in immune suppression in sepsis.[22] A summary of various factors is given in **Table 1**.

Common Pathogens

Intensive care units are a major source of infections around the globe. High prevalence of both primary and nosocomial infections across various ICUs in Europe and North America were reported by the European studies on prevalence of infections (EPIC 1 and EPIC 2).[23-25] Various studies from ICUs

TABLE 1: Types of anti-inflammatory response mechanism.

Mechanism	*Description*
Portal of entry	Portal of entry can be through natural orifice, through the in situ devices, translocation from the gut, or breach of skin or mucosa
Specific infection	Healthcare-associated infections (HAIs) in intensive care unit (ICU) under surveillance include catheter-associated urinary tract infection (CAUTI), hospital-acquired pneumonia (HAP), central line-associated bloodstream infection (CLABSI), surgical site infection (SSI), and *Clostridium difficile* infection (CDI)
Biofilm formation	Bacteria form biofilms, which protect them from immune attacks and antibiotics
Host factor	Immunosuppressed patients (malignancy, immunosuppressant use, and diabetes mellitus) have an increased risk of infection
Immune response	Infection triggers the innate and adaptive immune responses that can lead to release of pro-inflammatory markers
Immune dysregulation	Imbalance of the innate and adaptive immune systems, and imbalance between hyperinflammation response [systemic inflammatory response syndrome (SIRS)] and hypo-inflammation [compensatory anti-inflammatory response syndrome (CARS)] can lead to sepsis, multiorgan failure, and death
Endothelial dysfunction	Increased vascular permeability and micro-thrombosis cause capillary leak syndrome, tissue hypoxia, and disseminated intravascular coagulation (DIC)
Multidrug-resistant organisms (MDRO)	Microbes can develop resistance to multiple antibiotics leading to nonresolution of infection
Environmental factors	ICU settings promote infections due to high patient turnover, invasive procedures, and frequent antibiotic use

of different parts of India too have shown similar prevalence of infection.[26] Prolonged ICU stay, multiple comorbidities, and aging population are some known predisposing factors for infection in ICUs. The pattern of infection and the causative organisms are depicted in **Table 2.**[27]

CONCLUSION

The pathophysiology of infections in ICU is complex. The mechanism of infection depends on the host, the pathogen, and also on the environment. Once the pathogen has entered the body, it can trigger an immune response. The immune response when triggered leads to activation of leukocytes,

TABLE 2: Pattern of infection and causative organisms.

Community-acquired infections	***Causative organisms***
Community-acquired pneumonia (CAP)	• *Streptococcus pneumoniae, Klebsiella, Haemophilus influenzae, Mycoplasma pneumoniae, Pseudomonas aeruginosa*, and influenza virus are more common • *Staphylococcus aureus, Legionella*, and *Mycobacterium tuberculosis* are less common
Pyogenic meningitis	*Neisseria meningitidis, Streptococci, Haemophilus influenzae, Listeria monocytogenes*, and *Staphylococcus* species
Brain abscess	*Streptococcus viridans, S. aureus, Bacteroides, Fusobacterium*, and *Peptostreptococcus*
Peritonitis	Gram-negative enteric organisms
Pyogenic liver abscess	*Escherichia coli* and *Klebsiella*
Skin and soft-tissue infection	*S. aureus* [mostly methicillin-resistant *S. aureus* (MRSA)] *Enterococcus, Pseudomonas, Klebsiella, E. coli* (mostly extended-spectrum beta-lactamase producing]
Healthcare-associated infections	***Causative organisms***
Ventilator-associated pneumonia (VAP)	*Acinetobacter baumannii, Klebsiella pneumoniae, P. aeruginosa*, and *Staphylococcus aureus* (MRSA)
Catheter-related bloodstream infection (CRBSI)	Coagulase-negative Staphylococci, *S. aureus, Enterococcus*, and *Candida*
Catheter-associated urinary tract infection (CAUTI)	*E. coli, Klebsiella*, and *Candida*

release of various proinflammatory cytokines, activation of complement system, and development of a proinflammatory condition to clear the infection. However, in sepsis, uncontrolled proinflammatory response leads to coagulation disorder, vasodilatation, and capillary leakage, subsequently leading to SIRS. Several anti-inflammatory mechanisms are also activated to counterbalance the harmful effects of pro-inflammation and to restore homeostasis. The initial hyperinflammatory response in sepsis later leads to increased immune cell dysfunction and immune paralysis. The dysregulation or imbalance of these pro- and anti-inflammatory mechanisms can lead to multiorgan failure, septic shock, long-term complications, and both early and late mortality. Understanding the mechanism of infection and pathophysiology is equally important as identifying and managing the infections in the ICU.

REFERENCES

1. Sikora A, Zahra F. Nosocomial Infections. In: StatPearls [Internet]. Treasure Island (FL): StatPearls Publishing; 2025.
2. Pradhan NP, Bhat SM, Ghadage DP. Nosocomial infections in the medical ICU: A retrospective study highlighting their prevalence, microbiological profile and impact on ICU stay and mortality. J Assoc Physicians India. 2014;62(10):18-21.
3. Loubet P, Voiriot G, Houhou-Fidouh N, Neuville M, Bouadma L, Lescure FX, et al. Impact of respiratory viruses in hospital-acquired pneumonia in the intensive care unit: A single-center retrospective study. J Clin Virol. 2017;91:52-7.
4. Grund S, Roggendorf M, Schweiger B. Outbreak of influenza virus A/H1N1 in a hospital ward for immunocompromised patients. Arch. 2010;155(11):1797-802.
5. Flores-Mireles A, Hreha TN, Hunstad DA. Pathophysiology, treatment, and prevention of catheter-associated urinary tract infection. Top Spinal Cord Inj Rehabil. 2019;25(3):228-40.
6. Diaconu O, Siriopol I, Poloşanu LI, Grigoraş I. Endotracheal tube biofilm and its impact on the pathogenesis of ventilator-associated pneumonia. J Crit Care Med (Targu Mures). 2018;4(2):50-5.
7. Arunan B, Ahmed NH, Kapil A, Vikram NK, Sinha S, Biswas A, et al. Central line-associated bloodstream infections: effect of patient and pathogen factors on outcome. J Glob Infect Dis. 2023;15(2):59-65.
8. Mada PK, Alam MU. *Clostridioides difficile* infection. In: StatPearls [Internet]. Treasure Island (FL): StatPearls Publishing; 2025.
9. Ahn D, Prince A. Host-Pathogen Interface: Progress in understanding the pathogenesis of infection due to multidrug-resistant bacteria in the Intensive Care Unit. J Infect Dis. 2017;215(suppl 1):S1-S8.
10. Shishido SN, Varahan S, Yuan K, Li X, Fleming SD. Humoral innate immune response and disease. Clin Immunol. 2012;144(2):142-58.
11. van Vught LA, Klein Klouwenberg PM, Spitoni C, Scicluna BP, Wiewel MA, Horn J, et al. Incidence, risk factors, and attributable mortality of secondary infections in the intensive care unit after admission for sepsis. JAMA. 2016;315(14):1469-79.
12. Kumar S, Ingle H, Prasad DV, Kumar H. Recognition of bacterial infection by innate immune sensors. Crit Rev Microbiol. 2013;39(3):229-46.
13. Murphy K, Weaver C, Mowat A. Janeway's Immunobiology, 9th edition. New York: Garland Science; 2016.
14. Denning NL, Aziz M, Gurien SD, Wang P. DAMPs and NETs in sepsis. Front Immunol. 2019;10:2536.
15. Hotchkiss RS, Moldawer LL, Opal SM, Reinhart K, Turnbull IR, Vincent JL. Sepsis and Septic Shock. Nat Rev Dis Primers. 2016;2:16045.
16. Vénéreau E, Ceriotti C, Bianchi ME. DAMPs from cell death to new life. Front Immunol. 2015;6:422.
17. Hattori Y, Hattori K, Suzuki T, Matsuda N. Recent advances in the pathophysiology and molecular basis of sepsis-associated organ dysfunction: Novel therapeutic implications and challenges. Pharmacol Ther. 2017;177:56-66.
18. Evans CE. Hypoxia and HIF Activation as a possible link between sepsis and Thrombosis. Thromb J. 2019;17:16.
19. Boldt J, Papsdorf M, Rothe MA, Kumle B, Piper S. Changes of the hemostatic network in critically ill patients: Is there a difference between sepsis, trauma, and neurosurgery patients? Crit Care Med. 2000;28(2):445-50.

20. Osuchowski MF, Welch K, Siddiqui J, Remick DG. Circulating cytokine/inhibitor profiles reshape the understanding of the SIRS/CARS continuum in sepsis and predict mortality. J Immunol. 2006;177(3):1967-74.
21. Otto GP, Sossdorf M, Claus RA, Rödel J, Menge K, Reinhart K, et al. The late phase of sepsis is characterized by an increased microbiological burden and death rate. Crit Care. 2011;15(4):R183.
22. Torres LK, Pickkers P, van der Poll T. Sepsis-induced immunosuppression. Annu Rev Physiol. 2022;84:157-81.
23. Vincent JL, Bihari DJ, Suter PM, Bruining HA, White J, Nicolas-Chanoin MH, et al. The prevalence of nosocomial infection in intensive care units in Europe. Results of the European Prevalence of Infection in Intensive Care (EPIC) Study. EPIC International Advisory Committee. JAMA. 1995;274(8):639-44.
24. Richards MJ, Edwards JR, Culver DH, Gaynes RP. Nosocomial infections in medical intensive care units in the United States. National nosocomial infections surveillance system. Crit Care Med. 1999;27(5):887-92.
25. Vincent JL, Rello J, Marshall J, Silva E, Anzueto A, Martin CD, et al.; EPIC II Group of Investigators. International study of the prevalence and outcomes of infection in intensive care units. JAMA. 2009;302(21):2323-9.
26. Trivedi TH, Shejale SB, Yeolekar ME. Nosocomial pneumonia in medical intensive care unit. J Assoc Physicians India. 2000;48(11):1070-3.
27. Khilnani GC, Zirpe K, Hadda V, Mehta Y, Madan K, Kulkarni A, et al. Guidelines for Antibiotic Prescription in Intensive Care Unit. Indian Critical Care Med. 2019;23(Suppl 1):S1-S63.

3

CHAPTER

Standard Precautions of Infections in the Intensive Care Unit

Priyanka Patil, Sneha Johnson, Bhavna Sunil Ghewari

LEARNING OBJECTIVES

- Apply standard precautions—including hand hygiene, personal protective equipment (PPE) use, and aseptic practices—to prevent transmission via shared equipment and procedures.
- Identify how factors such as staff fatigue, high patient turnover, and overlooked routine practices can increase infection risk.
- Promote a culture of safety where infection prevention is a visible, shared responsibility embedded in daily intensive care unit (ICU) care.

INTRODUCTION

Infection prevention in the intensive care unit (ICU) is a critical component of patient safety. ICU patients are often immunocompromised and exposed to invasive procedures, making them highly susceptible to healthcare-associated infections (HAIs). Standard precautions are the cornerstone of infection control, designed to minimize the risk of pathogen transmission among patients and healthcare workers. This chapter provides a comprehensive guide to implementing standard precautions which are uniform practices that apply to all patients, regardless of suspected or confirmed infection status.

The application of standard precautions during patient care is determined by the nature of the healthcare worker (HCW)-patient interaction and the extent of anticipated blood, body fluid, or pathogen exposure.

For example, in ICU a procedure like oral care will require only clean gloves and a mask, whereas during an invasive procedure such as central line insertion, maximal sterile barrier precaution is needed, i.e., gown, mask, cap, gloves, etc., along with surgical hand hygiene. Thus, education and training on the principles and rationale for recommended practices are critical elements of standard precautions because they facilitate appropriate decision-making and promote adherence when HCWs are faced with new circumstances. Another example of the importance of the use of Standard Precautions in ICU is during emergency intubation when infectious agents may not be suspected, but later are identified [e.g., severe acute respiratory syndrome coronavirus 2 (SARS-CoV-2), Neisseria meningitidis, etc., which are respiratory borne pathogens). Standard precautions are also intended to protect patients by ensuring that healthcare personnel do not carry infectious agents to patients on their hands or via equipment used during patient care.[1]

CORE CONTENT

In an ICU setting, it is always advisable to assume that every person is potentially infected or colonized with an organism that could be transmitted and apply infection control practices during care delivery.[1]

Standard precautions include a group of infection prevention practices that apply to all patients, regardless of suspected or confirmed infection status, in any setting in which healthcare is delivered.

The elements of standard precautions include:[1-10]

- Hand hygiene
- Personal protective equipment (PPE)
- Respiratory hygiene
- Appropriate patient placement
- Cleaning and disinfection of the environment
- Handling of textiles, laundry, and waste
- Safe injection practices

Hand Hygiene

During healthcare delivery, avoid unnecessary touching of surfaces in close proximity to the patient to prevent both contamination of clean hands from environmental surfaces and transmission of pathogens from contaminated hands to surfaces.

Cleaning your hands reduces:

- The potential spread of deadly germs to patients including those resistant to antibiotics.
- The risk of healthcare personnel colonization or infection caused by germs received from the patient or the surrounding environment.

In ICU, every opportunity of Hand hygiene is equally important as explained in **Table 1**. The method of hand hygiene, hand wash, or hand rub will depend upon the gross organic matter on hand. For WHO Moment 2 and Moment 3, handwashing with soap and water is generally preferred, as these steps often involve procedures or exposures where the likelihood of organic soiling is higher.

When hands are visibly dirty, contaminated with proteinaceous material, or visibly soiled with blood or body fluids, wash hands with either a nonantimicrobial soap and water or an antimicrobial soap and water. If Hands are not visibly soiled use alcohol-based hand rub.

Technique: Refer to Chapter 5

Wash hands with non-antimicrobial soap and water or with antimicrobial soap and water if contact with spores (e.g., *Clostridium difficile* or *Bacillus*

TABLE 1: Indications for Hand Hygiene by World Health Organization (WHO).

WHO moments	*Examples from ICU setting*	*Default action*
Before touching a patient	Before shaking hands, before taking vitals (BP, pulse, and temperature), and before auscultating the chest or abdomen	ABHR (if hands are not visibly soiled)
Before clean or aseptic procedure	Before inserting a central line or foley catheter, before suctioning via endotracheal/tracheostomy tube, before dressing a central line or surgical wound, before preparing IV antibiotics or infusion, and before assisting in bedside sterile procedures (e.g., chest tube insertion)	ABHR preferred
After body fluid exposure risk	After emptying the foley catheter bag or chest drain, after handling blood samples or sputum containers, after cleaning vomitus or stool, after changing incontinence sheets or dressing with drainage, after assisting with wound irrigation	ABHR or hand wash (if visibly soiled)
After touching a patient	After repositioning or comforting the patient, after adjusting the oxygen mask or checking a peripheral line, after checking capillary refill or skin turgor, after physically supporting the patient during mobilization	ABHR
After touching a patient's surrounding	After adjusting ventilator settings or monitors, after touching IV stand, infusion pump, or bed remote, after handling the call bell, side rail, or medication cart, after touching patient files or bedside notes	ABHR
In addition, wash hands when visibly soiled, before eating or feeding patients, and after using the restroom		

(ABHR: alcohol-based hand rub; ICU: intensive care unit; WHO: World Health Organization)

anthracis) is likely to have occurred. The physical action of washing and rinsing hands under such circumstances is recommended because alcohols, chlorhexidine, iodophors, and other antiseptic agents have poor activity against spores.

Along with hand hygiene its equally important to not wear artificial fingernails or extenders since the staff duties include direct contact with patients at high risk for infection and associated adverse outcomes.

Washbasins in ICUs should have elbow or foot operated taps and be strategically situated for convenient access by HCWs. Washbasins designated for hand washing should be separate and not used to wash instruments.

Personal Protective Equipment

The selection of PPE is based on the nature of the patient interaction and/or the likely mode(s) of transmission. Ensure there is no contamination of clothing or skin while removing PPE. Discard PPE when leaving the patient's room and perform hand hygiene before meeting the next patient. Discard and replace PPE if it becomes damaged, soiled, or wet.

- *Gloves:* Health workers should:
    - Remember that wearing gloves is not a substitute for hand hygiene.
    - Wear gloves during activities that may involve exposure to blood and other body fluids, for contact precautions and in outbreak situations.
    - Remove gloves after caring for a patient—the same pair of gloves should not be worn for the care of more than one patient.
    - Change gloves between tasks and procedures if moving from a contaminated body site to another body site (noncontaminated) on the same patient.
    - Wear sterile gloves for aseptic procedures, such as catheter insertion, as part of maximal barrier precautions.
    - Do not reuse gloves after reprocessing or decontamination.
- *Gown:* Routine donning of gowns upon entrance to the ICU is not indicated but HCWs should:
    - Wear a gown to protect skin and prevent soiling of clothing during activities that are likely to generate splashes or sprays of blood, body fluids, secretions, or excretions. A waterproof apron should be worn over the gown if the gown is not fluid-resistant, and if splashing or spraying is anticipated.
    - Do not reuse gowns even for repeated contacts with same patient in ICU.
- *Medical masks:* Health workers should:
    - Wear a surgical mask to protect mucous membranes of the nose and mouth against splashes or sprays of body fluids, respiratory secretions, and chemicals.
    - This mask also helps to protect the sample from contamination which leads to false positive test results, e.g., during a lumbar puncture, if a medical mask is not worn, the CSF may get contamination with the HCW's saliva leading to a false positive *Streptococcus pneumoniae* (oral flora) result.
    - *Respirators:* Wear a respirator (e.g., N95) for protection from inhalation of airborne particles (<5 μm) and/or when performing aerosol-generating procedures. Examples of aerosol-generating procedures in ICU—tracheal intubation, noninvasive ventilation such as bi-level positive airway pressure, continuous positive airway pressure, tracheostomy, cardiopulmonary resuscitation, manual ventilation before intubation, bronchoscopy, sputum induction by using nebulized hypertonic saline, etc.
    - Do a fit test before using a respirator for the first time, and perform a seal check every time a respirator is used.
    - Replace the mask or respirator if it is damaged, visibly soiled or wet or if breathing becomes difficult.

- *Eye protection:*
  - Wear either eye protection (eye visor, goggles) or a face shield to protect mucous membranes of the eyes during activities that are likely to generate splashes or sprays of blood, body fluids, secretions, and excretions.
  - Ensure that goggles fit over and around the eyes or personal prescription lenses.
  - Ensure that a face shield covers the forehead, extends below the chin, and wraps around the side of the face. Face shields are more comfortable to wear with eyeglasses.

Respiratory Hygiene

- Health workers should apply source control measures for individuals with respiratory symptoms.
- Encourage patients and staff to use tissues or masks to cover their mouth and nose when coughing or sneezing as shown in **Figure 1**.
- Maintain spatial separation of at least one meter or 3 feet between patients.

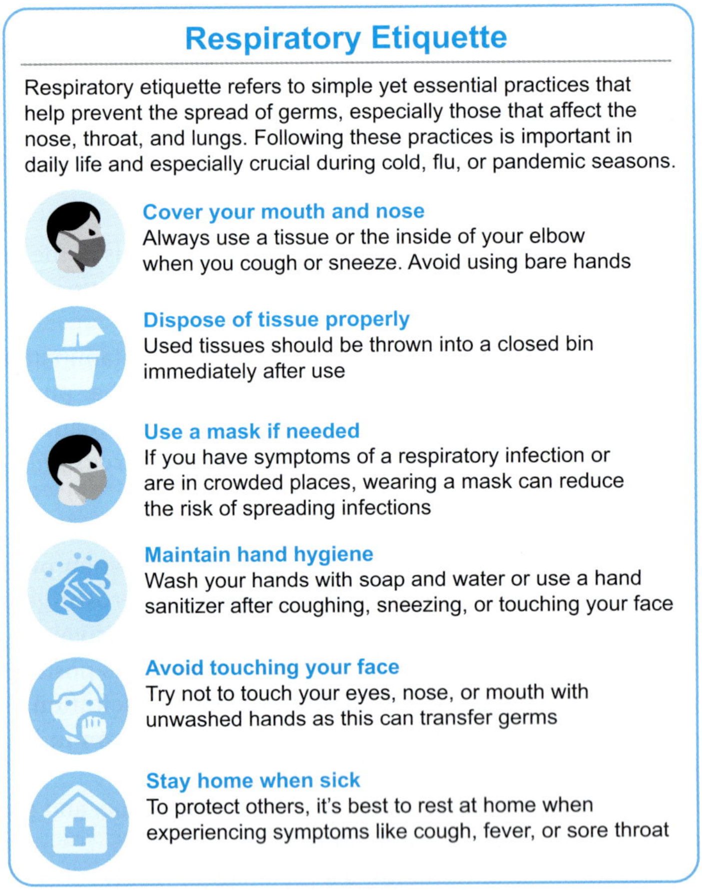

Fig. 1: Respiratory hygiene.

Appropriate Patient Placement

Appropriate patient placement is essential to prevent infection spread in hospitals. Whenever possible, place patients in *single rooms*—especially for those with contact, droplet, or airborne transmission risks. If single rooms are unavailable, *cohort* patients with the same infection, and maintain at least *1 meter (≈ 3 feet)* between beds. Decisions should factor in transmission mode, patient infectivity, and the vulnerability of others. In addition, applying standard precautions involves recognizing the need for specific isolation types and environmental controls:[1]

- *Barrier nursing* is used to prevent the spread of infection from patients with highly contagious diseases.
- *Protective (reverse barrier) nursing* is applied for *immunocompromised patients*, often in *positive-pressure rooms* to prevent entry of airborne pathogens.
- *Negative-pressure rooms* are essential for *airborne infections* (e.g., tuberculosis and measles), as they prevent contaminated air from escaping into adjacent areas.
- Use of *dedicated medical equipment* for isolated patients further limits cross-transmission.
- Continuous *education of HCWs and patients* about isolation measures strengthens adherence and enhances safety.

Cleaning and Disinfection of the Environment

- Establish policies and procedures for routine and targeted cleaning of environmental surfaces as indicated by the level of patient contact and degree of soiling.
- Clean and disinfect surfaces that are likely to be contaminated with pathogens, including those that are in close proximity to the patient (e.g., side tables) and frequently touched surfaces in the patient care environment (e.g., bed rails, door knobs, monitors, and syringe pumps), telephones in ICU.
- Do not use surface cleaning cloths from one ICU bed to another.
- Use US Environmental Protection Agency (EPA)-registered disinfectants that have microbiocidal (i.e., killing) activity against the pathogens most likely to contaminate the ICU environment. Use in accordance with manufacturer's instructions. Review the efficacy of in-use disinfectants when evidence of continuing transmission of an infectious agent (e.g., rotavirus, *C. difficile,* and norovirus) may indicate ineffectiveness to the in-use product and change to an effective disinfectant based on Centers for Disease Control and Prevention (CDC), USA guidelines.[1]
- Deal with spills of blood and body fluid/substance as soon as possible, in accordance with local protocols.[11]

Handling of Textiles, Laundry, and Biomedical Waste

- Handle-soiled linen and waste carefully (with minimal manipulation or agitation) to prevent personal contamination and transfer to other patients. Ensure there is minimum dispersion of aerosols from contaminated linen.
- Remove heavily-soiled material (e.g. feces) from linen, while wearing appropriate PPE, before placing it in the laundry bag.
- The bedside-soiled linen should be stored in a designated area, away from direct patient care and medication preparation area.
- Store clean linen in a clean, dry, closed cupboards to protect from dust, dirt, and pests.

Biomedical Waste Management[12]

- Effective biomedical waste management is legally mandated and essential for minimizing environmental contamination and reducing infection risk. Facilities must comply with the Bio-Medical Waste Management Rules, 2016 (amended 2019), and follow local State Pollution Control Board–approved protocols regarding segregation, collection, storage, transport, treatment, and disposal.
- *Segregation:* Separate waste at the point of generation into categories such as infectious, sharps, and general waste.
- *Color-coded containers **(Fig. 2)**:*
  Use appropriately labeled containers for different types of waste (e.g., yellow for infectious nonrecyclable waste, red for infectious recyclable waste, blue for glass material and metal implants, and white puncture proof containers for sharps).
- *Disposal:* Ensure timely removal and safe transportation of waste to designated temporary disposal sites within the premises.

Safe Injection Practices

Health workers should:

- Prepare injections in a clean workspace, where there is low risk of contamination from blood, body fluid, splashes, or sprays.

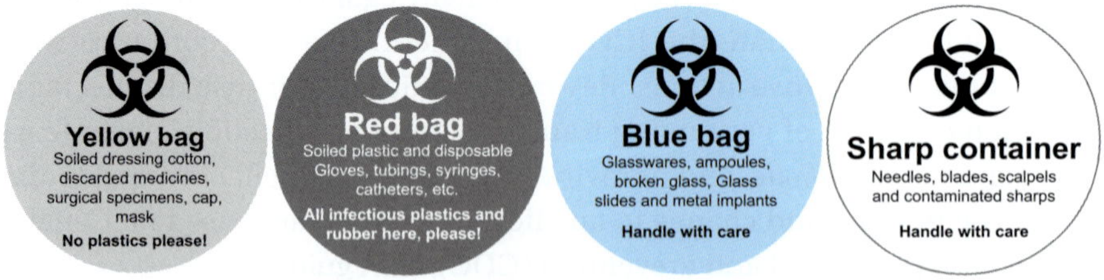

Fig. 2: Biomedical waste segregation color-coded *(For color version, see Plate 1)*.

- Perform hand hygiene prior to preparing the medication and touching the patient.
- Preferably use a sterile, safety-engineered syringe to avoid injuries to HCWs.
- Use a sterile medication vial and diluents.
- Always use a sterile syringe and needle to withdraw and reconstitute medications, and never leave a needle in the septum of a vial.
- Avoid use of multi-dose vials or, if used, dedicate the vial for single-patient use.
- Label each multidose vial (MDV) with the date it was first opened. Follow the manufacturer's discard instructions, discard immediately if sterility is in doubt, and dispose of it 28 days after opening—unless the vial label indicates a different timeframe.
- Before any invasive procedure, cleanse the skin using a suitable antiseptic, such as chlorhexidine or povidone-iodine, in a center-to-periphery motion. Allow the antiseptic to air-dry completely to reduce the risk of contamination and maximize its effectiveness.
- Provide a puncture-resistant sharps container for sharps disposal at the point of care for easy access not recap, bend, break, manipulate, or manually remove the needle from the syringe. Discard the sharps container when it is three quarters full, seal it, and store it in a secure area.
- *Scrub the hub:* Before any access, disinfect the hub with a 70% alcohol wipe for at least 5 seconds.[13]
- *Flush the line:* After connecting, flush with sterile saline to keep the catheter clear and reduce infection risk. These steps are essential to maintain asepsis and prevent catheter-related infections.

CONCLUSION

Standard precautions are backbone to prevent infection transmission in a high-risk environment like the ICU. They should be followed for every patient irrespective of their known or unknown infectious disease status. These precautions are critical to protecting both patients and HCWs in the ICU setting.

REFERENCES

1. Siegel JD, Rhinehart E, Jackson M, Chiarello L. 2007 Guideline for Isolation Precautions: Preventing Transmission of Infectious Agents in Health Care Settings. Am J Infect Control. 2007;35(10):S65-164.
2. CDC Infection Control. (2024). Standard Precautions for All Patient Care. [online] Available from https://www.cdc.gov/infection-control/hcp/basics/standard-precautions.html [Last accessed August, 2025].
3. WHO. 2022. Standard precautions for the prevention and control of infections: aide-memoire. [online] Available from https://iris.who.int/bitstream/

handle/10665/356855/WHO-UHL-IHS-IPC-2022.1-eng.pdf?sequence=1 [Last accessed August, 2025].

4. Centers for Disease Control and Prevention. (2024). Clinical safety: Hand hygiene for healthcare workers. [online] Available from https://www.cdc.gov/clean-hands/hcp/clinical-safety/index.html [Last accessed August, 2025].
5. Centers for Disease Control and Prevention (U.S.). (2005). Cover your cough, clean your hands after coughing or sneezing. [online] Available from https://stacks.cdc.gov/view/cdc/23304 [Last accessed August, 2025].
6. World Health Organization. (2009). WHO Guidelines on Hand Hygiene in Health Care. [online] Available from: https://www.who.int/publications/i/item/9789241597906 [Last accessed August, 2025].
7. CDC. (2024). Safe Injection Practices to Prevent Transmission of Infections to Patients. [online] Available from https://www.cdc.gov/injection-safety/hcp/clinical-guidance/index.html [Last accessed August, 2025].
8. Directorate General of Health Services Ministry of Health & Family Welfare, Central Pollution Control Board Ministry of Environment, Forest & Climate Change. (2016). Guidelines for Management of Healthcare Waste as per Biomedical Waste Management Rules, 2016. [online] Available from https://cpcb.nic.in/uploads/Projects/Bio-Medical-Waste/Guidelines_healthcare_June_2018.pdf [Last accessed August, 2025].
9. CDC Infection Control. (2024). CDC's Core Infection Prevention and Control Practices for Safe Healthcare Delivery in All Settings. [online] Available from https://www.cdc.gov/infection-control/hcp/core-practices/index.html [Last accessed August, 2025].
10. Rutala WA, Weber DJ. Disinfection and sterilization in health care facilities. *Infect Dis Clin North Am.* 2021;*35*(3):575-607.
11. National Centre for Disease Control (NCDC), Ministry of Health & Family Welfare. (2020). National Guidelines for Infection Prevention and Control in Healthcare Facilities, India. Section 5.3: "Blood and body substance spill management." [online] Available from https://cdn.who.int/media/docs/default-source/searo/india/antimicrobial-resistance/ipcguidelines-web-sep2020.pdf [Last accessed August, 2025].
12. Central Pollution Control Board, Ministry of Environment, Forest and Climate Change. Bio-Medical Waste Management Rules, 2016. G.S.R. 343(E), dated 28 March 2016; amended 16 March 2018 and 19 February 2019. Government of India. Available from: https://cpcb.nic.in/uploads/Projects/Bio-Medical-Waste/Bio-medical_Waste_Management_Rules_2016.pdf
13. Centers for Disease Control and Prevention (CDC). Guidelines for the Prevention of Intravascular Catheter-Related Infections. 2011; updated April 12, 2024.

2

SECTION

Infection Control Policies and Guidelines

Section Editor: *Aruna Poojary*

4

CHAPTER

Overview of Key Global Guidelines for Infection Control Policies

Poonam Gupta

LEARNING OBJECTIVES

Key global infection prevention and control guidelines:

- Hand hygiene.
- Surgical site infections.
- Core components of an IPC program.
- Environmental cleaning, disinfection and sterilization guidelines.
- *Clostridium difficile* infections.

INTRODUCTION

Healthcare-associated infections (HAIs) remain a significant global health challenge, leading to increased morbidity, prolonged hospital stays, and higher healthcare costs. The World Health Organization (WHO) estimates that 15% of hospitalized patients worldwide acquire at least one HAI, with rates up to 20 times higher in low- and middle-income countries (LMICs) compared to high-income countries (HICs) which is about 7%. Infection Prevention and Control (IPC) guidelines are essential tools in the fight against HAIs. These guidelines, developed by global health authorities, provide evidence-based recommendations to standardize and improve IPC practices across diverse healthcare settings. This chapter provides an overview of key global IPC guidelines that inform our local practices and strategies.

GLOBAL INFECTION RATES

Understanding global infection rates is crucial for contextualizing the importance of IPC guidelines. **Table 1** summarizes key infection types and their global incidence.

These infection rates underscore the need for robust IPC programs and adherence to established guidelines.[1]

TABLE 1: Infection rates global incidence.

Infection type	*Global incidence*	*Remarks*
Surgical site infections (SSI)	2–5% of surgical patients globally; higher in LMICs	• SSIs are the most common • HAIs in surgical patients
Catheter-associated UTIs (CAUTIs)	1.5–3.1 per 1,000 catheter-days	Rates vary by facility resources and staff training
Central line-associated BSIs (CLABSIs)	0.8–4.8 per 1,000 central	Especially high in ICUs with limited IPC programs
Ventilator-associated events (VAEs)	1–6 per 1,000 ventilator-days	Ventilator-associated pneumonia is the most severe category
Clostridium difficile infection (CDI)	2.56 per 1,000 admissions globally; higher in North America (4.85) and Europe (2.84)	Reflects antibiotic stewardship and environmental cleaning practices

(BSIs: bloodstream infections; HAIs: healthcare-associated infections; ICU: intensive care unit; IPC: infection prevention and control; LMIC: low- and middle-income countries; UTI: urinary tract infections)

KEY GLOBAL INFECTION PREVENTION AND CONTROL GUIDELINES

World Health Organization Guidelines on Hand Hygiene in Healthcare (2009, Updated 2022)[2]

Overview

Hand hygiene is the most effective measure to prevent the transmission of infections in healthcare settings. The World Health Organization (WHO) "Five Moments for Hand Hygiene" framework has become a standard teaching and monitoring tool in healthcare facilities.

Impact and Evidence of Effectiveness

Implementation of WHO hand hygiene strategies has led to significant improvements in compliance and infection rates:

- A large-scale intervention in Geneva showed that hand hygiene compliance increased from 48 to 66%, and methicillin-resistant *Staphylococcus aureus* (MRSA) infection rates declined by 50%.
- Studies in African and South Asian hospitals implementing WHO strategies noted reductions in neonatal sepsis and surgical site infections (SSIs).

World Health Organization "Five Moments for Hand Hygiene" Framework

A central innovation of the WHO guidance is the "Five Moments for Hand Hygiene" model. This framework simplifies decision-making for healthcare workers by identifying critical moments when hand hygiene should be performed:

1. *Before touching a patient:* To prevent transmission of pathogens to the patient.
2. *Before clean/aseptic procedures:* To protect the patient from harmful microbes, including their own flora.
3. *After body fluid exposure risk:* To protect oneself and the healthcare environment.
4. *After touching a patient*: To prevent spread to oneself and the environment.
5. *After touching patient surroundings:* To prevent indirect transmission via environmental surfaces.

This model is intended to reduce ambiguity and improve the timing and consistency of hand hygiene practices.

Preferred Methods and Techniques

The WHO recommends two primary methods for hand hygiene in clinical settings:

1. *Alcohol-based hand rub (ABHR):*
    - Preferred method when hands are not visibly soiled.
    - Must contain 60–80% alcohol to be effective.
    - Quick, effective, and well-tolerated by skin.
2. *Handwashing with soap and water:*
    - Required when hands are visibly dirty or contaminated with proteinaceous material (e.g., blood, bodily fluids).
    - Also necessary in outbreak settings involving *Clostridioides difficile* or norovirus, where alcohol alone may not be sufficient.

Both methods should follow WHO-recommended techniques, ensuring coverage of all hand surfaces for 20–40 seconds (ABHR) or 40–60 seconds (soap and water).

- *Surgical hand antisepsis,* an ABHR for duration of 2–3 minutes recommended.

ABHR should have:

- 60–80% alcohol content
- Have *broad-spectrum activity* (including against bacteria and viruses).
- Demonstrate *persistent antimicrobial effect.*
- Be tested according to *EN 12791* (European Standard) or equivalent the American Society for Testing and Materials (ASTM) standards.

World Health Organization Global Guidelines for the Prevention of Surgical Site Infection (2016)[3]

Overview

Surgical site infections are among the most common and preventable HAI. They can lead to prolonged hospital stays, increased antimicrobial resistance, and additional surgical interventions. In LMICs, the incidence of SSIs can be as high as 20% in certain surgical procedures.

Recognizing this global burden, the WHO released its first consolidated *Global Guidelines for the Prevention of Surgical Site Infection* in 2016. The document provides evidence-based recommendations that span the *entire surgical pathway*—from preoperative patient preparation to postoperative wound care.

The WHO guideline is structured into *29 recommendations*, divided into two major phases:

1. *Prevention measures in the preoperative and intraoperative period (23 recommendations)*
2. *Postoperative period (6 recommendations)*

Each recommendation is based on a systematic review of the best available evidence, rated using the GRADE (Grading of Recommendations Assessment, Development, and Evaluation) approach.

Key Preoperative Recommendations

- *Preoperative bathing or showering:* Patients should bathe or shower prior to surgery using either soap or antiseptic solution to reduce skin flora. There is no evidence that antiseptic solutions are more effective than plain soap.
- *Hair removal:* If hair must be removed, it should be done with clippers—not razors—and as close to the time of surgery as possible. Shaving increases the risk of skin abrasions and subsequent infection.
- *Antimicrobial prophylaxis:* Antibiotics should be administered within 120 minutes before surgical incision (preferably within 60 minutes) to ensure adequate tissue levels. Prophylaxis should not be continued after the end of surgery, except in specific clinical scenarios.
- *Patient decolonization:* For high-risk patients (e.g., carriers of *Staphylococcus aureus*), the use of mupirocin nasal ointment and chlorhexidine body wash may be considered.

Intraoperative Recommendations

- *Hand preparation for surgical team:* Use of an ABHR with persistent antimicrobial activity is recommended over traditional surgical scrubbing with antiseptic soap and water.
- *Use of sterile gloves and gowns:* Single-use, sterile surgical gloves and gowns are essential, with double gloving recommended for high-risk procedures.
- *Maintenance of normothermia:* Active warming devices should be used to maintain normal body temperature during surgery. Hypothermia is associated with higher SSI rates due to impaired immune function.

- *Control of blood glucose:* In both diabetic and nondiabetic patients, perioperative glucose levels should be controlled. Hyperglycemia increases the risk of infection due to immunosuppression and poor wound healing.
- *Use of appropriate surgical antiseptic agents:* Alcohol-based antiseptic solutions (e.g., chlorhexidine-alcohol) are preferred for skin preparation before incision. These agents reduce skin flora more effectively than aqueous solutions.

Postoperative Recommendations

- *Wound dressing management:* A sterile dressing should be used to cover the surgical site for 24–48 hours postoperatively. There is no added benefit to prolonged dressing beyond this period if the wound remains dry and uninfected.
- *Antibiotic stewardship:* Routine use of postoperative antibiotics in clean surgical procedures is not recommended. This reduces the risk of antimicrobial resistance and side effects.
- *Monitoring and wound care:* Regular assessment of the surgical wound for signs of infection is essential. Healthcare workers should be trained in recognizing early signs of SSI and managing them appropriately.

Implementation Tools and Support

To facilitate adoption, WHO developed several practical tools, including:

- *SSI prevention checklists* integrated into surgical safety programs.
- *Training modules* for surgical and nursing staff.
- *Multimodal improvement strategies,* aligning with the WHO's broader IPC framework.

Facilities are encouraged to integrate SSI surveillance into broader infection monitoring programs and use standardized case definitions, such as those from National Healthcare Safety Network (NHSN).

Key Elements

- Preoperative bathing or showering using soap or antiseptic.
- Appropriate surgical antimicrobial prophylaxis (timing, selection, and duration).
- Maintenance of perioperative normothermia and glycemic control.
- Effective sterilization of surgical instruments and use of sterile techniques.
- Appropriate postoperative wound care and dressing selection.

Relevance

These guidelines are critical for surgical teams aiming to reduce complications and improve surgical outcomes in both routine and high-risk procedures.

Their structured approach supports compliance through policy integration and operating room protocols.

World Health Organization Core Components of Infection Prevention and Control Programs (2016)[4]

Overview

This document outlines eight essential components that underpin effective IPC systems at the national and facility levels. These components are designed to be scalable and adaptable across all resource settings.

Key Elements

- IPC programs supported by national and facility-level structures.
- Evidence-based IPC guidelines.
- IPC education and training for healthcare workers.
- HAI surveillance systems using standardized definitions.
- Multimodal strategies for effective implementation.
- Monitoring and feedback mechanisms for IPC practices.
- Adequate staffing, infrastructure, and workload considerations.
- Institutional safety culture promoting IPC compliance.

Relevance

The framework serves as the foundation for any healthcare setting striving to establish or strengthen its IPC capacity. It has been especially valuable in countries initiating national IPC programs with WHO support.

World Health Organization Guidelines on Environmental Cleaning and Disinfection in Healthcare, Particularly for Resource-limited Settings (2019)[5]

Overview

Environmental cleaning plays a pivotal role in reducing microbial contamination and preventing HAIs, particularly those caused by multidrug-resistant organisms (MDROs). The WHO's environmental cleaning guidelines provide clear, risk-based protocols tailored to LMICs.

Key Elements

- Zoning of healthcare areas by risk level to guide cleaning frequency.
- Selection and appropriate use of cleaning agents (e.g., chlorine-based disinfectants).
- Standardized cleaning procedures and schedules.
- Training and supervision of environmental cleaning staff.
- Safe waste disposal and linen handling procedures.

Relevance

This guidance is critical in settings where advanced sterilization equipment or high-level disinfectants may be unavailable. By emphasizing practical, affordable, and impactful practices, it improves environmental hygiene even with limited resources.

Centers for Disease Control and Prevention Guidelines for Disinfection and Sterilization in Healthcare Facilities (2008, Updated 2017)[6]

Overview

Published by the U.S. Centers for Disease Control and Prevention (CDC), this guideline provides comprehensive recommendations for the cleaning and sterilization of medical instruments and surfaces.

Key Elements

- Classification of medical devices (critical, semicritical, and noncritical items).
- Appropriate cleaning and disinfection processes for each device type.
- Use of high-level disinfectants and sterilization methods (e.g., autoclaving, ethylene oxide).
- Recommendations for managing exposure incidents and monitoring process efficacy.
- Environmental infection control procedures for surfaces, rooms, and water systems.

Relevance

These protocols are widely referenced in hospitals globally, particularly for surgical, critical care, and outpatient services. They serve as a technical standard, especially in facilities where infection control committees oversee sterilization departments.

Centers for Disease Control and Prevention Guidelines National Healthcare Safety Network Surveillance Protocols[7]

Overview

The NHSN provides standardized methods for HAI surveillance, which supports quality improvement and benchmarking in healthcare facilities. While originally developed for U.S. hospitals, many international institutions use NHSN definitions and tools. CDC HAI progress reports give the latest benchmarks and have defined 2023 National HAI Benchmarks and 2024–2028 Reduction Targets.

Key Elements

- Surveillance definitions for key HAIs [e.g., central line-associated bloodstream infection (CLABSI), catheter-associated urinary tract infection (CAUTI), ventilator-associated pneumonia (VAP), SSI].
- Standardized data collection and reporting formats.
- Risk-adjusted benchmarking [standardized infection ratio (SIR)].
- Tools for antimicrobial use and resistance surveillance.

Relevance

Hospitals and health systems use NHSN protocols for internal performance monitoring and external reporting. Adoption of these standards enhances comparability of HAI data across regions and countries.

Association for Professionals in Infection Control and Epidemiology Guidelines and Resources on *Clostridoides difficile* Infection[8]

Overview

The Association for Professionals in Infection Control and Epidemiology (APIC) offers detailed recommendations for managing and preventing *C. difficile* infections in healthcare environments, which remain a major cause of morbidity and mortality globally.

Key Elements

- Early identification and isolation of suspected CDI cases.
- Contact precautions and use of personal protective equipment (PPE).
- Use of sporicidal disinfectants for environmental cleaning.
- Antibiotic stewardship programs to minimize unnecessary antimicrobial use.
- Education and training for staff and visitors.

Relevance

The APIC's guidance is instrumental for facilities dealing with CDI outbreaks or endemic cases. Their resources align with CDC and Society for Healthcare Epidemiology of America (SHEA) recommendations, offering comprehensive prevention bundles.[9,10]

CONCLUSION

The global burden of HAIs remains unacceptably high, particularly in resource-constrained environments. However, HAIs are largely preventable with effective IPC programs grounded in evidence-based guidelines. The global IPC-related guidance documents outlined in this chapter form the backbone of contemporary infection control efforts.

From WHO's comprehensive frameworks and hand hygiene campaigns to CDC's technical sterilization protocols and APIC's targeted CDI strategies, each resource offers specific tools and actions that are both practical and adaptable. Adoption of these guidelines supports:

- Standardization of IPC protocols across departments and facilities.
- Strengthening of institutional safety cultures.
- Monitoring compliance and performance through reliable surveillance.
- Improved patient outcomes and reductions in antimicrobial resistance.

Institutions should adopt these global standards into context-specific protocols, including local challenges, implementation pathways, and outcome measurements.

REFERENCES

1. World Health Organization. (2024). Global report on infection prevention and control. [Online] Available from https://www.who.int/publications/i/item/9789240103986 [Last accessed August, 2025].
2. World Health Organization. (2009, updated 2022). WHO Guidelines on Hand Hygiene in Health Care. [Online] Available from https://www.who.int/publications/i/item/9789241597906 [Last accessed August, 2025].
3. World Health Organization. (2016). Global Guidelines for the Prevention of Surgical Site Infection. [Online] Available from https://www.who.int/publications/i/item/9789241550475 [Last accessed August, 2025].
4. World Health Organization. (2016). Core Components for Infection Prevention and Control Programmes. [Online] Available from https://www.who.int/publications/i/item/9789241549929 [Last accessed August, 2025].
5. World Health Organization. (2019). Environmental cleaning procedures in health care facilities in resource limited settings. [Online] Available from https://iris.who.int/bitstream/handle/10665/366379/9789240051041-eng.pdf [Last accessed August, 2025].
6. Rutala WA, Weber DJ, Healthcare Infection Control Practices Advisory Committee (HICPAC). (2008). Guideline for Disinfection and Sterilization in Healthcare Facilities. Update June 2024. [Online] Available from https://www.cdc.gov/infection-control/media/pdfs/guideline-disinfection-h.pdf [Last accessed August, 2025].
7. National Healthcare Safety Network (NHSN). (2025). Patient safety component manual. [Online] Available from https://www.cdc.gov/nhsn/pdfs/pscmanual/pcsmanual_current.pdf [Last accessed August, 2025].
8. APIC. (2022). Guide to Preventing *Clostridium difficile* Infections. [Online] Available from https://apic.org/resources/topic-specific-infection-prevention/clostridium-difficile/ [Last accessed August, 2025].
9. Lessa FC, Bamberg WM, Beldavs ZG, Dumyati GK, Dunn JR, Farley MM, et al. Burden of *Clostridium difficile* Infection in the United States. New Engl J Med. 2015;372(9):825-34.
10. Angulo FJ, Furtado M, Gonzalez E, Zhang P, Kelly PH, Moïsi JC. Incidence of public health surveillance-reported *Clostridioides difficile* infections in thirteen countries worldwide: A narrative review. J Anaerobe. 2024;74:102878.

5 CHAPTER

Environmental Hygiene in Intensive Care Unit Settings

Gyanendra Agarwal, (Lt Col) Shibu Sasidharan, Smita Sharma, Yasmin Muhammed, Suryasnata Das

LEARNING OBJECTIVES

- Know the spectrum of action and specific qualities of antiseptics so that we can use them effectively.
- Know about various modalities of disinfection and their specific qualities that can be used to disinfect the environment around us in ICUs.
- By knowing these effective practices, we can help and guide other healthcare professionals (doctors and nurses), housekeeping, and general duty assistants in the work of infection control.

INTRODUCTION

Healthcare-associated infections (HCAIs) affect millions of patients worldwide.[1] HCAI leads to critical illness, prolonged hospital and ICU stays, financial and resource burden on the healthcare system, disability, and often leads to loss of life. The World Health Organization (WHO) in October 2005 launched "Clean Care is Safer Care," aimed at reducing HCAI worldwide.[1] The incidence of HCAI is significant in developed countries, that is, 5–15% of hospitalized patients and 9–37% of those admitted to intensive care units (ICUs).[1] In a developing country like ours, where there are numerous unfavorable factors such as overcrowding, poor hygiene, and sanitation facilities, a lack or shortage of basic healthcare infrastructure, limited financial resources, and inadequately trained staff, HCAI is a huge problem. HCAIs are more prevalent in the developing countries, with the highest prevalence in the ICUs, as endorsed by Mehta A, Rosenthal V, Detal study [HCAI incidence rate of 4.4% (9.06 infections per 1,000 ICU days)].[2] HCAIs are mostly due to multidrug-resistant organisms (MDROs), leading to the use of higher antibiotics for a longer duration.[3]

Environmental hygiene in the ICU is a critical component of infection prevention and control, directly impacting patient safety and clinical outcomes.[4-8] The ICU environment presents unique challenges due to the concentration of critically ill, immunocompromised patients who are at the highest risk for HAIs. Studies demonstrate that environmental contamination contributes to 20–40% of HAIs, with pathogens persisting on surfaces for extended periods and serving as reservoirs for cross-transmission.[9] The complex ICU ecosystem, characterized by high patient acuity, frequent invasive procedures, and intensive use of medical devices, necessitates stringent environmental controls to minimize infection risk.[8]

The environmental hygiene in the ICU involves comprehensive monitoring of surfaces, air, and water quality, along with rigorous disinfection of medical equipment and patient care items.[5] Evidence-based environmental hygiene practices have been shown to reduce HAI rates by up to 30% when implemented systematically.[9]

AIR QUALITY

The healthcare setting must have air changes, temperature, and humidity appropriate to the specific area requirements. ICU-specific air quality standards include:

- *Air changes per hour (ACH):* Minimum 6 ACH for general ICU areas, with at least two ACH of outside air.
- *Temperature control:* Maintained between 20 and 24°C (68–75°F) to optimize patient comfort and prevent condensation.
- *Relative humidity:* 30–60% to minimize microbial growth while preventing static electricity and respiratory irritation.
- *Filtration:* Minimum MERV 14 filters (equivalent to 90% efficiency) for general ICU areas.

PRESSURE DIFFERENTIALS AND INTENSIVE CARE UNIT-SPECIFIC REQUIREMENTS

Negative pressure airflow must be maintained in soiled areas, and positive pressure airflow must be maintained in clean areas and should be regularly monitored. Specific ICU applications include:

- *Isolation rooms:* Negative pressure with a minimum of 12 ACH (including 2 ACH outside air) for airborne infection isolation rooms housing patients with tuberculosis, measles, or varicella.
- *Protective environment rooms:* Positive pressure with 12 ACH for immunocompromised patients (bone marrow transplant and severe neutropenia).
- *Pressure monitoring:* Continuous monitoring with visual indicators (smoke tubes and electronic monitors) and alarm systems for pressure failures.
- *Anteroom requirements:* Properly designed air locks with pressure cascading from clean to dirty areas.

WATER QUALITY

Water quality represents a critical vulnerability in ICU settings that has precipitated numerous serious outbreaks affecting vulnerable patient populations.[8] The healthcare setting should be aware of the quality of its water supply and develop policies to address known problems.[5]

Major Intensive Care Unit Water-related Outbreak Examples

- *Legionella pneumophila* outbreaks in ICU water systems have resulted in pneumonia clusters with mortality rates exceeding 25%.
- *Pseudomonas aeruginosa* contamination of ICU tap water led to ventilator-associated pneumonia outbreaks with significant morbidity.
- *Acinetobacter baumannii* waterborne transmission resulted in multidrug-resistant infections in critically ill patients.

BIOFILM PREVENTION STRATEGIES

- *Regular flushing protocols:* Daily flushing of all water outlets, especially low-use taps, to prevent stagnation and biofilm development.
- *Splashback prevention:* Avoiding sinks with poor drainage that create splashback conditions, which can aerosolize contaminated water.
- *Outlet maintenance:* Regular removal, cleaning, descaling, or replacement of water outlets, hoses, and thermal mixing valves.
- *System design optimization:* Ensuring proper water flow velocity and direction to keep microorganisms in a planktonic state rather than allowing biofilm formation through stagnation.

TEMPERATURE-BASED DISINFECTION

- *Routine temperature management:* Hot water maintained >50°C (>122°F) and cold water <20°C (<68°F) to prevent *Legionella* growth.
- *Thermal shock treatment*: High-pressure steaming or hot water circulation >80°C (>176°F) for treating contaminated systems.
- *Mechanical intervention*: Physical scrubbing of accessible surfaces combined with chemical disinfection.

FILTRATION AND CHEMICAL CONTROL

- *Point-of-use filtration:* 0.2 µm filters on all water outlets in high-risk areas (immunocompromised patient rooms, respiratory therapy areas), noting this addresses symptoms but not root causes.
- *Chemical disinfection:* Chlorine or ozone treatment for system-wide biofilm control.[8]
- *Advanced disinfection:* Copper-silver ionization or UV disinfection for contaminated systems.

MONITORING AND TESTING

- *Regular microbiological testing:* Monthly testing for *Legionella*, *Pseudomonas*, and other waterborne pathogens in ICU water systems.
- *Ice machine management:* Regular cleaning and microbiological monitoring of ice machines, which have been implicated in ICU outbreaks.
- *Last resort measures*: Replacement or removal of problematic pipework when other interventions fail.

Risk Assessment Considerations

Intensive care unit patients with invasive devices (endotracheal tubes, central lines, and urinary catheters) face amplified risk from waterborne pathogens due to bypassed natural defense mechanisms and impaired immune responses.[9]

RATIONAL APPROACH TO ENVIRONMENTAL HYGIENE

Disinfection and sterilization of patient-care items and equipment can be done efficiently by classifying them as proposed by Earle H Spaulding.[4,5] Earle H Spaulding categorized disinfection and sterilization of patient-care items and equipment as critical, semicritical, and noncritical depending on the degree of risk for infection involved in use of the items **(Table 1)**.[4]

- *Critical items:* Critical items enter sterile tissue, e.g., vascular system, joints, abdomen, brain, etc., and hence have a high risk for infection if they are contaminated. For example, central venous catheter, guidewires, tracheostomy tube, surgical instruments, urinary catheters, etc. Most of the items in this category are purchased as sterile and of single use or to be sterilized with steam. Heat-sensitive objects can be treated with ethylene oxide (EtO) or hydrogen peroxide gas plasma.[5] 7.5% stabilized hydrogen peroxide, 7.35% hydrogen peroxide with 0.23% peracetic acid, 0.2% peracetic acid, or 0.08% peracetic acid with 1.0% hydrogen peroxide.[5] Liquid chemical sterilant reliably produce sterility only if cleaning precedes treatment and if proper guidelines are followed regarding concentration, contact time, temperature, and pH.[5]
- *Semicritical items:* These are in contact with mucous membranes where commensal flora are present. Semicritical items should be free

TABLE 1: Spaulding's classification.

Spaulding category	*Medical device contacts*	*Reprocessing requirement*	*Examples*
Critical	Sterile tissue or the bloodstream	Items must be sterilized (all microbial life eliminated)	Surgical instruments used in ICU procedures; central-line insertion kits
Semicritical	Mucous membranes or nonintact skin	Requires high-level disinfection (kills most pathogens except spores)	Reusable ventilator nebulizer, bronchoscopes
Noncritical	Intact skin only	Needs low- or intermediate-level disinfection	Bed rails, bedside monitors, tables, floors, and stethoscopes

from all microorganisms. But small numbers of bacterial spores are permissible.[4] These include respiratory therapy, anesthesia equipment, endoscopes, laryngoscope blades, etc. Glutaraldehyde, hydrogen peroxide, orthophthalaldehyde, and peracetic acid with hydrogen peroxide are Food and Drug Administration (FDA) approved for high-level disinfection.[5]

- *Noncritical items:* Noncritical items are those that come in contact with intact skin but not mucous membranes.[4] Alcohols (60–95%), chlorines, iodophors (Nonantiseptic formulations), phenolics, or quaternary ammonium compounds (QUATs) are used for LLD.[5] Noncritical patient care items (such as bedpans, blood pressure cuffs, crutches, and computers).

TERMS

The terms that we need to understand before learning about how to disinfect our ICU environment:[5]

- *Cleaning:* Cleaning is the physical removal of foreign material such as dust, soil, and organic material-like blood, secretions, excretions, and microorganisms, rather than killing microorganisms. It is done with water, detergents, and mechanical action.[8]
- *Contact time:* Contact time is defined time for which surfaces of the medical device are exposed to a chemical or thermal disinfection process to achieve the appropriate level of disinfection.[5]
- *Decontamination:* Decontamination is the process of cleaning, followed by the inactivation of microorganisms, so that the object is safe for handling.[8]
- *Disinfection:* Disinfection is the inactivation of microorganisms. It does not destroy bacterial spores.[5] There are three levels of disinfection.
- *Low-level disinfection (LLD):* LLD is required for noninvasive medical equipment and some environmental surfaces. LLD processes destroy bacteria, viruses, and some fungi. It does not destroy mycobacteria and spores.[5]
- *Intermediate-level disinfection (ILD):* ILD is required for noncritical medical equipment/devices. ILD processes destroy most bacteria, some fungi, and certain types of viruses. It does not destroy bacterial spores.[5]
- *High-level disinfection (HLD):* HLD is required for semicritical medical equipment/devices. HLD processes destroy vegetative bacteria, mycobacteria, fungi, and enveloped (lipid) and nonenveloped (nonlipid) viruses, but not necessarily bacterial spores.[5]
- *Sterilization:* Sterilization is required for critical medical equipment/devices. Sterilization results in the destruction of all forms of microbial life, including bacteria, viruses, spores, and fungi.[5]

FACTORS AFFECTING THE EFFICACY OF DISINFECTION AND STERILIZATION

- *Microbial load and location of microorganisms:* Medical equipment/devices must be thoroughly cleaned before disinfection, as reducing the number of microorganisms reduces the contact time required for disinfection.[5] Surfaces in direct contact with the disinfectant/sterilint will only be disinfected, so there must be no air pockets, and the equipment must be completely immersed for the entire exposure period.[5]
- *Innate resistance of microorganisms:* Some microorganisms have intrinsic resistance to some disinfectants.[5] Prions are most resistant, followed by bacterial spores, coccidia (e.g., *Cryptosporidium*), mycobacteria (e.g., *Mycobacterium tuberculosis*), nonlipid or small viruses (e.g., poliovirus and coxsackievirus), fungi (e.g., *Aspergillus* and *Candida*), vegetative bacteria (e.g., *Staphylococcus* and *Pseudomonas*), and lipid or medium-size viruses [e.g., herpes and human immunodeficiency virus (HIV)].[5]
- *Concentration and potency of disinfectants:* The higher the concentration of disinfectant, the greater its efficacy and the shorter the time necessary to achieve microbial kill.[5] This also affects material compatibility.
- *Physical and chemical factors:* Temperature, pH, relative humidity, and water hardness affect the disinfection process.[5]
- *Organic and inorganic matter:* Organic matter (such as serum, blood, and pus) can interfere with the disinfection process by acting as a physical barrier or by reacting itself with the disinfectant.[5] Removing inorganic contaminants by cleaning makes the disinfection process more effective.
- Contact time.[5]
- *Biofilms:* Biofilms are microbial communities that are tightly attached to surfaces and make the disinfection process harder.[5] Newer decontamination methods, chlorine and monochloramines, can effectively inactivate biofilm bacteria. Cleaning also helps remove biofilms.[5]

MULTIDRUG-RESISTANT ORGANISMS SUSCEPTIBILITY TO DISINFECTANTS

Bacteria develop "reduced susceptibility" or "increased tolerance" to disinfectant by chromosomal gene mutation or form plasmids or transposons, just like antibiotics.[7] Reduced susceptibility does not mean resistance to disinfectant, as concentrations used in disinfection still greatly exceed the cidal level. Multidrug-resistant pathogens (i.e., *Enterococcus, P. aeruginosa, Klebsiella pneumoniae, Escherichia coli, S. aureus*, and *Staphylococcus epidermidis*) are equally susceptible to disinfectants as antibiotic-sensitive strains.[7]

MEDICAL EQUIPMENT AND PATIENT CARE ITEMS STERILIZATION AND DISINFECTION IN INTENSIVE CARE UNIT

Surface cleaning: The frequency of surface cleaning in various areas of the hospital is based on the risk for infection in those areas.[10] ICU is categorized as a high-risk area, hence cleaning of floors and all the surfaces is recommended three-hourly or whenever visibly dirty **(Table 2)**.[10]

The Central Sterile Services Department (CSSD) is an integrated department in healthcare facilities that provides sterilized medical devices, equipment, and consumables for patient care.[6] CSSD keeps a record of the effectiveness of cleaning, disinfection, and sterilization processes. Sterilization and HLD are done at CSSD. Medical care equipment and patient care items requiring LLD are cleaned and disinfected by housekeeping, general duty assistants, and nursing under the supervision of the nursing team leader **(Table 3)**.

ENVIRONMENTAL CLEANING AND DISINFECTION

Introduction

Environmental cleaning and disinfection are critical in an ICU due to the high vulnerability of patients and the potential for HCAIs.[8] The environment, especially high-touch surfaces in patient rooms such as bedrails, over-bed tables, and nursing call bells, as well as reusable medical equipment such as deep vein thrombosis (DVT) pumps, glucometers, and stethoscopes,

TABLE 2: Frequency of surface cleaning based upon the risk involvement of that area.[10]

Status	*Area*	*Frequency of cleaning*
Very high-risk area	OT, BMT, ICUs, isolation rooms, chemotherapy, and bronchoscopy room	Cleaning of floor and all surfaces every 3 hours or whenever visibly dirty
High-risk area	Dialysis, laboratory, pharmacy, labor room, endoscopy room, radiation oncology, laundry, emergency room	Cleaning of floor and all surfaces every shift, i.e., morning, evening, and night, or whenever visibly dirty
Significant risk	Wards, kitchen, visitors waiting areas, OPDs, mortuary, EHC, radiology department, cafeteria, physiotherapy, laundry	Cleaning of floor and all surfaces twice daily, i.e., morning and evening
Low risk	Administrative areas, medical records	Cleaning

(BMT: bone marrow transplant; EHC: emergency health care; ICU: intensive care unit; OPD: outpatient department; OT: operation theater)

TABLE 3: Medical care equipment and patient care items requiring low-level disinfection.

Items	*Method*	*Frequency*	*Responsibility*	*Comment*
Floors	1% hypochlorite after wet mopping with detergent	Minimum thrice a day, and after spillage	Housekeeping	Quaternary ammonium compound (QAC) based disinfectants can be used. Frequency according to the healthcare area
Bed pens	1% hypochlorite to be used after thorough cleaning	After each use	Housekeeping to carry out. Nursing to supervise	Individual separate plans for each patient
Blood gas machines	Alcohol wiping	Daily	Housekeeping to carry out. Nursing to supervise	If contaminated or visibly soiled, wipe with 1% hypochlorite. Responsibility of biomedical engineering during repair and maintenance
Blood pressure cuffs	Sponge the cuff with a damp cloth. If soiled, remove bladder and wipe the cover with alcohol-based disinfectant	Daily	Nursing	In the ICU, dedicated cuffs are used
Cardiac monitors	Alcohol spray/wipe	Daily	Nursing	
Crash carts	Quaternary ammonium wiping	Daily and after soiling	Housekeeping to carry out the pharmacy to supervise	Include wheels
Dressing trolleys	Quaternary ammonium wiping	Daily and after soiling	Housekeeping to carry out. Nursing to supervise	Include wheels. If contaminated or visibly soiled, wipe with 1% hypochlorite
Medication cupboard (bedside)	Detergent wiping	Daily	Housekeeping to carry out nursing to supervise	

Contd...

Contd…

Items	*Method*	*Frequency*	*Responsibility*	*Comment*
Food trolleys	Detergent wiping/wash	Daily	Housekeeping to carry out. Food and beverage staff to supervise	
Gas cylinders	Detergent wiping	Daily	Housekeeping to carry out the engineering to supervise	
Hand rub holders	Detergent wiping	Daily	Housekeeping to carry out nursing to supervise	
Hand-wash stations	• *Sinks:* Thoroughly cleaned and scrubbed with detergent • *Taps:* Cleaned thoroughly with detergent	Daily	Housekeeping to carry out nursing to supervise	Plugholes and overflow should be checked daily
IV stands	Detergent wiping	Daily and after soiling	Housekeeping to carry out nursing to supervise	Include wheels
Linen trolleys	Detergent wiping	Daily and after soiling	Laundry to carry out nursing/ engineering supervision	Include wheels. If contaminated or visibly soiled, wipe with 1% hypochlorite
Mattresses	Wiped with QAC-based disinfectant in between patients. Whenever contaminated, disinfect with 1% hypochlorite	Use low-level disinfectants in between patients	Housekeeping to carry out Nursing supervision	Mattresses would be immediately replaced if they become torn or in need of repair
Medication refrigerators	Detergent wiping	Daily	Nursing to carry out pharmacy supervision	
Medication trolleys	Detergent wiping	Daily and after soiling	Housekeeping to carry out nursing supervision	Include wheels

Contd…

Contd...

Items	*Method*	*Frequency*	*Responsibility*	*Comment*
Suction equipment	Detergent wiping	Daily and after soiling	Housekeeping to carry out, nursing to supervise	
Oxygen saturation probes (reusable)	Detergent wiping	Daily and after soiling	Nursing to carry out and supervise	Whenever soiled, disinfect with alcohol
Flow sensor	Preferably autoclave flow sensor at 121°C or 134°C. • *Step 1:* Wash with detergent and water • *Step 2:* Dip in orthophthalaldehyde for 15–20 minutes • *Step 3:* Rinse with sterile water and dry it, store following sterile precautions	After each of us	Nursing to carry out and supervise	Whenever soiled, disinfect
Pillow	Laundered daily	Daily	Housekeeping to carry out nursing to supervise	If contaminated with blood/body fluids, these would be disinfected by 1% hypochlorite and replaced. All pillows should have nonpermeable covers
Sample collection trolleys	Detergent wiping	Daily and after soiling	Housekeeping to carry out phlebotomists supervise	If contaminated with blood/body fluids, 1% hypochlorite is to be used
Scrub station	• *Sinks:* Thoroughly cleaned and scrubbed with detergent. • *Taps:* Cleaned thoroughly with detergent	Daily and after soiling	Housekeeping to carry out nursing supervision	If sensor-based, daily maintenance is to be ensured. Plugholes and overflow should be checked daily
Stretcher	Detergent wiping followed by the use of 1% hypochlorite	Daily and after soiling	Housekeeping to carry out engineering to supervise	Include wheels

Contd...

Contd...

Items	*Method*	*Frequency*	*Responsibility*	*Comment*
Syringe pumps	Alcohol wiping	Daily and after soiling	Nursing to carry out	
Toilet seats	Detergent wash followed by phenolic disinfectant/ hypochlorite	Daily and after soiling	Housekeeping	
Ventilator/Anesthesia equipment (Re-usable)	Quaternary ammonium compound wiping	Daily and after soiling	Nursing/Paramedical to carry out	
Waste trolleys	Detergent wash for household waste and 1% hypochlorite/ phenolic disinfectant for all contaminated waste	Daily and after soiling	Housekeeping to carry out	Include wheels
Weighing machine	Detergent wiping	Daily and after soiling	Nursing/paramedical—where nursing is not available/front office	If contaminated/soiled, wash with detergent and then wipe with 70% alcohol
Wheelchairs	Detergent wiping, and in case of soiling with a quaternary ammonium compound	Daily and after soiling	Housekeeping to carry out engineering supervision	Include wheels
Computer/ keyboards	Detergent wiping	Daily	Housekeeping/nursing/front-office/area in charge of IT supervise	When grossly contaminated with blood, body-fluids, use 70% isopropyl alcohol after switching off
Fax/photocopiers/ printers/screens/ telephones/ television	Detergent wiping	Daily	Housekeeping/area in charge	

moved between rooms, plays a crucial role in the transmission of HCAIs and multidrug-resistant organisms (MDROs).[9] Along with standard precautions, environmental cleaning and disinfection are important pillars of infection risk prevention in an ICU healthcare setting.[11]

Importance of Environmental Cleaning and Disinfection

- *Prevention of transmission of HAIs:* Contaminated surfaces and equipment are major sources of MDROs, and proper cleaning and disinfection help break the chain of infection by reducing the bioburden of microorganisms such as *Clostridioides difficile*, methicillin-resistant *Staphylococcus aureus* (MRSA), and vancomycin-resistant *Enterococcus* (VRE).[9]
- *Reduction of pathogen reservoirs in a healthcare setup:* The high-touch surfaces and shared medical equipment can harbor the microorganisms, and effective cleaning and disinfection minimize these reservoirs, reducing the risk of cross-contamination.[11,12]
- *Improve patient recovery outcomes:* A clean environment contributes to lowering the chances of secondary infections, hence improved patient recovery.[13]
- *Safety for healthcare workers:* Disinfected environments reduce occupational exposure risks for healthcare workers who frequently come into contact with contaminated surfaces.[11]

Common Pathogens and Their Survival

Usually, dry conditions are conducive for the persistence of gram-positive cocci, such as coagulase-negative *Staphylococcus* spp., in healthcare setting surfaces, while moist and soiled environments encourage the growth and survival of gram-negative bacilli.[9] Fungal spores are commonly found in dust, and fungi have a predilection to survive in moist and fibrous materials.[9]

Environmental sampling of surfaces around hospital patients has shown that certain pathogens are released into the hospital environment and tend to remain in the environment for variable periods **(Table 4)**.[9]

TABLE 4: Survival of hospital pathogens on dry hospital surfaces.[9]

Organism	*Survival time*
Clostridium difficile (spores)	>5 months
Acinetobacter spp.	3 days to 11 months
Pseudomonas aeruginosa	6 hours to 16 months
Klebsiella spp.	2 hours to >30 months
Enterococcus spp. including VRE	5 days to >46 months
Staphylococcus aureus, including MRSA	7 days to >12 months

Environmental Cleaning Strategies

Several interconnected environmental cleaning strategies play a role in the process, such as the type and quality of cleaning products and methods used, cleaning techniques, education and training, auditing and feedback, and effective communication **(Box 1)**.[11,12]

Environmental cleaning should be prioritized in high-risk areas, with the risk stratification of each ICU determined by factors such as the types of patients, types of pathogens, equipment used, and the nature of the rooms, such as isolation rooms.[11]

Disinfection is most effective when pathogens have been removed from the surface or equipment through cleaning, as residual surface bioburden and dirt can reduce the efficacy of disinfectants.[8] Disinfection can be performed either after a cleaning process or, in some cases, can be performed simultaneously with cleaning.[8] Various disinfectants and disinfection methods are available, including alcohols, aldehydes, amines, chlorine and chlorine compounds, oxidative agents (such as hydrogen peroxide and peracetic acid), phenols, quaternary ammonium compounds, and ultraviolet-C (UV-C) light.[8]

The use of disinfection measures in a cleaning intervention should be based on a risk assessment.[11] Before applying disinfectants in the ICU, it is important to evaluate their compatibility with the materials to prevent any corrosion or damage.

The use of clean cloths, wipes, mops, buckets, and sponges is critical to a good cleaning and disinfection process in the ICU.[14] It is essential to follow the manufacturer's instructions for preparing dilutions and ensuring the proper contact time of the disinfectant to guarantee the effectiveness of the process **(Tables 5 and 6)**.[14]

BOX 1: Focus areas for cleaning.

High-touch surfaces:
- Bed rails
- IV poles and pumps
- Ventilator controls
- Monitors and touch screens
- Door handles and light switches
- Call bells

Patient-care equipment:
- Stethoscopes
- Thermometers
- Blood pressure cuffs
- Portable imaging devices

Common areas:
- Medication preparation areas
- Nurse stations
- Nursing station phones

TABLE 5: Factors to consider when selecting a cleaning product or method.[14]

Factor	*Considerations*
Health and safety	Health and safety considerations include evaluating ergonomic factors and identifying any potential risks associated with the preparation and application of cleaning and disinfection protocols. It is essential to wear the appropriate personal protective equipment (PPE) when handling chemicals for cleaning and disinfection
Preparation	Adequate time must be allocated for preparing the necessary solutions and setting up the area for disinfection. Solutions should be freshly prepared each day or more frequently, based on the manufacturer's instructions. Additionally, mop water must be discarded and replaced with fresh detergent solution between rooms (including bathrooms). Ensure that sufficient supplies are available for the entire cleaning process. In high-risk areas, use single-use disposable cloths or change reusable cleaning cloths between each patient room/bed space.
Contact time	Ensure that the disinfectant's wet-contact time—the duration it needs to remain on a surface for effective disinfection—adheres to the manufacturer's guidelines
Reprocessing	Cleaning cloths must be replaced between patient rooms and bathrooms to prevent cross-contamination. Mop heads should be either single-use or removable for daily laundering and should be changed between rooms, including bathrooms. Color-coded equipment can be used to clearly differentiate between cleaning zones. Disposable wipes impregnated with disinfectants can be used
Storage	After use, cleaning cloths and mop heads should be washed with detergent and dried. They should be stored in sealed containers to maintain hygiene. Mop buckets should be cleaned and stored in a dry condition
Compatibility	Verify that the cleaning product is compatible with the materials or equipment being cleaned
Efficacy	The effectiveness of the cleaning product should be assessed, including its spectrum of activity and sporicidal properties if necessary
Cleaning frequency	A thorough cleaning schedule should be created, outlining the equipment to be cleaned, the cleaning frequency, and the individuals responsible for each task, accompanied by a checklist. A daily cleaning plan and a terminal cleaning schedule (after each ICU bed is vacated) should be developed based on the specific risks associated with the ICU

TABLE 6: Cleaning practices.[15]

Type	*Frequency*	*Points to remember*
Daily cleaning	Thrice every shift and as needed	• *Clean and disinfect:* High-touch surfaces (only outside of neonatal incubator when occupied) • *Clean:* Floors with neutral detergent and water • *Last clean of the day:* Clean low-touch surfaces. Clean low-touch surfaces before high-touch surfaces, and clean patient areas before patient toilets. Use chlorine-releasing disinfectants in rooms contaminated with *Clostridium difficile* spores
Terminal cleaning	At discharge/ transfer	• *Clean and disinfect*: – High-touch surfaces – Low-touch surfaces – Floors • Discard used personal care items (e.g., cups and dishes) for reprocessing or disposal • Remove facility-provided linens for reprocessing or disposal • Inspect windowpanes; if soiled, clean the blinds on-site and remove curtains for laundering • Reprocess all reusable (noncritical) patient care equipment • Clean and disinfect all low- and high-touch surfaces, including areas that may have been inaccessible during occupancy (e.g., patient mattress, bedframe, top shelves, and vents), and the floors • Scrub and disinfected handwashing sinks

SURVEILLANCE METHODS

- *Visual inspection*:[16]
    - Observing cleanliness visually to identify any visible dirt, stains, or residues.
    - Checking adherence to cleaning protocols through checklists.
- *Cleaning and microbial monitoring*:[16]
    - *Swab testing*: Collecting samples from surfaces to detect microbial presence, especially during outbreaks.
    - *ATP testing*: Measuring adenosine triphosphate (ATP) as an indicator of organic material or microbial contamination.
    - *Ultraviolet light-detectable fluorescent (UV/F) surface markers*: The placement of transparent, UV light-visible markers on surfaces before terminal cleaning allows for easier identification and confirmation of cleaning effectiveness.

    - *Air sampling*: Checking for airborne pathogens or contaminants in case of new commissioning of ICU, after major maintenance work.
- *Audits*:[17]
    - Periodic audits to review cleaning schedules and processes.
    - Maintaining and reviewing records of cleaning frequency, methods, and personnel responsible.
- *Technology integration*:[13]
    - Use of automated cleaning systems and sensors to monitor cleaning effectiveness.
    - Data analysis to identify trends and potential problem areas.

CONCLUSION

Environmental hygiene in ICU settings is a critical component of comprehensive infection prevention and control strategies. The implementation of evidence-based cleaning and disinfection protocols, guided by Spaulding's classification system, significantly reduces healthcare-associated infections and improves patient outcomes. Proper management of air quality, water systems, and environmental surfaces, combined with appropriate use of disinfectants and regular surveillance, creates a safer environment for critically ill patients. Success in environmental hygiene requires a multidisciplinary approach involving housekeeping staff, nursing personnel, infection control teams, and engineering services working collaboratively. Regular training, adherence to standardized protocols, systematic auditing, and continuous quality improvement are essential to maintaining optimal environmental hygiene standards. As multidrug-resistant organisms continue to pose challenges in healthcare settings, meticulous attention to environmental hygiene remains a fundamental pillar in protecting our most vulnerable patients in intensive care units.

REFERENCES

1. HCAI World Alliance for Patient Safety. The Global Patient Safety Challenge 2005-2006 Clean Care is Safer Care. Geneva: World Health Organization; 2005.
2. Mehta A, Rosenthal VD, Mehta Y, Chakravarthy M, Todi SK, Sen N, et al. Deviceassociated nosocomial infection rates in Intensive Care Units of seven Indian cities. Findings of the international nosocomial infection control consortium (INICC). J Hosp Infect. 2007;67(2):168-74.
3. Mukhopadhyay C. Infection Control in Intensive Care Units. Infection control in intensive care units. Indian J Respir Care. 2018;7(1):14-21.
4. Spaulding EH. Chemical disinfection of medical and surgical materials. In: Lawrence C, Block SS (Eds). Disinfection, sterilization, and preservation. Philadelphia: Lea & Febiger; 1968. pp. 517-31.
5. Rutala WA, Weber DJ; Healthcare Infection Control Practices Advisory Committee. Guideline for Disinfection and Sterilization in Healthcare

Facilities. [Online] Available from https://www.cdc.gov/infection-control/hcp/disinfection-and-sterilization/index.html [Last accessed October, 2025].

6. Best Practices for Cleaning, Disinfection and Sterilization of Medical Equipment/Devices in All Health Care Settings, 3rd edition. Provincial Infectious Diseases Advisory Committee on Infection Prevention and Control (PIDAC-IPC).
7. Rutala WA, Stiegel MM, Sarubbi FA, Weber DJ. Susceptibility of antibiotic-susceptible and antibiotic-resistant hospital bacteria to disinfectants. Infect Control Hosp. Epidemiol. 1997;18(6):417-21.
8. Centers for Disease Control and Prevention (CDC). Environmental cleaning procedures. [Online]. Available from https://www.cdc.gov/infection-control/media/pdfs/Guideline-Disinfection-H.pdf [Last accessed October, 2025].
9. Otter JA, Yezli S, Salkeld JA, French GL. Evidence that contaminated surfaces contribute to the transmission of hospital pathogens and an overview of strategies to address contaminated surfaces in hospital settings. Am J Infect Control. 2013;41(5 Suppl):S6-11.
10. Ministry of Health and Family Welfare, Government of India. National guidelines for infection prevention and control in healthcare facilities. New Delhi: Ministry of Health and Family Welfare [Online]. Available from https://www.ncdc.mohfw.gov.in/wp-content/uploads/2024/03/83538105781625557301.pdf [Last accessed October, 2025].
11. Assadian O, Harbarth S, Vos M, Knobloch JK, Asensio A, Widmer AF. Practical recommendations for routine cleaning and disinfection procedures in healthcare institutions: a narrative review. 2021;113:104-14.
12. Mitchell BG, White N, Farrington A, Allen M, Page K, Gardner A, et al. Changes in knowledge and attitudes of hospital environmental services staff: the Researching Effective Approaches to Cleaning in Hospitals (REACH) study. Am J Infect Control. 2018;46(9):980e5.
13. Browne K, Mitchell BG. Multimodal environmental cleaning strategies to prevent healthcare-associated infections. Antimicrob Resist Infect Control. 2023;12(1):83.
14. Centers for Disease Control and Prevention. Appendix B2: Cleaning and Disinfection in Healthcare Settings. CDC. [Online] Available from https://www.cdc.gov/healthcare-associated-infections/hcp/cleaning-global/appendix-b2.html [Last accessed October, 2025].
15. Ziegler MJ, Babcock HH, Welbel SF, Warren DK, Trick WE, Tolomeo P, et al. Stopping Hospital Infections With Environmental Services (SHINE): A Cluster-randomized Trial of Intensive Monitoring Methods for Terminal Room Cleaning on Rates of Multidrug-resistant Organisms in the Intensive Care Unit. Clin Infect Dis. 2022;75(7):1217-23.
16. Luick L, Thompson PA, Loock MH, Vetter SL, Cook J, Guerrero DM. Diagnostic assessment of different environmental cleaning monitoring methods. Am J Infect Control. 2013;41(8):751-2. doi: 10.1016/j.ajic.2012.09.019. Epub 2013 Feb 4. PMID: 23380380.
17. Centers for Disease Control and Prevention. Environmental Cleaning for Prevention of Healthcare-Associated Infections. [Online] Available from https://www.cdc.gov/healthcare-associated-infections/media/pdfs/environmental-cleaning-RLS-508.pdf [Last accessed October, 2025].

6

CHAPTER

Education and Training for Intensive Care Unit Staff

Pradeep Kumar Bhatia, Sadik Mohammed

LEARNING OBJECTIVES

- Educate and regularly train healthcare professionals to adopt and practice infection prevention and control (IPC) guidelines to help prevent hospital-acquired infections.
- Include three core components in IPC education:
  - Teaching IPC principles
  - Providing training to correctly implement related protocols
  - Evaluating competency
- Equip healthcare professionals with essential knowledge and skills to improve compliance with IPC protocols and enhance patient outcomes.

INTRODUCTION

The high-risk nature of the intensive care unit (ICU) patients, combined with their vulnerability to acquiring hospital-acquired infections (HAIs) necessitate stringent adherence to infection prevention and control (IPC) protocols. According to the World Health Organization (WHO) global survey on the implementation of IPC at the healthcare facility level, only 35.7% of facilities in low-income countries met at least 50% of the WHO IPC minimum requirements, and a mere 0.6% met all of them.[1]

The IPC practices ensure a safe environment for both patients and staff. Organizational support is required for IPC to be effective at the clinical level. The organizational support includes employing sufficient healthcare workers and their education and training to deliver safe care, and fostering a culture where staff learn from mistakes, prioritize patients, practice transparency, and are equipped to address patient needs. However, sustained behavior change also requires supportive workplace conditions, proper motivation, and opportunities for continuous improvement.[2]

When staff members are well-informed about infection risks and prevention measures, they are more likely to take ownership of their roles in safeguarding patient health. This culture of accountability extends to patients and visitors, who can be educated on infection prevention practices, enhancing their participation in their care and further reducing the risk of infections. Many of the recent guidelines have identified education as an important aspect of the prevention and control of HAIs.[1,3,4]

This chapter explores the importance of regular training for ICU staff on infection control policies and strategies to improve compliance and knowledge retention among healthcare professionals.

CORE CONTENT

Being an evidence-based discipline, the IPC requires adherence to standardized and validated principles grounded in research. It demands the acquisition of specialized knowledge and practical skills. Education in IPC includes three distinct components: teaching the principles of IPC, training to correctly implement related protocols, and evaluating competency.

Important points to remember:

Education in infection prevention and control includes three distinct components:
1. Teaching the principles of IPC
2. Training to correctly implement related protocols
3. Evaluating competency

Teaching

Education through various means imparts knowledge about the correct practices and also helps to update the existing knowledge according to the changing scenarios. Establishing the right culture early in a healthcare worker's career is essential for getting things right.

Comprehensive Orientation for New Staff

Orientation programs are essential for familiarizing new employees with the facility's specific infection prevention protocols and procedures. These sessions ensure that all staff members have a clear understanding of their roles, responsibilities, and expectations related to infection control.

As part of a global strategy to enhance IPC practices, a comprehensive framework for an accredited in-service education curriculum was introduced following the 75th World Health Assembly. This framework adopts a people-centered approach, emphasizing safety and effectiveness across all roles in healthcare settings spanning pre- and postgraduate and in-service training.[5] The development of an in-service curriculum aims to define the competencies essential for IPC, focusing on current healthcare professionals. This curriculum facilitates the creation, development, and delivery of an educational program that equips all healthcare professionals with the knowledge and skills needed to effectively apply IPC principles in healthcare delivery. It highlights the importance of incorporating evidence-based IPC practices as a fundamental part of initial induction and annual in-service training. This ensures that every healthcare team member, from clinical staff to support personnel, is well-versed and confident in implementing IPC measures.

Important points to remember: Establishing the right culture early in a healthcare worker's career is essential for getting things right. From the undergraduate level to internship and ongoing professional development, education is key in fostering a mindset focused on error prevention and continuous learning.

Teaching and learning strategies should align with specific principles **(Table 1)**. Some of the most practiced methods are quasi-experimental settings where control and target groups are subjected to both didactic and practical sessions, scenario-based simulation training, face-to-face seminars, delivered by nurses on an annual basis, e-learning followed by a questionnaire and focused group discussions, and computer-assisted learning in infection control education.[6-10]

The IPC programs by WHO outlines the principles, recommendations, and minimum standards for IPC education and training. At the national level, it highlights the need for policies ensuring that all healthcare professionals receive IPC training, the development of an approved national IPC curriculum aligned with guidelines, and a monitoring and evaluation system to assess the effectiveness of IPC education and training.[11] Three distinct competency levels (foundational, intermediate, and advance), each including specific proposed IPC technical content, have been suggested **(Table 2)**. In addition to the foundational competencies, the health professionals working in clinical areas where invasive procedures are performed require advance competencies. The technical contents under advance competency relevant for ICU staff include prevention of central catheter-associated bloodstream infection (CRBSI), ventilator-associated pneumonia (VAP), surgical site infection (SSI), and other specific HAIs as well as concepts of antimicrobial stewardship.[12]

TABLE 1: Principles that should underpin the choice of teaching and learning approaches.

S. No.	*Principle*	*Comment*
1.	Inclusivity	The approach should support all individuals to engage and enable learning in a manner that most suits them
2.	Accessibility	It should be made available and accessible to all
3.	Authenticity	It should reflect "real-world" practice
4.	Collaboration	It should support group work so that participants can share experiences, learn from each other, and practice working with new people
5.	Engagement	It should engage participants actively in learning and reflecting on their practice

TABLE 2: Competency levels (foundational, intermediate, and advance) including specific proposed infection prevention and control (IPC) technical content.[4]

Foundational	*Intermediate*	*Advanced*
• General concepts of microbiology • Chain of transmission • Overview of HAI epidemiology • General concepts of standard precautions (hand hygiene, respiratory etiquette, PPE, environmental cleaning, waste management) • General concepts of transmission-based precautions • Prevention of infection among healthcare professionals, including the role of occupational health and safety, vaccinations, and postexposure evaluations and follow-up	• *Standard precautions:* Deep dive (risk assessment, management of reusable medical equipment/devices, linen management, prevention of needle stick injury, aseptic technique, patient placements) • *Transmission-based precautions:* Deep dive • Multimodal strategies for IPC interventions • General concepts of AMR prevention and antimicrobial stewardship. • Peripheral vascular catheter-associated bloodstream infection prevention • CAUTI prevention. • General principles of HAI surveillance and monitoring of IPC indicators	• The WHO core components and minimum requirements of IPC programs • Healthcare facility-built environment, infrastructure and building requirements to support IPC • Medical device reprocessing • CRBSI prevention • VAP prevention • SSI prevention • Other specific HAI prevention • Additional concepts of antimicrobial stewardship • The role of leadership in IPC • Importance and basic principles of HAI and AMR surveillance and feedback • Facility outbreak investigation and response • Importance and basic principles of monitoring of IPC indicators and feedback • Cost of HAIs and cost effectiveness of IPC interventions

(AMR: antimicrobial resistance; CAUTI: catheter-associated urinary tract infection; CRBSI: central catheter-associated bloodstream infection; HAI: healthcare associated infection; IPC: infection prevention and control; PPE: personal protective equipment; SSI: surgical site infection; VAP: ventilator-associated pneumonia; WHO: World Health Organization)
Source: Adapted from World Health Organization, 2024.[4]

Training

Learners often prefer experiential and practical learning scenarios, supplemented by opportunities for independent study, enabling engagement

TABLE 3: Competencies, every healthcare professional must be trained.

S. No.	*Competency*
1.	Hand hygiene
2.	Respiratory hygiene and cough/sneeze etiquette
3.	When and how to perform the appropriate level of precautions (standard and transmission-based precautions)
4.	Selection and use of personal protective equipment
5.	Aseptic technique
6.	Managing blood and body substance spills
7.	Managing blood or body substance exposure (appropriate to their role)
8.	Principles of environmental cleaning and reprocessing reusable medical devices (appropriate to their role)
9.	Where to find information on other aspects of infection prevention and control in the practice

at their own convenience. All staff must receive training in the required competencies and demonstrate proficiency within a reasonable timeframe after starting their roles **(Table 3)**. Training must occur during staff induction, within the first 3 months of employment and at least once a year thereafter or whenever need arises (whichever is earlier). Until competency is demonstrated, tasks should be performed under supervision when necessary. Training activities should be designed flexibly and creatively to address learner needs and achieve planned objectives across diverse learning contexts (e.g., group or individual settings, classrooms or work units, and online platforms).

Important points to remember: To ensure correct implementation of IPC related protocols, training sessions focusing on experimental and practical scenarios with an opportunity for independent learning must be held during staff induction and within the first 3 months of employment.

Role of Technology

Technology plays a vital role in advancing education and training for infection prevention by offering innovative and accessible solutions.

Online learning platforms and mobile applications: These tools provide flexible training opportunities, enabling healthcare professionals to learn at their own pace and revisit materials as needed. This flexibility supports continuous education and ensures that staff can stay updated on best practices without disrupting their schedules.[13]

Simulation technology: Practical, scenario-based training can significantly enhance the application of infection control techniques. Simulations allow healthcare workers to practice implementing infection prevention measures, such as isolation precautions, in a controlled, risk-free environment. These exercises help reinforce learning and boost confidence in real-life situations.[6]

Virtual reality (VR) and augmented reality (AR) enhance training by creating immersive, realistic scenarios. These technologies allow healthcare workers to practice infection control measures in a controlled environment, improving their skills and readiness for real-world challenges.[6]

Electronic health records (EHRs): EHRs are valuable for monitoring and improving infection prevention efforts. By analyzing data from EHRs, healthcare organizations can track compliance with infection control protocols, identify trends in infection rates, and pinpoint areas requiring targeted education and training interventions.

By leveraging these technological advancements, healthcare organizations can create more effective and engaging training programs, ultimately improving infection prevention practices and patient safety.

Evaluating Competency

The coordinator should evaluate and document staff members' education and competency in IPC. Regular audits of competencies and education can help identify additional training needs. Employers may also maintain a registry of staff training and task competencies related to IPC, tailored to the requirements of each staff member's role.

BARRIERS TO EFFECTIVE EDUCATION

Despite the critical role of education and training in infection prevention, several barriers can limit their effectiveness.

Staff turnover: High turnover rates in ICUs can lead to inconsistent training levels.

Resource limitations: Budget and staffing constraints may limit training opportunities. Support from hospital administration and external funding sources must be sought to sustain training initiatives.

Time constraints: Healthcare professionals often face demanding schedules and high patient-to-staff ratios, leaving little time for training. With direct patient care taking precedence, participation in educational sessions may be deprioritized, resulting in knowledge gaps and inconsistent adherence to infection control protocols. Offering flexible training schedules and concise modules help in minimizing disruptions.

Variability in training quality: The effectiveness of educational programs can be compromised by inconsistencies in their quality and relevance. Some training programs may lack depth or fail to address the specific requirements of various healthcare settings. For instance, IPC in acute care facilities differ significantly from those in long-term care settings, necessitating tailored training approaches.

Resistance to change: A reluctance to adopt new practices or guidelines is a common challenge. Healthcare professionals accustomed to established routines may resist changes, especially if they are unclear about the rationale or benefits of new infection prevention measures.

To overcome these barriers, training programs should be designed to accommodate busy schedules, offer context-specific content, needs based, and include strategies to address resistance by presenting clear evidence of the effectiveness of updated practices.

Important points to remember:

Barriers to effective training of ICU staff in IPC include:

- High staff turnover
- Resource limitation
- Time constraints
- Variability in training
- Resistance to change

STRATEGIES FOR IMPROVING COMPLIANCE AND KNOWLEDGE RETENTION[14]

Structured Training Programs

There must be comprehensive training modules that cover key infection control policies, such as hand hygiene, aseptic techniques, and isolation precautions. The incorporation of scenario-based simulations enhances practical understanding of the subject.

Ongoing Refresher Courses

Continuous education is critical to keeping healthcare professionals informed about the latest infection prevention guidelines, research, and advancements. Regular in-service training, workshops, and continuing education programs help maintain awareness and adaptability, especially in response to the evolving nature of infectious diseases and challenges like antibiotic resistance.[15,16]

The ongoing professional development develops a mindset focused on error prevention and continuous learning.[17,18] This approach not only instills effective IPC practices but also encourages openness to innovative ideas that enhance safety.

Periodic refresher courses must be scheduled to reinforce key concepts and introduce updates in guidelines. The use of interactive methods such as quizzes and group discussions would engage staff.

Ongoing Education and Targeted Training

Research consistently demonstrates that ongoing education and training in infection prevention significantly reduce infection rates. For instance, a recent systematic review revealed that healthcare facilities with well-established education and training programs reported lower rates of HAIs compared to those without such initiatives.[17] This evidence underscores a strong link between staff education and improved patient safety outcomes.

Additionally, targeted training interventions, such as hand hygiene campaigns, have shown measurable success in enhancing compliance and reducing infection rates. Implementing a comprehensive hand hygiene program significantly reduced the incidence of nosocomial infections. These findings highlight the importance of continuous education in reinforcing fundamental infection prevention practices.[13,19]

Leveraging Technology

Utilization of e-learning platforms and mobile applications for on-the-go training helps in increasing compliance. Incorporating VR simulations provide immersive learning experiences.

Feedback Mechanisms

Establish channels for staff to provide feedback on training programs. Use feedback to tailor content to address knowledge gaps and practical challenges.

Mentorship Programs and Peer Learning

Pair less experienced staff with mentors to foster a culture of continuous learning. Encourage peer-led sessions where staff share best practices and insights. Mentors provide guidance, share practical tips, and support their mentees in adopting best practices, and creating a collaborative and informed workforce.

Auditing

Conduct regular audits to assess compliance with infection control protocols. Share audit results with staff and use them to identify areas needing improvement.

Incentives and Recognition

Implement reward systems to acknowledge staff who excel in infection control practices. Recognition boosts morale and motivates others to prioritize adherence to guidelines.

CONCLUSION

Education and training are vital components of effective infection control in ICUs. Regular, well-structured training programs not only enhance staff knowledge and skills but also contribute to improved patient outcomes by reducing the incidence of HAIs. By adopting innovative strategies and addressing challenges proactively, healthcare organizations can foster a culture of compliance and continuous learning, ensuring the highest standards of patient care. While challenges such as time constraints and resistance to change may hinder the effectiveness of training, advancements in technology provide innovative solutions to support these efforts. The proven impact of ongoing education on infection rates highlights its critical role in enhancing patient safety and delivering high-quality care in healthcare settings.

REFERENCES

1. World Health Organization. (2024). Global report on infection prevention and control 2024: executive summary. World Health Organization. [Online] Available from https://doi.org/10.2471/B09195 [Last assessed August, 2025].
2. MoHFW. (2020). National Guidelines for Infection Prevention and Control in Healthcare Facilities. [Online] Available from https://ncdc.mohfw.gov.in/wp-content/uploads/2024/07/National-Guidelines-for-IPC-in-HCF-final1.pdf [Last assessed August, 2025].
3. National Health and Medical Research Council. (2019). Australian Guidelines for the Prevention and Control of Infection in Healthcare, Canberra. [Online] Available from https://www.nhmrc.gov.au/about-us/publications/australian-guidelines-prevention-and-control-infection-healthcare-2019 [Last assessed August, 2025].
4. World Health Organization. (2024). Infection prevention and control in-service education and training curriculum. [Online] Available from https://www.who.int/publications/i/item/9789240094123 [Last assessed August, 2025].
5. World Health Organization. (2019). Minimum requirements for infection prevention and control programmes. [Online] Available from https://iris.who.int/handle/10665/330080 [Last assessed August, 2025].
6. Mikkelsen J, Reime MH, Harris AK. Nursing students' learning of managing cross-infections–scenario-based simulation training versus study groups. Nurse Educ Today. 2008;28(6):664-71.
7. Cheng SM, Melanee EC, Rawson B. Infection prevention and control learning preferences of nurses sampled at a teaching hospital. Can J Infect Control. 2008;23(3):165-6. 168-71.
8. Reime MH, Harris A, Aksnes J, Mikkelsen J. The most successful method in teaching nursing students infection control – E-learning or lecture? Nurse Educ Today. 2008;28(7):798-806.
9. Bryce E, Yassi A, Maultsaid D. E-learning of infection control: it's contagious. Can J Infect Cont. 2008;23(4):28-32.
10. Columbine AM, Wharrad HJ. Using computer technology to deliver an infection control update on hand hygiene. British Journal of Infection Control. 2016;8(3):14-9.

11. World Health Organization. (2020). Core competencies for infection prevention and control professionals. [Online] Available from https://iris.who.int/handle/10665/335821 [Last assessed August, 2025].
12. Houghton C, Meskell P, McCarthy G. The impact of educational interventions on healthcare-associated infections in the hospital setting: A systematic review. J Hosp Infect. 2018;99(4):371-80.
13. Luangasanatip N, Hongsuwan M, Limmathurotsakul D, Lubell Y, Lee AS, Harbarth S, et al. Comparative efficacy of interventions to promote hand hygiene in hospital: systematic review and network meta-analysis. BMJ. 2015;351:h3728.
14. Alhumaid S, Al Mutair A, Al Alawi Z, Alsuliman M, Ahmed GY, Rabaan AA, et al. Knowledge of infection prevention and control among healthcare workers and factors influencing compliance: a systematic review. Antimicrob Resist Infect Control. 2021;10(1):86.
15. Davis D, O'Brien MA, Freemantle N, Wolf FM, Mazmanian P, Taylor-Vaisey A. Impact of formal continuing medical education: do conferences, workshops, rounds, and other traditional continuing education activities change physician behavior or health care outcomes? JAMA. 1999;282(9):867-74.
16. O'Brien MA, Rogers S, Jamtvedt G, Oxman AD, Odgaard-Jensen J, Kristoffersen DT, et al. Educational outreach visits: effects on professional practice and health care outcomes. Cochrane Database Syst Rev. 2007;2007(4):CD000409.
17. Safdar N, Abad C. Educational interventions for prevention of healthcare-associated infection: a systematic review. Crit Care Med. 2008;36(3):933-40.
18. Ward DJ. The role of education in the prevention and control of infection: a review of the literature. Nurse Educ Today. 2011;31(1):9-17.
19. Neo JRJ, Sagha-Zadeh R, Vielemeyer O, Franklin E. Evidence-based practices to increase hand hygiene compliance in health care facilities: an integrated review. Am J Infect Control. 2016;44(6):691-704.

7

CHAPTER Multidose Vial Policy

Shripad Taklikar, Rachana Ambarkar

LEARNING OBJECTIVES

- Handling of multidose vials.
- Adherence to injection safety.

INTRODUCTION

Administration of injections is the most common procedure in any health care setting. Every year, billions of injections are administered worldwide. The vast majority are given in therapeutic care. Immunization accounts for around 5% of all injections, and the remaining percentage is associated with transfusion of blood and blood products, intravenous administration of drugs and fluids, and administration of injectable contraceptives.

The World Health Organization (WHO) defines a safe injection as one that does not harm the recipient, does not expose the provider to avoidable risk, and does not result in waste that is dangerous to the community.[1]

Safe injection practices must be followed to prevent transmission of infections in health care settings, including intensive care units (ICUs), wards, ambulatory care, and home care.[2-4]

Injection safety comprises a set of infection prevention and control (IPC) measures implemented during the administration of injections to ensure safety for patients, healthcare personnel (HCP), and others.

All the healthcare institutes use single-dose as well as multidose vials (MDVs) for vaccines and medications. The medications can be utilized as oral formulations, injectables, skin, and topical medications. The microbial contamination rates of MDVs range from 0% to 27%.[5] The prevalence of vial contamination was lower than that in studies conducted in India (25%) and South Africa (6.4%).[6-8]

CORE CONTENT

Definitions[3]

A single-dose vial (SDV) is approved for use on a single patient for a single procedure or injection.

An MDV is recognized by its United States Food and Drug Administration (US FDA)-approved label. Although MDVs can be used for more than one patient when aseptic technique is followed, ideally, even MDVs are used for only one patient.[3]

Single-dose vials and MDVs can come in any shape or size. One should not assume that a vial is an SDV or MDV based on size or volume of medication. It is advisable to check the manufacturer's instructions and label.

Multidose vials are associated with reduced economic costs and environmental waste. However, these vials are prone to bacterial contamination, and their use has been reported to be a potential source of infections in different studies.[1] Various factors might affect the quality and sterility of medication present in these vials and are as follows: (1) Number of withdrawals made from the vial; (2) sterility of the techniques employed by HCP; (3) injection of environmental air into the vial during extraction; (4) duration of use and storage; (5) storage conditions, such as temperature and exposure to sun; and (6) presence of preservatives.[7] Most of the reported outbreaks associated with MDVs have been related directly to poor aseptic techniques, such as lack of hand hygiene, improper handling while administering the same solution to more than one patient, and entering a vial with a used syringe and needle and leaving the needle in the stopper.[6,7]

Hospitals use MDVs for cost reduction and to avoid wastage of drugs. Medications included xylocaine, insulin, heparin, vaccines, and miscellaneous agents are available as MDVs. The hospital must include the MDV policy in the Infection Control Manual and Nursing Manual. There should be adequate training on this policy and the monitoring tool for the MDV policy. MDVs typically contain an antimicrobial preservative to help limit the growth of bacteria.

Transmission of infection via contaminated MDVs has been well documented, and contamination with red blood cells raises concerns about the potential for transmission of bloodborne pathogens, such as hepatitis B, hepatitis C, and human immunodeficiency virus (HIV).[5,8-12]

Vonberg et al.[13] described that in 49.2% of 130 drug-related outbreaks, the use of MDV was reported. Smet et al.[14] identified an outbreak of Burkholderia cepacia bloodstream infections traced to the use of Ringer's lactate solution as MDV for catheter flushing in Cambodia.

Unlike MDVs, SDVs typically lack an antimicrobial preservative. Do not save leftover medication from these vials. Discard the SDV after every use.

Single- or MDVs are prone to bacterial contamination after improper handling and can be potential reservoirs of microorganisms that could be transmitted to the patient through the parenteral route.

Preparing Multidose Injections

- *Area for preparation of multidose injections:* Ensure there is a separate area allocation for injection preparation to avoid contamination.

- Prepare the area by cleaning as per the disinfection policy of the hospital or 70 % alcohol. Allow to dry.
- It is advisable to prepare multidose injections in a laminar flow to protect the product.
- Health care workers to perform hand hygiene.

- *Assemble all necessary materials needed*:
  - Sterile syringe and needles.
  - Reconstitution solutions such as sterile water and specific diluents as per the manufacturer's instructions.
  - Alcohol swabs
  - Sharp container
- *Labeling*: After reconstitution of an MDV, label the final medication container with the label as shown in **Box 1**.
- *Reconstitution:* If reconstitution of an MDV is essential, then:
  - Disinfect the rubber septum of the vial with 70% alcohol and allow it to dry.
  - Use a sterile syringe and needle to withdraw the diluent from the ampoule or vial.
  - Then insert the needle into the rubber septum of the MDVvial.
  - Inject the necessary amount of reconstitution solution.
  - Mix the contents of the vial thoroughly until all visible particles have dissolved.
  - After reconstituting the contents of a multidose vial, remove the needle and syringe and discard them immediately as a single unit into a sharp container.
  - Labeling should be mentioned here also.
- *Ready to use MDVs:* In case the MDV is to be used for a single patient. They should be labeled with the following, as given in **Box 2**.

BOX 1: Label the final medication container.

- Date of preparation
- Time of preparation
- Final concentration
- Expiry date and time after reconstitution
- Name of person
- Signature
- Not to be used beyond "MM/DD/YY."

BOX 2: The multidose vial (MDV) is to be used for a single patient.

- Name of patient
- Unique health identification (UHID) number
- MDV date and time of first piercing
- MDV to be used before: Name of person piercing the vial
- Signature

- *Administering injections:* When administering an injection
    - Check the medication chart to ensure proper drug, corresponding patient's name, and dosage.
    - Perform hand hygiene.
    - Clean the top of the vial with 70% alcohol using a swab or cotton ball and allow it to dry.
    - Using a sterile syringe and needle, withdraw the medication from the ampoule or vial.
    - Follow aseptic techniques at all times.
- *Ensuring sterility and safety of MDV use:*
    - Ensure a new sterile needle and syringe assembly is used for every access.
    - In order to minimize contamination of the vial's content, needles must not be left in the diaphragms between uses.
    - All MDVs containing parenteral medications are to be labeled with a NOT to be used beyond date at the time of opening.
    - Once punctured, MDVs must be assigned a beyond-use date of 28 days or the manufacturer's expiration date, whichever is earlier.
    - Vaccines are not exempt from the 28-day limit.[12]
    - For topical agents such as eye drops/ear drops/anesthetic solutions, ensure that the nozzles do not touch the patients' eyes/skin to avoid contamination with patients' flora.
    - An MDV should will be discarded if beyond expiry date on the vial.
    - As part of inventory management in the clinical area, a list of MDVs being used should be available in the treatment room, along with the mention of their expiry dates **(Table 1)**.
- *Discard of MDV:*
    - An MDV will be discarded.
        - When empty.
        - When suspected or visible contamination or particulate matter is present
        - When efficacy deterioration is suspected
        - When the rubber septum is damaged or appears to be leaking
        - When it is stored outside of the manufacturer's recommendations in terms of temperature and duration.

TABLE 1: Inventory management in the clinical area.

MDV name	*Single patients or multiple patients*	*Name of the patient if single*	*Storage temperature*	*Date of expiry*
Insulin	Single	Bar code label of Mr XYZ	2–8°C	DD/MM/YY
2% lignocaine	Multiple	-	Room temperature	DD/MM/YY

- *Reporting:*
    - Any staff member who becomes aware of injection safety risks, errors, and adverse events must report as per institutional policy.
    - If unsafe injection and infection control practices are observed, any affected patient should be notified, assessed for potential harm, and tested for blood-borne pathogens.
    - There should be a high degree of suspicion for outbreaks in case there is a sudden rise in the number of uncommon infections observed in a hospital setting. In such a scenario, each facility shall report clusters of infection or other adverse events to higher administrative authorities.

TECHNOLOGY INTERVENTION

There are devices now available that allow safer access of MDV vials. These allow direct syringe access and have a high-efficiency particulate air (HEPA) filter within to ensure sterile aspiration. It reduces the risk of contamination as well as the risk of needle stick injury to Health Care Professionals **(Fig. 1)**.[15]

This is a needle-free dispensing pin used for safe and efficient withdrawal and injection of fluids, particularly medications, from vials and semirigid containers.

The benefits are:

- *Needle-free design:* Minimizes the risk of needlestick injuries for healthcare professionals and patients.
- *Integrated air filter:* A 0.45 µm bacteria-retentive air filter helps prevent contamination of the medication from room air during preparation and multiple withdrawals.
- *Integrated air channel:* This automates pressure balancing, increasing efficiency during withdrawals and injections and eliminating the need for manual pressure release techniques.

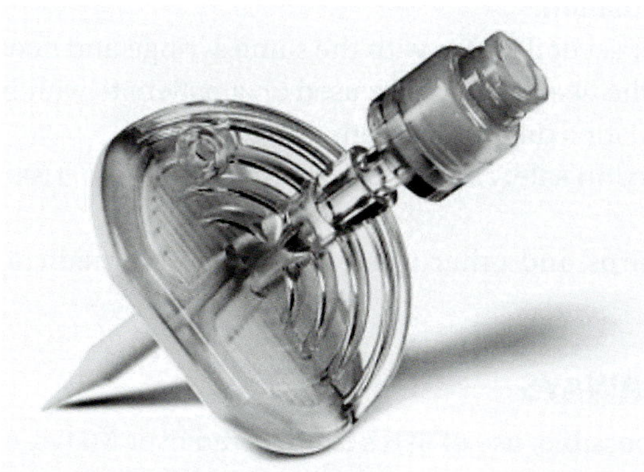

Fig. 1: Dispensing pins.

- *Snap cap:* Reduces touch contamination by allowing users to handle the device away from the critical Luer connection, and the tight-sealing cap prevents cap loss and leakage.
- *Universal compatibility:* Can be used with standard medication vials and Luer-Lock and Luer-Slip connections.

Many studies indicate that technology interventions need not always be expensive when cost-benefit, patient safety, and HCP safety are considered.

PRACTICAL TOOLS

Checklists[2]

- Always prepare MDV injections away from patient care spaces in a clean designated area, e.g., treatment room.
- Perform hand hygiene before touching the vial.
- Check the label to make sure it is an MDV.
- Check to make sure the vial is not expired or "beyond use."
- Look and see if any precipitation or discoloration of the drug is visible.
- Use new, sterile needles and syringes for every dose.
- Disinfect the vial stopper with an alcohol prep pad every time.
- Make sure the top is dry before puncturing it with the needle.
- After accessing, write the date and time on the label. Or use a tally mark.
- Follow the manufacturer's instructions for storage.
- Never pool doses (combine partial doses from multiple vials to make one dose for patients).

IMPORTANT POINTS TO REMEMBER

- Do not allow the needle to touch any surface.
- Do not reuse the needle or syringe.
- Do not touch the diaphragm after disinfection with 70% alcohol (isopropyl alcohol or ethanol).
- Do not enter several MDVs with the same syringe and needle.
- Do not use the needle or syringe used on a patient to withdraw medication from the vial for a different patient.
- Follow injection safety to avoid harm to the patient, risk for health care workers.
- Discard sharps and other waste as per the biomedical waste (BMW) guidelines.

KEY TAKEAWAYS

- Whenever possible, use of SDVs is preferred over MDVs, especially when medications are administered to multiple patients.[3]
- Use SDVs for parenteral medications whenever possible.

- If MDVs must be used, both the needle or cannula and the syringe used to access the MDV must be sterile.
- Do not keep MDVs in the immediate patient area and store them in accordance with the manufacturer's recommendations; discard if sterility is compromised or questionable.
- MDVs require a specific set of safety procedures that are:
  - Different from those for SDVs or MDVs used. With only one patient.

CONCLUSION

Adherence to safe injection and infusion practices is very important to prevent outbreaks of infection in health-care settings. Continuous healthcare professional training on infection control and safe injection and infusion practices should be encouraged. Frequent infection control audit is mandatory to ensure compliance with safe injection and infusion practices.

REFERENCES

1. World Health Organization. Injection Safety Aide Memoire, WHO 2000. [Online] Available from https://cdn.who.int/media/docs/default-source/integrated-health-services-%28ihs%29/injection-safety/aidememoire-injection-safety.pdf [Last accessed August, 2025].
2. Centers for disease control and prevention. (2024). Questions about multi dose vials. [Online] Available from https://www.cdc.gov/injectionsafety/ providers/provider_faqs_multivials.html [Last accessed August, 2024].
3. Centers for disease control and prevention. (2024). Safe Infection Practices to Prevent Transmission of Infections to Patients. [Online] Available from https://www.cdc.gov/injectionsafety/pr oviders/provider_faqs_multivials.html [Last accessed August, 2024].
4. Kottapalli P, Podduturi NCR, Aswini G, Jyothi S, Naveen A. Safe injection, infusion and medication-vial practices at a tertiary care centre: a quality improvement initiative. GMS Hyg Infect Control. 2023;18:Doc03.
5. Melnyk PS, Shevchuk YM, Conly JM, Richardson CJ. Contamination study of multiple-dose vials. Ann Pharmacother. 1993;27(3):274-78.
6. Bhatia M, Mishra B, Loomba PS, Dogra V. A pilot study for evaluation of knowledge and common practises of nursing staff regarding use of multidose injection vials and their microbial contamination rate in a super-specialty hospital. J Educ Health Promot. 2018;7:120.
7. Van den Heever A, Scribante J, Perrie H, Lowman W. Microbial contamination and labelling of self-prepared, multi-dose phenylephrine solutions used at a teaching hospital. South Afr J AnaesthAnalg. 2016;22(6):175-9.
8. Chen Y, Wu P, Shiea J, Lo LH, Wu YC, Kuo HK. Evaluation of the sterility, stability, and efficacy of bevacizumab stored in multiple-dose vials for 6 months. J Ocul Pharmacol Ther. 2009;25(1):65-70.
9. Lin S, Lay PC, Hughes LF, Bass R. The safety of multi-dose vials in allergy immunotherapy. Otolaryngol Head Neck Surg. 2008;139(2):195-7.

10. Morgan G. Microbial growth in a mixture of hyperbaric bupivacaine and fentanyl prepared in a multi-dose syringe in the operating theatre environment. S Afr J Anaesth Analg. 2010;16(2):17-21.
11. Arrington ME, Gabbert KC, Mazgaj PW, Wolf MT. Multidose vial contamination in anesthesia. Am Assoc Nurs Anesthetists J. 1990;58(6):462-6.
12. https://www.paho.org/en/documents/magnet-multi-dose-open-vial-policy-who-prequalified-vaccines accessed on 25.11.2025
13. Vonberg RP, Gastmeier P. Hospital-acquired infections related to contaminated substances. J Hosp Infect. 2007;65(1):15-23.
14. De Smet B, Veng C, Kruy L, Kham C, van Griensven J, Peeters C, Ieng S, et al. Outbreak of Burkholderia cepacia bloodstream infections traced to the use of Ringer lactate solution as multiple-dose vial for catheter flushing, Phnom Penh, Cambodia. Clin Microbiol Infect. 2013;19(9):832-7.
15. Braun Sharing Enterprise. Product Monograph, Minispike. [Online] Available from https://catalogs.bbraun.com/en-01/p/PRID00009236/mini-spike-filter-mini-spike-filter-v-mini-spike-filter-micro-tip?bomUsage=overview [Last accessed August, 2025].

8 CHAPTER

Significance of Device Days and Recommended Usage Durations

Monalisa Mishra, Debottam Gangopadhyay

LEARNING OBJECTIVES

After completing this chapter, the reader will be able to:

- Define device days and explain their relevance in ICU infection surveillance and quality improvement.
- Describe the relationship between invasive devices and healthcare-associated infections (HAIs) in critically ill patients.
- Identify recommended usage durations for common ICU devices, including central venous catheters, urinary catheters, endotracheal tubes, peripheral IV cannulas, arterial lines, PICCs, and chest tubes.
- Calculate device days and device utilization ratios (DUR) using standardized methods.
- Interpret infection rates expressed per 1,000 device days and understand their importance in benchmarking and performance evaluation.
- Recognize the role of multidisciplinary teams in optimizing device use and preventing device-associated infections.
- Apply evidence-based strategies such as insertion and maintenance bundles, daily device necessity assessments, and early removal protocols to reduce device-associated harm.
- Use surveillance data and electronic health record (EHR) tools to identify trends, guide interventions, and enhance patient safety in critical care settings.

INTRODUCTION

Patients admitted to the intensive care unit (ICU) with multiple underlying health conditions often require interventions such as mechanical ventilation, inotropic support, central lines, urinary catheters, and parenteral nutrition. These invasive measures increase their vulnerability to healthcare-associated infections (HAIs). The ICU environment, often colonized by multidrug-resistant (MDR) organisms, poses a heightened risk of opportunistic infections, particularly in the presence of such devices. Device-associated (DA) HAIs, especially those leading to bloodstream infections and sepsis, are a significant contributor to prolonged hospitalization, increased demands on barrier nursing and patient isolation, higher morbidity and mortality rates, rising healthcare costs, and decreased bed availability.[1]

Device days refer to the total number of days a medical device, such as a central venous catheter (CVC), urinary catheter, or ventilator, is used by patients typically in the ICU. This metric plays a crucial role in infection control, quality improvement, and benchmarking efforts in critical care. By correlating infections with device days, healthcare providers can assess and monitor infection rates trends in relation to device use. Device days serve as a denominator for calculating device-associated infections (e.g., infections per 1,000 device days), allowing comparisons across units, institutions, and healthcare systems.[1] This standardization helps identify outliers and areas requiring targeted interventions. Also, tracking device days helps evaluate the impact of infection prevention strategies, such as bundle implementation, hand hygiene compliance, and early device removal protocols.[2]

RECOMMENDED USAGE DURATIONS

Central Venous Catheters

Central venous catheters are critical for administering medications, fluids, and parenteral nutrition, particularly in critically ill patients. However, they pose a high risk of central line-associated bloodstream infections (CLABSI), with the risk increasing over time. Guidelines emphasize that CVCs should remain in place only as long as clinically necessary, with daily assessments of necessity.[3] Strict adherence to aseptic insertion and maintenance techniques are recommended to reduce infection risks. Additionally, removing the catheter promptly once no longer needed is crucial. Routinely changing CVCs at frequent intervals is also not advised.

Urinary Catheters

Urinary catheters, while commonly used for accurate urine output monitoring and managing urinary retention, significantly increase the risk of catheter-associated urinary tract infections (CAUTI). Current guidelines recommend removing urinary catheters within 24–48 hours postoperatively for most surgical patients or as soon as they are no longer indicated.[4] Alternatives such as bladder scanning or intermittent catheterization can help reduce unnecessary catheter usage. Adherence to sterile insertion and maintenance techniques along with daily evaluation is pivotal in minimizing CAUTI risk.

Endotracheal Tubes

Endotracheal tubes (ETTs) are vital for mechanical ventilation in critically ill patients, but prolonged intubation is associated with ventilator-associated pneumonia (VAP) and airway injury. Evidence supports daily assessments for extubation readiness through sedation interruptions and spontaneous breathing trials.[5] For patients requiring extended mechanical ventilation beyond 7–10 days, early tracheostomy may be considered to reduce complications.[5]

Other Devices

Peripheral intravenous catheters (PIVCs) are widely used but carry risks of infection and thrombophlebitis. Recent evidence has shifted away from routine replacement every 72–96 hours, recommending replacement only when clinically indicated or when complications such as occlusion or infection occur.[6] Regular site inspections and aseptic techniques during insertion and care are essential.

Arterial lines, used for continuous blood pressure monitoring and blood gas sampling, should be maintained only as long as necessary.[6] Prolonged use increases the risk of infection and thrombosis, underscoring the importance of daily necessity assessments and strict aseptic care. Similarly, peripherally inserted central catheters (PICCs) are suitable for intermediate to long-term use but require weekly reassessment for necessity and careful maintenance to prevent deep vein thrombosis (DVT) and infections.

Chest tubes, often used to manage pneumothorax or pleural effusions, should be removed promptly once the clinical indication resolves. Prolonged placement increases infection risk and patient discomfort.

Optimization of device utilization within the ICU represents pivotal components of patient safety and quality of care, necessitating a multidisciplinary team approach. The undue prolongation or unwarranted employment of medical devices, such as CVCs, urinary catheters, and ETTs, substantially increases the potential for adverse events, encompassing nosocomial infections, thrombosis, and mechanical trauma. Multidisciplinary input, integrating the expertise of physicians, nurses, infection control team, and respiratory therapists, are instrumental in attenuating these risks through the application of rigorously evidence-based interventions and the routine re-evaluation of device necessity. Mechanisms such as standardized protocols, procedural checklists, and algorithmic decision-making for device deployment and withdrawal serve to ensure uniformity in practice and improve guideline adherence. In the context of urinary catheterization, the prioritization of alternative methodologies—including intermittent catheterization or the utilization of external devices such as condom catheters—is advocated to mitigate the incidence of CAUTI. For patients reliant on mechanical ventilation, the institution of daily spontaneous breathing trials alongside sedation interruptions is imperative for gauging extubation readiness, thereby diminishing the incidence of VAP. Additionally, early tracheostomy emerges as a viable consideration for patients projected to require extended ventilatory support, in alignment with the recommendations of the Society of Critical Care Medicine (SCCM).[7]

Calculating Device Days for Intensive Care Unit Patients

Calculating device days is a critical metric in ICU management, enabling healthcare teams to monitor and evaluate device utilization rates and associated complications. A "device day" represents one calendar day during which a patient has a specific device in place, such as a CVC, urinary catheter, or ETT. The calculation of device days involves counting each day a device remains in use for every patient within the ICU. For example, if five patients have a urinary catheter in place for 3 days, this accounts for 15 device days.[8]

Accurate tracking of device days is essential for calculating infection rates, such as CAUTI or CLABSI, expressed as infections per 1,000 device days. This measurement provides a standardized means to compare infection rates across units, institutions, and benchmarks.[7] Data collection typically relies on daily monitoring of medical records, nursing flow sheets, or automated electronic health record (EHR) systems. Ensuring consistency in the method of documentation is critical for reliable data.

Device Utilization Ratio

A device utilization ratio (DUR) measures how often a specific device, like a ventilator or catheter, is used in relation to the total number of patient days. It helps assess exposure to devices and identify potential risks of device-associated infections and other harms.[9]

How to calculate DUR: The ratio is calculated by dividing the number of device days (days a patient has a device) by the total number of patient days at a facility. For example, if a hospital has 1,000 patient days and 250 of those days involve a device, the device utilization ratio would be 0.25.

Device day calculations are integral to quality improvement initiatives and infection prevention programs. By analyzing trends, multidisciplinary teams can identify patterns of prolonged device usage and develop targeted interventions, such as implementing reminder systems or adherence to removal protocols. Regular audits and feedback sessions using device day metrics foster accountability and drive the adoption of best practices, ultimately enhancing patient safety and care quality.

Device-associated infections, such as CLABSI and CAUTI, represent significant challenges in ICU care. Surveillance of these infections serves as a cornerstone for monitoring patient safety and improving healthcare quality. The systematic collection and analysis of data on infection rates, typically expressed as events per 1,000 device days, enable institutions to assess performance and identify trends over time.

Benchmarking is a critical component of this process, allowing healthcare facilities to compare their infection rates against national or international standards, such as those established by the Centers for Disease Control and Prevention's (CDC) National Healthcare Safety Network (NHSN).

Surveillance data play an instrumental role in guiding infection prevention strategies. For instance, rising CLABSI rates may prompt institutions to revisit central line insertion protocols, ensure compliance with maintenance bundles, and provide targeted staff training. Similarly, CAUTI surveillance might drive the adoption of alternatives to indwelling catheters, such as intermittent catheterization or external devices, and reinforce timely catheter removal practices.

Advanced technologies have further enhanced the precision and utility of infection surveillance. EHR and automated surveillance systems facilitate real-time data collection and analysis, allowing for early identification of infection trends or potential outbreaks. Machine learning algorithms and predictive analytics are emerging tools that enable risk stratification and resource allocation, optimizing the efficiency of infection prevention efforts.

Benchmarking also supports institutional accountability and compliance with regulatory requirements. Healthcare facilities are often mandated to report infection rates to public health agencies or accreditation bodies, ensuring transparency and fostering competition to achieve better outcomes. Regular feedback to clinical teams, coupled with visual dashboards or performance scorecards, motivates adherence to preventive measures and sustains improvements over time.[8]

CONCLUSION

The surveillance and benchmarking of infections such as CLABSI and CAUTI are integral to enhancing ICU care quality. By leveraging device day data, multidisciplinary collaboration, and advanced analytics, healthcare facilities can achieve significant reductions in infection rates, improving patient outcomes and setting new standards for excellence in infection control.[10]

In the constantly evolving healthcare environment, maintaining vigilance in monitoring and preventing infections, particularly those associated with medical devices, is essential in ICUs. As a critical hub for patient care, ICUs require robust systems focused on infection surveillance and prevention to address these challenges effectively.[10]

REFERENCES

1. Khan ID, Basu A, Kiran S, Trivedi S, Pandit P, Chattoraj A. Device-associated healthcare-associated infections (DA-HAI) and the caveat of multiresistance in a multidisciplinary intensive care unit. Med J Armed Forces India. 2017;73(3):222-31.
2. Septimus EJ, Moody J. Prevention of device-related healthcare-associated infections. F1000Res. 2016;5:F1000.
3. Marschall J, Mermel LA, Fakih M, Hadaway L, Kallen A, O'Grady NP, et al. Strategies to prevent central line-associated bloodstream infections in acute care hospitals: 2014 Update. Infect Control Hosp Epidemiol. 2014;35(7):753-71.
4. Hooton TM, Bradley SF, Cardenas DD, Colgan R, Geerlings SE, Rice JC, et al.; Infectious Diseases Society of America. Diagnosis, prevention, and treatment of

catheter-associated urinary tract infection in adults: 2009 International Clinical Practice Guidelines from the Infectious Diseases Society of America. Clin Infect Dis. 2010;50(5):625-63.

5. Klompas M, Branson R, Eichenwald EC, Greene LR, Howell MD, Lee G, et al.; Society for Healthcare Epidemiology of America (SHEA). Strategies to prevent ventilator-associated pneumonia in acute care hospitals: 2014 update. Infect Control Hosp Epidemiol. 2014;35(8):915-36.
6. Mehta Y, Gupta A, Todi S, Myatra SN, Samaddar DP, Patil V, et al. Guidelines for prevention of hospital acquired infections. Indian J Crit Care Med. 2014;18(3):149-63.
7. O'Grady NP, Alexander E, Alhazzani W, Alshamsi F, Cuellar-Rodriguez J, Jefferson BK, et al. Society of Critical Care Medicine and the Infectious Diseases Society of America Guidelines for Evaluating New Fever in Adult Patients in the ICU. Crit Care Med. 2023;51(11):1570-86.
8. Saint S, Greene MT, Krein SL, Rogers MA, Ratz D, Fowler KE, et al. A program to prevent catheter-associated urinary tract infection in acute care. N Engl J Med. 2016;374(22):2111-9.
9. Abrantes-Figueiredo JI, Ross JW, Banach DB. Device utilization ratios in infection prevention: process or outcome measure? Curr Infect Dis Rep. 2018;20(5):8.
10. Gade N, Burri R, Sujiv A, Mishra M, Pradeep BE, Debaje H, et al. Promoting patient safety: Exploring device-associated healthcare infections and antimicrobial susceptibility pattern in a multidisciplinary intensive care units. Cureus. 2023;15(12):e50232.

9

CHAPTER

Effective Surveillance Strategies and Reporting of Infections in Intensive Care Units

(Lt Col) Shibu Sasidharan, Yasmin Muhammed

LEARNING OBJECTIVES

- Healthcare-associated infections (HAIs) affect ICU patients at rates 5–10 times higher than general hospital wards, accounting for ~25% of all HAIs despite ICUs representing only 5-10% of hospitalized patients.
- The evolution from NNIS to NHSN represents a major advancement in surveillance methodology, with NHSN now serving over 37,000 healthcare facilities globally.
- Ventilator-associated event (VAE) surveillance provides objective criteria but remains controversial regarding correlation with traditional VAP definitions.
- Central line-associated bloodstream infection (CLABSI) surveillance requires careful differentiation between primary and secondary BSIs.
- Electronic surveillance systems can reduce workload by up to 90% while maintaining high sensitivity and specificity.
- Standardized infection ratio (SIR) enables risk-adjusted comparisons but has limitations in adequacy.
- Resource constraints and data quality issues remain fundamental barriers to effective surveillance implementation.
- Surveillance data must drive targeted interventions - surveillance alone does not prevent infections.
- International harmonization faces challenges due to different healthcare systems and regulatory frameworks.

INTRODUCTION

Healthcare-associated infections (HAIs) represent one of the most significant patient safety challenges globally, with intensive care units (ICUs) bearing a disproportionate burden. According to the World Health Organization (WHO), HAIs affect hundreds of millions of patients worldwide annually, with ICU patients experiencing infection rates 5–10 times higher than general hospital wards.[1] Despite representing only 5-10% of hospitalized patients, ICU patients account for approximately 25% of all HAIs.[2]

Recent surveillance data reveal concerning trends. The European Centre for Disease Prevention and Control (ECDC) estimates that >3.5 million cases of HAI occur in the European Union and European Economic Area each year, leading to >90,000 deaths.[3] The COVID-19 pandemic further exacerbated this burden, with ICU HAI rates increasing substantially during 2020–2021.[4,5] The global burden varies significantly by economic setting, with low- and middle-income countries experiencing pooled overall HAI prevalence of 15.5% compared to 5–15% in high-income countries.[6]

The economic impact is also substantial. In Europe alone, HAIs are estimated to cause approximately 2.5 million disability-adjusted life years (DALYs), a burden exceeding the cumulative burden of other infections including influenza and tuberculosis.[3] In the United States, the cost of treating major HAIs is estimated at billions of dollars annually.[7] Furthermore, HAIs constitute 71% of cases of infections with antibiotic-resistant bacteria, making surveillance and prevention critical for both patient safety and antimicrobial stewardship efforts.[3]

EVOLUTION OF SURVEILLANCE SYSTEMS

The landmark 1985 Centers for Disease Control and Prevention (CDC) Study established the foundation of modern ICU infection Surveillance on the Efficacy of Nosocomial Infection Control (SENIC), which demonstrated that 32% of HAIs were preventable with effective surveillance and control programs.[8] This study provided crucial evidence that hospitals with organized infection surveillance and control programs, including trained infection control physicians and nurses, experienced significantly lower infection rates.

The evolution from the National Nosocomial Infections Surveillance (NNIS) system to the current National Healthcare Safety Network (NHSN) represents a major advancement in surveillance methodology. Launched in 2005, NHSN now serves over 37,000 healthcare facilities and provides the most comprehensive HAI tracking system globally.[9] In Europe, the transition from the Hospitals in Europe Link for Infection Control through Surveillance (HELICS) network to the current HAI-Net program coordinated by ECDC has standardized surveillance across member states.[10]

Methodological advances have included the shift from whole-hospital to targeted surveillance, development of standardized definitions enabling interfacility comparisons, integration of process and outcome measures, and implementation of risk adjustment methodologies. The introduction of electronic surveillance systems and automated case detection algorithms represents the most recent evolutionary phase, potentially reducing surveillance workload by up to 90% while maintaining high sensitivity and specificity.[11]

CURRENT SURVEILLANCE DEFINITIONS AND METHODOLOGIES

Nondevice-associated Infections in ICU Surveillance

Hospital-acquired Pneumonia (Nonventilator Associated)

Nonventilator hospital-acquired pneumonia (NV-HAP) affects patients developing pneumonia >48 hours after admission without mechanical ventilation. NHSN criteria require new radiographic infiltrates plus clinical signs (fever, leukocytosis, and purulent sputum) with antimicrobial therapy initiation.[43] Radiographic interpretation remains subjective, particularly in patients with underlying cardiopulmonary conditions.

Risk factors include advanced age, immunosuppression, prolonged hospitalization, and recent antibiotic exposure.[44] Surveillance challenges include distinguishing from community-acquired pneumonia, aspiration pneumonitis, and ensuring consistent radiographic interpretation. Many facilities implement chest imaging review protocols to improve diagnostic consistency.

Primary Bloodstream Infections

Primary bloodstream infection (BSI) (noncentral line associated) requires positive blood cultures with no identifiable infection source within the surveillance period. The challenge lies in accurate source attribution, as ICU patients frequently have multiple potential sources.[45] NHSN secondary BSI attribution extends from 2 days before to 1 day after blood culture collection.

Risk factors include immunosuppression, malignancy, neutropenia, and multiple invasive procedures. Microbiology often differs from device-associated infections, with higher rates of gram-positive organisms, particularly coagulase-negative staphylococci requiring careful contaminant interpretation.

Healthcare-associated Urinary Tract Infection (Noncatheter Associated)

Noncatheter urinary tract infections (UTIs) present unique challenges in distinguishing healthcare-associated from community-acquired infections. NHSN symptomatic UTI criteria require compatible signs/symptoms plus positive urine culture, but symptom assessment can be challenging in critically ill, sedated patients.[46]

ICU-specific risks include recent urological procedures, immunosuppression, and diabetes. Contaminated specimens frequently lead to misdiagnosis, necessitating careful collection method evaluation. Asymptomatic bacteriuria presents particular challenges, as guidelines discourage treatment in most populations, but ICU patients may have altered symptom presentation.[47]

Clostridioides Difficile Infection

Clostridioides difficile infection (CDI) rates are significantly higher in ICUs than general populations. NHSN surveillance includes healthcare-associated CDI >3 days after admission, community-onset healthcare-associated CDI within 28 days of exposure, and recurrent CDI within 8 weeks.[24]

ICU risk factors include broad-spectrum antibiotics, proton pump inhibitors, advanced age, and immunosuppression. Spores survive standard cleaning and persist for months on surfaces.[48] Nucleic acid amplification tests increase sensitivity but may detect colonization rather than infection. Two-step testing algorithms combining glutamate dehydrogenase screening with toxin detection improve specificity.

Multidrug-resistant Organism Surveillance

Multidrug-resistant organism (MDRO) surveillance encompasses active screening for colonization and passive surveillance for clinical infections. Priority organisms include methicillin-resistant *Staphylococcus aureus* (MRSA), vancomycin-resistant enterococci (VRE), carbapenem-resistant *Enterobacterales* (CRE), carbapenem-resistant *Acinetobacter* and *Pseudomonas*, and *Candida auris*.[49]

Active surveillance involves routine screening through nasal/rectal cultures to detect asymptomatic colonization, enabling early identification and contact precautions. However, this requires significant laboratory resources. Risk-based screening may provide better resource utilization than universal screening.[50]

Molecular epidemiology through whole genome sequencing enables discrimination between endemic strains and outbreak-associated transmission, identifying clusters before apparent through traditional methods.[51]

Skin and Soft Tissue Infections

Healthcare-associated skin and soft tissue infections (SSTIs) in ICUs include nonprimary surgical site infections (SSIs), pressure ulcer-associated infections, and device site infections. ICU patients face unique risks through prolonged immobilization, pressure exposure, multiple devices, and altered nutritional status.[52]

Surveillance challenges include distinguishing healthcare-associated from community-acquired infections and determining infection versus colonization in chronic wounds. Microbiology often reflects ICU environmental organisms with higher MRSA, VRE, and gram-negative bacteria rates.

Integration and Implementation Challenges

Nondevice infection surveillance requires integration with device-associated programs through coordinated case finding, shared risk assessment, and unified prevention strategies. Resource allocation presents challenges, as these infections require more subjective clinical assessment compared to device-associated infections with objective criteria.[27]

Electronic surveillance systems have limited capability due to reliance on clinical interpretation rather than objective data. Integration with antimicrobial stewardship offers intervention opportunities—CDI surveillance guides antibiotic decisions, MDRO surveillance informs contact precautions, and primary BSI surveillance identifies procedure modification opportunities.

Quality improvement initiatives should encompass both device and nondevice infections. Bundled interventions may address multiple types simultaneously, such as antimicrobial stewardship reducing both CDI and MDRO transmission.[53]

Reporting and Benchmarking Challenges

Current reporting systems emphasize device-associated infections due to objective definitions and standardized calculations. Nondevice infections present benchmarking challenges due to definitional variability, case mix differences, and varying surveillance intensity.[29]

International comparison remains problematic due to fundamental differences between CDC/NHSN and European surveillance approaches.[39,40] WHO standardization efforts may help address these disparities. Future surveillance involves greater antimicrobial resistance integration, enhanced molecular epidemiology, and automated systems processing clinical narrative data.

Device-associated Infections in ICU Surveillance

Ventilator-associated Pneumonia and Ventilator-associated Events

The transition from traditional ventilator-associated pneumonia (VAP) surveillance to ventilator-associated event (VAE) surveillance in 2013 represented a paradigm shift in methodology.[12] The VAE algorithm uses objective criteria based on sustained increases in ventilator settings after a period of stability, eliminating the subjectivity inherent in pneumonia diagnosis. The three-tier VAE system comprises ventilator-associated condition (VAC), defined as sustained increase in fraction of inspired oxygen (FiO_2) or positive end-expiratory pressure (PEEP) after at least 2 days of stability; infection-related VAC (IVAC), which includes VAC plus temperature abnormality or white blood cell count abnormality and new antimicrobial agent; and possible/probable VAP (PVAP), consisting of IVAC plus purulent respiratory secretions and/or positive culture.[41,42]

However, significant controversy persists regarding this approach. Studies demonstrate variable correlation between VAE and traditional VAP, with critics arguing that VAE may miss clinically important pneumonias while capturing noninfectious complications.[13] The ECDC maintains traditional clinical pneumonia definitions, creating challenges for international benchmarking.[14-16]

Central Line-associated Bloodstream Infections

Central line-associated bloodstream infection (CLABSI) surveillance definitions have remained relatively stable overtime, requiring a central line in place for >2 calendar days, laboratory-confirmed BSI meeting NHSN criteria, and no other identifiable source of infection.[17,18] The NHSN 2024 update continues to refine secondary BSI attribution criteria while maintaining core diagnostic elements.

CRITICAL DEFINITIONAL CHALLENGES FOR ACCURATE CASE CLASSIFICATION

Distinguishing CLABSI from Secondary BSI

Secondary BSI attribution concept: The most complex aspect of CLABSI surveillance involves determining whether a BSI is primary (CLABSI) or secondary to another infection site. NHSN establishes a specific attribution period during which infection preventionists must systematically review for any qualifying infections that could serve as the source.

General secondary BSI sources include:

- UTIs
- Pneumonia (including ventilator-associated)
- Surgical site infections
- Skin and soft tissue infections
- Other documented infection sites with appropriate microbiological confirmation

Organism matching principle: For a BSI to be considered secondary, organisms from the blood culture must match organisms identified from the suspected source site according to NHSN matching criteria.

Clinical guidance for teams:

- Document all potential infection sources thoroughly in medical records.
- Obtain appropriate cultures from suspected infection sites.
- Communicate clinical suspicion of infection sources to the infection prevention team.
- Coordinate culture timing when clinically appropriate.[19]

Common Skin Contaminants and True Pathogen Determination

Skin contaminant concept: NHSN recognizes that certain organisms commonly found on skin may represent contamination rather than true infection. These organisms require additional criteria to be considered true pathogens.

General Approach

- Multiple positive blood cultures with the same organism strengthen the case for true infection.
- Clinical signs and symptoms (fever, chills, hypotension) support pathogenicity.
- Single positive cultures of skin contaminants require careful clinical correlation.

Clinical Best Practices

- Draw multiple blood culture sets when CLABSI is suspected.
- Document exact timing and sites of blood culture collection.
- Record clinical signs and symptoms at time of culture collection.
- Ensure proper skin antisepsis before blood culture collection.

Mucosal Barrier Injury Laboratory-confirmed Bloodstream Infection

Mucosal barrier injury laboratory-confirmed bloodstream infection (MBI-LCBI) concept: This surveillance category recognizes that certain BSIs in immunocompromised patients with MBI may be unavoidable despite optimal central line care. It was developed primarily for oncology and hematopoietic stem cell transplant populations.

General Framework

- Applies to patients with both central lines and qualifying MBI
- Limited to specific organisms likely to originate from gastrointestinal sources
- Requires documentation of qualifying underlying conditions
- Tracked separately from standard CLABSI rates

Clinical Considerations

- Document MBI and underlying conditions clearly.
- Maintain optimal central line care regardless of MBI-LCBI eligibility.
- Communicate patient immunocompromised status to infection prevention teams.

SURVEILLANCE IMPLEMENTATION PRINCIPLES

Documentation requirements:

- Central line insertion date and maintenance
- Blood culture collection details
- Clinical presentation and symptoms
- Potential secondary infection sources
- Relevant patient risk factors

Quality assurance approach:

- Systematic review of potential secondary sources
- Careful evaluation of organism significance
- Appropriate application of special surveillance categories
- Regular multidisciplinary case review

Prevention integration: Accurate classification enables targeted prevention strategies. Different CLABSI types may require different prevention approaches, emphasizing the importance of precise surveillance categorization.

Catheter-associated Urinary Tract Infections

Catheter-associated urinary tract infection (CAUTI) surveillance requires an indwelling urinary catheter for >2 calendar days, symptoms or signs compatible with UTI, and positive urine culture with no more than two species of organisms, at least one with 10^5 CFU/mL or more. Recent NHSN updates excluding nonbacterial pathogens as sole causative agents resulted in substantial changes to reported rates, highlighting how definitional modifications impact surveillance data.[20] CAUTI remains among the most common HAIs, though often with less severe outcomes than other device-associated infections.[21]

Surgical Site Infections

Surgical site infection surveillance in ICU patients requires special considerations given the complexity of postoperative care. The NHSN SSI criteria include superficial incisional infections within 30 days, deep incisional infections within 30–90 days depending on implant presence, and organ/space infections within 30–90 days. Risk stratification uses the NHSN risk index incorporating wound class, American Society of Anesthesiologists (ASA) Physical Status Classification System score, and procedure duration. However, ICU-specific factors such as emergency surgery, multiple procedures, and immunosuppression may not be adequately captured by traditional risk indices.[22]

Postdischarge surveillance is critical as 60% of SSIs manifest after hospital discharge. Methods include surgeon surveys, patient questionnaires, and administrative data review, though optimal approaches remain debated.[23] The challenge of postdischarge surveillance is particularly acute in resource-limited settings where patient follow-up may be incomplete. Electronic health record integration and patient-reported outcome systems offer promising approaches for improving detection of SSIs.

Clostridioides Difficile Infection Surveillance

Clostridioides difficile infection (CDI) surveillance in ICUs requires particular attention given the high-risk environment and vulnerable patient population.

The NHSN CDI surveillance framework categorizes infections based on timing and location of symptom onset. Healthcare facility-onset (HO-CDI) includes cases with symptom onset on day 4 or later of admission, while community-onset healthcare facility-associated (CO-HCFA) CDI captures cases occurring within 4 weeks of discharge from a healthcare facility. ICUs typically experience CDI rates 2–3 times higher than general wards, reflecting intensive antibiotic use and patient acuity.

Surveillance definitions require either a positive nucleic acid amplification test (NAAT) or toxin test for C. difficile, combined with clinical symptoms of diarrhea (≥3 unformed stools in 24 hours). The challenge lies in distinguishing true infection from colonization, as NAAT testing's high sensitivity may detect asymptomatic carriers. Two-step testing algorithms combining glutamate dehydrogenase (GDH) antigen screening with confirmatory toxin testing improve specificity but may miss some true infections.

Laboratory-identified (LabID) event reporting simplifies surveillance by using positive laboratory results as proxies for infection, reducing subjective clinical assessment. However, this approach may overestimate true infection burden by including colonized patients tested inappropriately. Facilities must balance simplified surveillance methodology with clinical accuracy, often supplementing LabID surveillance with clinical review of positive cases.

CDI surveillance data drives multiple quality improvement initiatives including antimicrobial stewardship interventions, environmental cleaning protocols, and diagnostic stewardship to reduce inappropriate testing. Integration with antimicrobial use data enables identification of high-risk antibiotic exposures and opportunities for de-escalation. Given CDI's substantial morbidity, mortality, and recurrence risk, robust surveillance remains essential for prevention efforts in ICU settings.

Microbiological Considerations in ICU Surveillance

ICUs are consistently dominated by a limited spectrum of high-risk organisms. Gram-negative bacilli (*Klebsiella pneumoniae, Acinetobacter baumannii,* and *Pseudomonas aeruginosa*) account for a substantial proportion of HAIs. Among gram-positive pathogens, *S. aureus*, especially methicillin-resistant strains (MRSA), and *Enterococcus* species, including *VRE*, are of particular concern. Opportunistic fungi, notably *Candida* species, further complicate the infection landscape, especially in the context of catheter-associated bloodstream infections.

Concurrently, CDI has emerged as a formidable nosocomial pathogen, constituting a principal etiology of healthcare-associated diarrhea, particularly among patients subjected to protracted ICU admissions and extensive broad-spectrum antimicrobial regimens that disrupt the commensal intestinal microbiota.[24] The inherent capacity of *C. difficile* to form resilient spores, persist in the healthcare environment, and propagate nosocomial outbreaks substantially augments the complexity of infection prevention in critical care contexts, underscoring the imperative for stringent environmental decontamination protocols and judicious antimicrobial stewardship.

Robust surveillance is intrinsically linked to dependable microbiological support. Blood cultures remain the cornerstone of diagnosing BSIs; however, their utility is contingent on meticulous aseptic collection technique, appropriate blood volume, and prompt processing to reduce false positives due to contamination. Advances in diagnostic microbiology, including the use of matrix-assisted laser desorption/ionization time-of-flight mass spectrometry (MALDI-TOF MS) for rapid organism identification and syndromic multiplex polymerase chain reaction (PCR) panels, have significantly enhanced diagnostic turnaround times and precision. Nonetheless, the effectiveness of these technologies hinges on stringent sampling protocols and reliable transport logistics to ensure the integrity and timeliness of results.

The ICU setting increasingly confronts the challenge of emerging resistant pathogens. The rise of *C. auris*, with its notable multidrug resistance and remarkable environmental persistence, has been linked to several healthcare-associated outbreaks worldwide. Equally concerning is the emergence of colistin-resistant gram-negative bacteria and CRE, both of which severely constrain available therapeutic options. These developments amplify the imperative for continuous microbiological surveillance, prompt detection, and rigorous containment measures.

A particular microbiological complexity in ICU surveillance arises from the propensity of many device-associated pathogens to form biofilms on indwelling catheters and other invasive devices. Biofilm formation confers significant protection against both host immune defenses and antimicrobial agents, rendering infections recalcitrant to treatment and eradication. This reality reinforces the principle that invasive devices should be employed judiciously and removed at the earliest opportunity when no longer clinically indicated.[25]

Maintaining the quality of microbiological surveillance necessitates adherence to well-established laboratory performance benchmarks. Blood culture contamination rates should ideally not exceed 3%, and laboratories should strive to report positive culture results within 48–72 hours. Participation in accredited external quality assurance programs remains vital to ensuring sustained diagnostic accuracy, laboratory competence, and alignment with national standards. An effective ICU surveillance system is fundamentally dependent upon the rigor and reliability of its microbiological underpinnings. A nuanced understanding of pathogen prevalence, antimicrobial resistance patterns, diagnostic best practices, and laboratory quality indicators enables timely, targeted interventions that are critical for reducing the burden of preventable infections in critically ill patients.

Technology and Automation in Surveillance

Electronic surveillance represents the most significant advancement in HAI detection efficiency. A systematic review of automated surveillance systems found pooled sensitivity of 85.9% (95% CI 77.9–91.9%) and specificity of 91.3% (95% CI 83.2–96.4%) across different HAI types.[26] These systems leverage natural language processing for unstructured clinical notes, machine learning algorithms for risk prediction, real-time alerting systems, automated device-day calculations, and integration of multiple data sources including laboratory, pharmacy, and radiology systems.

Implementation challenges remain substantial despite the clear benefits. Recent surveys indicate that adoption of electronic surveillance systems varies significantly, with barriers including cost, IT infrastructure requirements, and data standardization issues.[27] However, facilities with electronic systems report 61–85% reduction in surveillance workload while maintaining or improving case detection accuracy. The transition to electronic surveillance requires significant upfront investment in technology and training but yields long-term benefits in efficiency and data quality.

Advanced analytics capabilities enable predictive modelling and early outbreak detection. Machine learning algorithms can identify patterns suggesting increased infection risk, allowing for targeted preventive interventions. Natural language processing extracts relevant information from clinical notes, radiology reports, and discharge summaries, capturing infections that might be missed by traditional laboratory-based surveillance. Integration with clinical decision support systems enables real-time feedback to clinicians, promoting adherence to prevention bundles and timely intervention for suspected infections.

Reporting Systems and Quality Measures

Modern HAI reporting has evolved from voluntary internal quality improvement to mandatory public reporting in many jurisdictions. The NHSN serves as the backbone for US reporting, with data used for Centers for Medicare and Medicaid Services (CMS), CMS Hospital-acquired Condition Reduction Program, Quality Reporting Programs, state mandatory reporting requirements, and public reporting on *Care Compare* (care.cms.gov). This multipurpose use of surveillance data has increased the stakes for accurate reporting while also raising concerns about gaming and data manipulation.

The standardized infection ratio (SIR) enables risk-adjusted comparisons using 2015 baseline data. However, significant limitations exist including exclusion of data failing quality checks, variations in surveillance intensity, and challenges in risk adjustment adequacy.[28] The SIR methodology assumes that the baseline population and current population are comparable, which may not hold true given changes in patient acuity, diagnostic practices, and prevention interventions overtime.

In Europe, HAI-Net provides standardized surveillance protocols and annual reporting, though participation remains voluntary in many countries. The system emphasizes both outcome indicators such as infection rates and process indicators including compliance with prevention practices.[29] This dual approach recognizes that process measures may be more actionable for quality improvement while outcome measures remain important for accountability and benchmarking.

Electronic health record systems enable some facilities to automate certain quality measure calculations, potentially reducing manual chart review burden for infection preventionists.[27] Patient-reported outcomes have gained recognition as important quality indicators across various healthcare domains, though their specific application in infection prevention remains limited.

Current HAI reporting focuses primarily on process measures such as prevention bundle compliance and outcome measures including SIRs. Cost-effectiveness analyses of infection prevention interventions provide additional context for quality improvement prioritization, though standardized methodologies for such assessments remain under development. The integration of multiple data sources, including laboratory, pharmacy, and clinical documentation systems, offers potential for more comprehensive surveillance approaches.

However, challenges persist in implementing advanced quality measurement systems, including data standardization, interoperability between different electronic systems, and validation of automated surveillance methods. Future developments in healthcare quality measurement will require careful evaluation to ensure they improve rather than complicate infection surveillance and prevention efforts.

Implementation Challenges and Solutions

Resource constraints represent a fundamental barrier to effective surveillance implementation. Surveillance activities consume approximately 44% of infection preventionist time, with many facilities reporting inadequate staffing.[30] The recommended ratio of one infection preventionist per 100 beds is achieved by less than half of US hospitals. This staffing shortage is particularly acute in smaller hospitals and resource-limited settings where infection preventionists may have multiple competing responsibilities.

Data quality issues compound the challenge of effective surveillance. Inter-rater reliability for HAI determination remains problematic, with studies showing moderate agreement for complex definitions.[31] Training programs and automated validation checks partially address these challenges, but the subjective nature of many surveillance definitions continues to introduce variability. Standardized training curricula, certification programs, and regular competency assessments help improve data quality but require ongoing investment.

Organizational barriers often impede surveillance program success. Critical success factors include executive leadership support, physician champions, multidisciplinary engagement, integration with quality improvement infrastructure, and regular feedback to frontline staff. The Comprehensive Unit-based Safety Program (CUSP) model demonstrates how cultural transformation combined with technical interventions achieves sustainable improvements.[32] This model emphasizes the importance of addressing both technical and adaptive challenges in infection prevention, recognizing that sustainable change requires more than just implementing new protocols.[38]

Areas of Controversy and Ongoing Research

The transition from traditional VAP to VAE surveillance continues to generate debate among infection prevention professionals.[33] While VAE criteria provide more objective metrics, some facilities have chosen to maintain both surveillance methods to address different quality improvement needs.

International surveillance harmonization faces inherent challenges due to different healthcare systems, regulatory frameworks, and surveillance capabilities across countries. The CDC/NHSN and European surveillance approaches reflect these underlying differences in healthcare delivery and regulatory requirements.

Technology integration in surveillance systems progresses incrementally, with facilities implementing electronic data capture and automated reporting systems where feasible. However, validation of new surveillance technologies requires careful evaluation against established surveillance standards.

GLOBAL GUIDELINES COMPARISON

Centers for Disease Control and Prevention/National Healthcare Safety Network (United States)

The CDC's NHSN serves as the primary HAI surveillance system in the United States.[9] Federal regulations require certain healthcare facilities to participate in NHSN reporting, including hospitals participating in Medicare and Medicaid programs. The system provides standardized surveillance definitions and risk adjustment calculations for HAIs.

National Healthcare Safety Network implementation requires dedicated personnel for data collection, validation, and reporting. Facilities must invest in training, data management systems, and ongoing surveillance activities.

Smaller hospitals may face particular challenges in allocating sufficient resources for comprehensive surveillance programs.

The system's standardized definitions have influenced surveillance approaches in other countries, though the extent and specifics of international adoption vary by region and healthcare system. Implementation outside the US context may require modifications to accommodate different healthcare structures, reporting requirements, and available resources.

The European Centre for Disease Prevention and Control/ Healthcare-associated Infection-Net (Europe)

The European approach through HAI-Net emphasizes flexibility and adaptation to diverse healthcare systems across member states. The system offers both light and standard protocol options, allowing countries to choose surveillance intensity based on available resources. The current HAI-Net ICU protocol (version 2.2) provides standardized definitions while recognizing national implementation variations.[14] Strengths include flexibility for national adaptation, emphasis on process indicators alongside outcome measures, and mechanisms for cross-border collaboration. Limitations include voluntary participation in many countries, which may lead to selection bias, and annual reporting cycles that limit real-time surveillance capabilities. The heterogeneity of implementation across European countries creates challenges for meaningful comparisons but reflects the reality of diverse healthcare systems and resources.

WHO Guidelines

The WHO surveillance framework represents a significant advancement in global standardization efforts, providing simplified definitions designed for implementation across diverse resource settings.[34] Key features include resource-stratified recommendations recognizing different capability levels, minimum dataset requirements focusing on essential elements, simplified microbiological criteria reducing laboratory dependence, and integration with antimicrobial resistance surveillance to address interconnected threats. The WHO approach acknowledges that perfect surveillance is less important than consistent, sustainable surveillance that can drive local improvement efforts.

INDIAN CONTEXT

National Framework

India's HAI surveillance faces challenges common to many low- and middle-income countries, including resource constraints, infrastructure limitations, and the need for context-appropriate surveillance methods.[35,36] Healthcare systems must balance comprehensive surveillance goals with practical implementation realities in diverse healthcare settings.

The country has undertaken efforts to strengthen infection prevention and control through systematic surveillance initiatives, recognizing the interconnected challenges of HAIs and antimicrobial resistance.[35,37] These efforts acknowledge that surveillance systems must be adapted to local healthcare delivery contexts and available resources.

Healthcare facility accreditation programs and quality improvement initiatives have influenced infection prevention practices in some institutions, though implementation varies significantly across different healthcare sectors and geographic regions.[35] The development of sustainable surveillance approaches continues to evolve as healthcare systems work to balance comprehensive monitoring with resource availability.

Surveillance Challenges

Major challenges in the Indian context reflect both resource limitations and systemic issues.[35,36] Limited dedicated infection control staff means surveillance often becomes an additional duty for already overburdened clinical staff. Inadequate laboratory infrastructure, particularly in smaller cities and rural areas, limits the ability to confirm infections microbiologically. Manual data collection systems predominate, increasing workload and limiting analytical capabilities. High patient-to-nurse ratios, sometimes exceeding 1:20 in general wards, compromise both infection prevention practices and surveillance quality. The lack of systematic postdischarge surveillance means many infections, particularly SSIs, go undetected and unreported.

Indian Evidence

Recent multicenter studies from India reveal concerning infection rates that highlight the urgent need for strengthened surveillance and prevention efforts. A prospective surveillance study conducted across a network of Indian hospitals documented substantial variations in HAI rates across facilities.[54] Device-associated infection rates showed considerable variation between institutions, reflecting differences in patient populations, prevention practices, and surveillance methodologies.

The Lancet Global Health study by Mathur et al. provided comprehensive data on bloodstream and UTIs across multiple Indian healthcare facilities, demonstrating the burden of HAIs in this setting.[55] A separate study focusing on VAP surveillance using modified definitions adapted for the Indian context further illustrated the challenges of implementing standardized surveillance in diverse healthcare environments.[56]

High antimicrobial resistance rates compound these challenges, with carbapenem resistance exceeding 50% in common pathogens such as *Klebsiella pneumoniae* and *Acinetobacter baumannii*.[37] This resistance pattern increases mortality, length of stay, and treatment costs while limiting therapeutic options. The convergence of elevated infection rates and antimicrobial resistance creates a particularly challenging environment for Indian ICUs, emphasizing the critical importance of prevention efforts.

Successful Adaptations

Indian facilities have developed innovative approaches to overcome resource constraints and implement effective surveillance. Simplified surveillance definitions reduce laboratory dependence while maintaining clinical relevance. Mobile phone-based data collection systems leverage widespread smartphone availability to enable real-time data capture. Task-shifting to bedside nurses/link nurses distributes surveillance responsibilities while building infection prevention awareness among frontline staff. Focus on high-impact interventions such as hand hygiene and bundle implementation maximizes benefit from limited resources. Public-private partnerships for training expand capacity building beyond what government resources alone could achieve.

These adaptations demonstrate that effective surveillance is possible even in resource-limited settings when approaches are tailored to local contexts. The key lies in identifying essential surveillance elements that drive improvement while acknowledging constraints. Success stories from Indian facilities provide models for other low- and middle-income countries facing similar challenges.

FUTURE DIRECTIONS

Technological Advances

Emerging technologies are poised to transform surveillance capabilities in the coming decade. 5G-enabled real-time monitoring will enable continuous data streaming from multiple devices, providing unprecedented granularity in infection risk assessment. Internet of medical things (IoMT) integration will automate data collection from ventilators, infusion pumps, and other devices, reducing manual documentation burden. Quantum computing may enable complex modelling of transmission dynamics and outbreak prediction beyond current capabilities. Advanced visualization dashboards will make surveillance data more accessible and actionable for frontline staff. Automated outbreak detection algorithms will identify clusters faster than traditional methods, enabling rapid intervention.

Precision Prevention

The future of infection prevention lies in personalized approaches based on individual risk factors. Genomic risk profiling may identify patients with increased susceptibility to specific infections, enabling targeted prevention strategies. Microbiome analysis could guide decisions about prophylactic antibiotics and decolonization protocols. Individual colonization patterns assessed through rapid diagnostics will inform isolation and prevention strategies. Real-time risk scoring combining multiple data streams will enable dynamic adjustment of prevention interventions. Targeted decolonization strategies based on resistance patterns and patient factors will replace broad-based approaches, potentially reducing selection pressure for resistance.

Global Initiatives

International collaboration continues to evolve with several key developments shaping the future landscape. WHO Global Action Plan implementation drives standardization while respecting local contexts. Integration of HAI and antimicrobial resistance surveillance recognizes these interconnected challenges require coordinated responses. Climate change adaptation strategies acknowledge that rising temperatures and extreme weather events may alter infection risks and require surveillance system modifications. Pandemic preparedness incorporation ensures surveillance systems can rapidly adapt to emerging threats. South-South collaboration networks facilitate knowledge exchange between countries facing similar resource constraints, providing more relevant solutions than traditional North-South technology transfer models.

CONCLUSION

Effective HAI surveillance in ICUs requires a delicate balance between standardization for benchmarking and flexibility for local adaptation. While technological advances offer unprecedented opportunities for efficient, accurate surveillance, fundamental challenges persist in resource allocation, definitional harmonization, and implementation sustainability. The evidence clearly demonstrates that surveillance alone does not prevent infections; rather, surveillance data must drive targeted interventions and quality improvement efforts.

Success in HAI surveillance and prevention depends on several critical factors. Leadership commitment and culture change create the foundation for sustainable programs. Adequate resources for surveillance infrastructure, including both human resources and technology, enable high-quality data collection. Meaningful use of surveillance data for improvement, rather than mere compliance, drives actual infection reduction. Integration with broader patient safety initiatives recognizes that infection prevention cannot occur in isolation. Continuous adaptation to emerging threats, whether new organisms, resistance patterns, or care delivery models, ensures surveillance remains relevant.

The evidence strongly supports that comprehensive surveillance coupled with evidence-based interventions can prevent 35–55% of HAIs, potentially saving thousands of lives and billions in healthcare costs annually. This preventable fraction has remained relatively stable over decades, suggesting both the continued potential for improvement and the challenges in achieving zero infections. As we advance into an era of precision medicine and digital health, surveillance systems must evolve while maintaining focus on the ultimate goal—protecting vulnerable ICU patients from preventable infections. The path forward requires continued innovation balanced with attention to implementation science, ensuring that advances in surveillance technology translate into improved patient outcomes across all healthcare settings.

REFERENCES

1. Allegranzi B, Bagheri Nejad S, Castillejos GG, Kilpatrick C, Kelley E, Mathai E; Clean Care is Safer Care Team. Report on the burden of endemic health care-associated infection worldwide. Geneva: World Health Organization; 2011.
2. Vincent JL, Rello J, Marshall J, Silva E, Anzueto A, Martin CD, et al. International study of the prevalence and outcomes of infection in intensive care units. JAMA. 2009;302(21):2323-9.
3. European Centre for Disease Prevention and Control. Healthcare-associated infections. Stockholm: ECDC; 2024.
4. Weiner-Lastinger LM, Pattabiraman V, Konnor RY, Patel PR, Wong E, Xu SY, et al. The impact of coronavirus disease 2019 (COVID-19) on healthcare-associated infections in 2020: A summary of data reported to the National Healthcare Safety Network. Infect Control Hosp Epidemiol. 2022;43(1):12-25.
5. European Centre for Disease Prevention and Control. Healthcare-associated infections acquired in intensive care units-Annual Epidemiological Report for 2020. Stockholm: ECDC; 2023.
6. Allegranzi B, Bagheri Nejad S, Combescure C, Graafmans W, Attar H, Donaldson L, et al. Burden of endemic health-care-associated infection in developing countries: systematic review and meta-analysis. Lancet. 2011;377(9761):228-41.
7. Zimlichman E, Henderson D, Tamir O, Franz C, Song P, Yamin CK, et al. Health care-associated infections: a meta-analysis of costs and financial impact on the US health care system. JAMA Intern Med. 2013;173(22):2039-46.
8. Haley RW, Culver DH, White JW, Morgan WM, Emori TG, Munn VP, et al. The efficacy of infection surveillance and control programs in preventing nosocomial infections in US hospitals. Am J Epidemiol. 1985;121(2):182-205.
9. Centers for Disease Control and Prevention. National Healthcare Safety Network (NHSN). Atlanta: CDC; 2024.
10. European Centre for Disease Prevention and Control. Healthcare-Associated Infections Surveillance Network (HAI-Net). Stockholm: ECDC; 2023.
11. van Mourik MS, van Duijn PJ, Moons KG, Bonten MJ, Lee GM. Accuracy of administrative data for surveillance of healthcare-associated infections: a systematic review. BMJ Open. 2015;5(8):e008424.
12. Klompas M. Complications of mechanical ventilation—the CDC's new surveillance paradigm. N Engl J Med. 2013;368(16):1472-5.
13. Fan Y, Gao F, Wu Y, Zhang J, Zhu M, Xiong L. Does ventilator-associated event surveillance detect ventilator-associated pneumonia in intensive care units? A systematic review and meta-analysis. Crit Care. 2016;20(1):338.

14. European Centre for Disease Prevention and Control. Surveillance of healthcare-associated infections and prevention indicators in European intensive care units: HAI-Net ICU protocol, version 2.2. Stockholm: ECDC; 2017.
15. Shi Z, Xie H, Wang P, Zhang Q, Wu Y, Chen E, et al. Oral hygiene care for critically ill patients to prevent ventilator-associated pneumonia. Cochrane Database Syst Rev. 2016;10(10):CD008367.
16. Klompas M, Speck K, Howell MD, Greene LR, Berenholtz SM. Reappraisal of routine oral care with chlorhexidine gluconate for patients receiving mechanical ventilation: systematic review and meta-analysis. JAMA Intern Med. 2014;174(5):751-61.
17. Centers for Disease Control and Prevention. Bloodstream Infection Event (Central Line-Associated Bloodstream Infection and Non-central Line Associated Bloodstream Infection). Atlanta: CDC; 2024.
18. Pronovost P, Needham D, Berenholtz S, Sinopoli D, Chu H, Cosgrove S, et al. An intervention to decrease catheter-related bloodstream infections in the ICU. N Engl J Med. 2006;355(26):2725-32.
19. Ista E, van der Hoven B, Kornelisse RF, van der Starre C, Vos MC, Boersma E, et al. Effectiveness of insertion and maintenance bundles to prevent central-line-associated bloodstream infections in critically ill patients of all ages: a systematic review and meta-analysis. Lancet Infect Dis. 2016;16(6):724-34.
20. Centers for Disease Control and Prevention. Urinary Tract Infection (Catheter-Associated Urinary Tract Infection [CAUTI] and Non-Catheter-Associated Urinary Tract Infection [UTI]) Events. Atlanta: CDC; 2024.
21. Meddings J, Rogers MA, Krein SL, Fakih MG, Olmsted RN, Saint S. Reducing unnecessary urinary catheter use and other strategies to prevent catheter-associated urinary tract infection: an integrative review. BMJ Qual Saf. 2014;23(4):277-89.
22. Centers for Disease Control and Prevention. Surgical Site Infection Event (SSI). Atlanta: CDC; 2024.
23. Woelber E, Schrick EJ, Gessner BD, Evans HL. Proportion of surgical site infections occurring after hospital discharge: a systematic review. Surg Infect (Larchmt). 2016;17(5):510-9.
24. McDonald LC, Gerding DN, Johnson S, Bakken JS, Carroll KC, Coffin SE, et al. Clinical Practice Guidelines for *Clostridium difficile* Infection in Adults and Children: 2017 Update by the Infectious Diseases Society of America (IDSA) and Society for Healthcare Epidemiology of America (SHEA). Clin Infect Dis. 2018;66(7):987-94.
25. Maldiney T, Pineau V, Neuwirth C, Ouzen L, Eberl I, Jeudy G, et al. Endotracheal tube biofilm in critically ill patients during the COVID-19 pandemic : description of an underestimated microbiological compartment. Sci Rep. 2022;12(1):22389. doi: 10.1038/s41598-022-26560-w. PMID: 36575298; PMCID: PMC9794690.
26. Freeman R, Moore LS, García Álvarez L, Charlett A, Holmes A. Advances in electronic surveillance for healthcare-associated infections in the 21st century: a systematic review. J Hosp Infect. 2013;84(2):106-19.
27. Hebden JN. Ratios of infection preventionists are associated with hospital-acquired infection rates in acute care hospitals in the United States. Am J Infect Control. 2023;51(3):350-2.

28. Centers for Disease Control and Prevention. The NHSN Standardized Infection Ratio (SIR). Atlanta: CDC; 2023.
29. European Centre for Disease Prevention and Control. Point prevalence survey of healthcare-associated infections and antimicrobial use in European acute care hospitals—protocol version 6.1. Stockholm: ECDC; 2023.
30. Stone PW, Pogorzelska-Maziarz M, Reagan J, Merrill JA, Sperber B, Cairns C, et al. Impact of laws aimed at healthcare-associated infection reduction: a qualitative study. BMJ Qual Saf. 2015;24(10):637-44.
31. Stevens JP, Silva G, Gillis J, Novack V, Talmor D, Klompas M, et al. Automated surveillance for ventilator-associated events. Chest. 2014;146(6):1612-8.
32. Pronovost PJ, Watson SR, Goeschel CA, Hyzy RC, Berenholtz SM. Sustaining reductions in central line-associated bloodstream infections in intensive care units in Michigan. Am J Med Qual. 2011;26(1):24-33.
33. Klompas M, Kleinman K, Murphy MV. Descriptive epidemiology and attributable morbidity of ventilator-associated events. Infect Control Hosp Epidemiol. 2014;35(5):502-10.
34. World Health Organization. Surveillance of health care-associated infections at national and facility levels: practical handbook. Geneva: WHO; 2024.
35. Swaminathan S, Prasad J, Dhariwal AC, Guleria R, Misra MC, Malhotra R, et al. Strengthening infection prevention and control and systematic surveillance of healthcare associated infections in India. BMJ. 2017;358:j3768.
36. Mathur P. Surveillance of healthcare-associated infections in low- and middle-income countries: an Indian perspective. J Patient Saf Infect Control. 2018;6(1):6-8.
37. Walia K, Ohri VC, Madhumathi J, Ramasubramanian V. Establishing Antimicrobial Resistance Surveillance & Research Network in India: Journey so far. Indian J Med Res. 2019;149(2):164-79.
38. O'Boyle C, Jackson M, Henly SJ. Staffing requirements for infection control programs in US health care facilities: Delphi project. Am J Infect Control. 2002;30(6):321-33.
39. Cassini A, Plachouras D, Eckmanns T, Abu Sin M, Blank HP, Ducomble T, et al. Burden of six healthcare-associated infections on European population health: estimating incidence-based disability-adjusted life years through a population prevalence-based modelling study. PLoS Med. 2016;13(10):e1002150.
40. Mitchell BG, Fasugba O, Cheng AC, Gregory V, Koerner J, Collignon P, et al. Chlorhexidine versus saline in reducing the risk of catheter associated urinary tract infection: A cost-effectiveness analysis. Int J Nurs Stud. 2019;97:1-6.
41. Suetens C, Latour K, Kärki T, Ricchizzi E, Kinross P, Moro ML, et al. Prevalence of healthcare-associated infections, estimated incidence and composite antimicrobial resistance index in acute care hospitals and long-term care facilities: results from two European point prevalence surveys, 2016 to 2017. Euro Surveill. 2018;23(46):1800516.
42. Magill SS, O'Leary E, Janelle SJ, Thompson DL, Dumyati G, Nadle J, et al. Changes in prevalence of health care-associated infections in U.S. hospitals. N Engl J Med. 2018;379(18):1732-44.
43. Kalil AC, Metersky ML, Klompas M, Muscedere J, Sweeney DA, Palmer LB, et al. Management of Adults With Hospital-acquired and Ventilator-associated Pneumonia: 2016 Clinical Practice Guidelines by the Infectious Diseases Society of America and the American Thoracic Society. Clin Infect Dis. 2016 Sep

1;63(5):e61-e111. doi: 10.1093/cid/ciw353. Epub 2016 Jul 14. Erratum in: Clin Infect Dis. 2017 May 1;64(9):1298. doi: 10.1093/cid/ciw799. Erratum in: Clin Infect Dis. 2017 Oct 15;65(8):1435. doi: 10.1093/cid/cix587. Erratum in: Clin Infect Dis. 2017;65(12):2161. doi: 10.1093/cid/cix759. PMID: 27418577; PMCID: PMC4981759.

44. Sopena N, Sabria M. Multicenter study of hospital-acquired pneumonia in non-ICU patients. Chest. 2005;127(1):213-9.
45. Goto M, Al-Hasan MN. Overall burden of bloodstream infection and nosocomial bloodstream infection in North America and Europe. Clin Microbiol Infect. 2013;19(6):501-9.
46. Hooton TM, Bradley SF, Cardenas DD, Colgan R, Geerlings SE, Rice JC, et al. Infectious Diseases Society of America. Diagnosis, prevention, and treatment of catheter-associated urinary tract infection in adults: 2009 International Clinical Practice Guidelines from the Infectious Diseases Society of America. Clin Infect Dis. 2010;50(5):625-63. doi: 10.1086/650482. PMID: 20175247.
47. Nicolle LE, Gupta K, Bradley SF, Colgan R, DeMuri GP, Drekonja D, et al. Clinical practice guideline for the management of asymptomatic bacteriuria: 2019 update by the Infectious Diseases Society of America. Clin Infect Dis. 2019;68(10):e83-e110.
48. Weber DJ, Anderson D, Rutala WA. The role of the surface environment in healthcare-associated infections. Curr Opin Infect Dis. 2013;26(4):338-44.
49. Magiorakos AP, Srinivasan A, Carey RB, Carmeli Y, Falagas ME, Giske CG, et al. Multidrug-resistant, extensively drug-resistant and pandrug-resistant bacteria: an international expert proposal for interim standard definitions for acquired resistance. Clin Microbiol Infect. 2012;18(3):268-81.
50. Derde LP, Cooper BS, Goossens H, Malhotra-Kumar S, Willems RJL, Gniadkowski M, et al. Interventions to reduce colonisation and transmission of antimicrobial-resistant bacteria in intensive care units: an interrupted time series study and cluster randomised trial. Lancet Infect Dis. 2014;14(1):31-9.
51. Kwong JC, McCallum N, Sintchenko V, Howden BP. Whole genome sequencing in clinical and public health microbiology. Pathology. 2015;47(3):199-210.
52. Stevens DL, Bisno AL, Chambers HF, Dellinger EP, Goldstein EJ, Gorbach SL, et al. Practice guidelines for the diagnosis and management of skin and soft tissue infections: 2014 update by the Infectious Diseases Society of America. Clin Infect Dis. 2014;59(2):e10-52.
53. Baur D, Gladstone BP, Burkert F, Carrara E, Foschi F, Döbele S, et al. Effect of antibiotic stewardship on the incidence of infection and colonisation with antibiotic-resistant bacteria and *Clostridium difficile* infection: a systematic review and meta-analysis. Lancet Infect Dis. 2017;17(9):990-1001.
54. Mathur P, Ningombam A, Soni KD, Aggrawal R, Singh KV, Samanta P, et al. Surveillance of ventilator associated pneumonia in a network of Indian hospitals using modified definitions: A pilot study. Lancet Reg Health Southeast Asia. 2024;28:100450.
55. Mathur P, Malpiedi P, Walia K, Srikantiah P, Gupta S, Lohiya A, et al; Indian Healthcare Associated Infection Surveillance Network collaborators. Health-care-associated bloodstream and urinary tract infections in a network of hospitals in India: a multicentre, hospital-based, prospective surveillance study. Lancet Glob Health. 2022;10(9):e1317-25.
56. Murhekar MV, Kumar CG. Health-care-associated infection surveillance in India. Lancet Glob Health. 2022;10(9):e1222-3.

3

SECTION

Device-related Infections and Prevention Strategies

Section Editor: *Nishant Kumar*

10

CHAPTER Ventilator-associated Infections

Nishant Sahay, Rajesh Kumar

LEARNING OBJECTIVES

- Know, about the different ventilator-associated events (VAE), including ventilator-associated pneumonia (VAP).
- Discuss the pathogenesis and risk factors of VAP.
- Diagnose VAE, including VAP.
- Discuss strategies to prevent VAP (via the Bundle approach).

INTRODUCTION

Placing a critically ill person on a ventilator is vitally important for the survival of the patient. The reported in-hospital mortality in patients on ventilators in an intensive care unit (ICU) ranges from 23 to 51%.[1,2] Positive pressure ventilation is an unphysiological way of breathing, and the machine induces many adverse effects on patients. In an ICU, pulmonary infections are often present, even before patients are placed on a ventilator, and thus these patients may not strictly be considered to have ventilator-associated infections or ventilator-associated pneumonia (VAP). In fact, most of the definitions suggested for VAP are ambiguous, do not provide a valid, reliable definition of this condition, and are neither sensitive nor specific to identify it. These rely on chest radiographs, where the reporting is subjective and highly variable, because the image presented to the clinician can have many variations in exposure, rotation, etc.

To help solve the dilemma of diagnosis of the gamut of adverse consequences of placing a patient on a ventilator, the Centre for Disease Control United States of America (CDC USA) convened a meeting of many stakeholders to propose a new approach for surveillance of ventilator-associated events (VAE). This group suggested three definition tiers within the VAE algorithm to encompass ventilator-associated conditions (VAC), infection-related ventilator-associated complications (IVAC), and possible VAP (PVAP).

PATHOBIOLOGY OF VENTILATOR-ASSOCIATED INFECTIONS, INCLUDING VENTILATOR-ASSOCIATED PNEUMONIA

The pathobiology of ventilator-associated infections, is complex and multifactorial, involving alterations in protective airway defenses, changes in microbiological flora, and immune responses of critically ill patients, all brought about by the ventilator. Incidence rates are influenced by factors such as diagnostic criteria, preventative measures, and patient and geographical variations.[3]

Risk Factors for Ventilator-associated Infections

Microaspiration despite the presence of an endotracheal tube (ETT) is one of the primary risk factors for ventilator-associated infections, including VAP. ETT breaches the natural protective barriers of the upper airway, allowing direct access to the tracheobronchial tree. Although the high-volume low-pressure cuff of the ETT minimizes gross aspiration, it does not prevent microaspiration.[4] Microaspiration can occur due to pooled secretions, loss of cuff pressure, or ETT movement. The oropharynx, nasal sinuses, and stomach can serve as reservoirs for these secretions, which may leak below the cuff and lead to silent microaspirations. ETT also causes epithelial damage and impairs cough, swallowing, and mucociliary clearance. These protective mechanisms are further compromised by ICU interventions such as sedation, paralysis, and positive pressure ventilation. Although these interventions are necessary for patient management, they can lead to respiratory muscle weakness, mucociliary dysfunction, reduced airway humidification, and clearance of secretions.

Bacterial biofilm formation on the ETT surface is another critical aspect of the VAP pathobiology. Biofilms are present in 95% of mechanically ventilated patients and act as reservoirs for infectious microorganisms. These microorganisms can be dislodged and enter the distal airways, leading to VAP. Biofilm formation occurs within hours of intubation, and the risk of VAP increases with the duration of mechanical ventilation.

Microbiology of Ventilator-associated Pneumonia

Ventilator-associated pneumonia is often polymicrobial with an increasing prevalence of antibiotic-resistant bacteria. The most common pathogens include gram-negative bacteria such as *Klebsiella*, *Acinetobacter*, *Pseudomonas*, and *Escherichia coli*, as well as some gram-positive species, such as *Staphylococcus aureus* and *Enterococci*. *Candida* colonization is also a concern, as it poses a risk for fungal VAP.

Ventilator-associated pneumonia may have an early or a late-onset. Early onset VAP occurs within 48–96 hours of ICU admission and is typically caused by antibiotic-sensitive bacteria and thus has a better prognosis. In contrast, the late-onset VAP, which occurs after 96 hours, is often associated with multidrug-resistant (MDR) pathogens and higher morbidity and mortality.[5] Factors such as preadmission immunosuppression, prior antibiotic use, and recent hospitalization increase the risk of MDR infections.[5,6]

Recent studies have raised concerns about the possible etiology of fungal pathogens. *Aspergillus* infection may be seen in up to 12% of non-neutropenic patients. Additionally, reactivation of viruses, such as cytomegalovirus, herpes simplex virus-1, and Epstein–Barr virus, has been observed in patients with bacterial pneumonia, further complicating the clinical picture.[7]

The Lung Microbiome and Ventilator-associated Pneumonia

The lung microbiome, once thought to be sterile, is now recognized as a diverse ecosystem that plays a crucial role in the maintenance of immune homeostasis. Dysbiosis of lung microbiota can occur during critical illness owing to factors such as prior antibiotic use, mechanical ventilation, and dietary changes. Dysbiosis is linked to an increased risk of complications, such as VAP.

During VAP, the lung microbiota is overwhelmed, resulting in low microbial diversity and a high microbial burden. Innate immune response in the lungs is critical for combatting infections. Alveolar macrophages (AMs) serve as the first line of defense against respiratory pathogens, maintaining alveolar homeostasis and orchestrating the immune response through cytokine activity.

When pathogenic microbes overwhelm local immune defenses, AMs and epithelial cells release additional cytokines, facilitating the recruitment of neutrophils to the infection site. In cases of VAP with positive bacterial cultures, neutrophils are recruited to the lungs, leading to phagocytosis, degranulation, and formation of neutrophil extracellular traps (NETs). NETs contain antimicrobial peptides that can kill invading pathogens.

Localized Inflammation and Biotrauma

Critical illness is characterized by a complex interplay between inflammation and immunosuppression. Mechanical ventilation can induce localized inflammatory responses known as biotrauma, which may increase the risk of VAP. Identifying the causal mediators of inflammation and their contributions to VAP is clinically challenging.

Some studies have shown significant increases in pulmonary biomarkers, such as interleukin-1 beta (IL-1β), IL-8, matrix metalloproteinase-8 (MMP-8), MMP-9, and human neutrophil elastase (HNE), in patients with VAP.[8] Although neutrophils play a vital role in the innate immune response, the release of NETs can also contribute to persistent inflammation.

Persistent inflammation can lead to lung injury and increase the risk of mortality. The simultaneous presence of pro-inflammatory and immunosuppressive states complicates the clinical management of VAP, making it essential to develop targeted therapeutic strategies that address both aspects of the immune response.[9]

DIAGNOSIS

To incriminate the ventilator as a cause for the pneumonia, it is important to ensure true ventilator association with the deterioration in oxygenation. Many times, there can be a pre-existing condition, which has deteriorated after initiation of ventilation. A period of stability or an initial improvement after placing a patient on a ventilator, has thus been suggested to define ventilator-associated complications, including pneumonia. The National Healthcare Safety Network of the USA came up with a three-tier ventilator-associated events (VAE) Surveillance Algorithm in January 2025.

Ventilator-associated Condition

After a period of stability or improvement on the ventilator, if the patient deteriorates and demonstrates an increase in daily minimum FiO_2 of ≥0.20 (20 points) over the daily minimum FiO_2 and sustained for ≥2 calendar days, or there is an increase in daily minimum positive end-expiratory pressure (PEEP) values of ≥3 cm water over the daily minimum PEEP over the baseline period, sustained for ≥2 calendar days, it is indicative of a ventilator associated condition.

Infection-related Ventilator-associated Complication

Infection is suspected if on or after the third day of mechanical ventilation, and within 2 calendar days before or after the onset of worsening oxygenation, patient temperature is >38°C or <36°C, or white blood cell count ≥12,000 cells/mm^3 or ≤4,000 cells/mm^3 and a new antimicrobial agent(s) is started and is continued for ≥4 days.

Possible Ventilator-associated Pneumonia

On or after calendar Day 3 of mechanical ventilation, and within 2 calendar days before or after the onset of worsening oxygenation, if any ONE of the following criteria is met, possible VAP is suspected.

- *Criterion 1:* Positive culture of one of the following specimens, meeting quantitative or semiquantitative thresholds without requirement for purulent respiratory secretions:
  - Endotracheal aspirate, ≥10^5 colony-forming unit (CFU)/mL or corresponding semiquantitative result.
  - Bronchoalveolar lavage, ≥10^4 CFU/mL or corresponding semiquantitative result.
  - Lung tissue, ≥10^4 CFU/g or corresponding semiquantitative result.
  - Protected specimen brush, ≥10^3 CFU/mL or corresponding semiquantitative result.
- *Criterion 2:* Purulent respiratory secretions (defined as secretions from the lungs, bronchi, or trachea that contain ≥ 25 neutrophils and ≤10 squamous

epithelial cells per [low power field (LPF) × 100] *PLUS* organism identified from one of the following specimens:

- Sputum
- Endotracheal aspirate
- Bronchoalveolar lavage
- Lung tissue
- Protected specimen brush

- *Criterion 3:* One of the following positive tests:
  - Organism identified from pleural fluid (where specimen was obtained during thoracentesis or within 24 hours of chest tube placement; pleural fluid specimens collected after a chest tube is repositioned or from a chest tube in place > 24 hours are not eligible for PVAP).
  - *Lung histopathology, defined as:* (1) Abscess formation or foci of consolidation with intense neutrophil accumulation in bronchioles and alveoli, (2) evidence of lung parenchyma invasion by fungi (hyphae, pseudohyphae, or yeast forms), and (3) evidence of infection with the viral pathogens listed below based on results of immunohistochemical assays, cytology, or microscopy performed on lung tissue.
  - Diagnostic test for *Legionella* species.
  - Diagnostic test on respiratory secretions for influenza virus, respiratory syncytial virus, adenovirus, parainfluenza virus, rhinovirus, human metapneumovirus, and coronavirus.

Prevention Strategies for Ventilator-associated Pneumonia

Implementing effective prevention strategies can reduce mechanical ventilation duration, ICU stay, mortality, antibiotic usage, and overall healthcare costs. Key prevention strategies include minimizing intubation, optimizing sedation, promoting physical activity, and maintaining hygiene. As per West Yorkshire Critical Care Operational Delivery Networks 2016, eight elements have been arranged as part of a VAP prevention Bundle and may be found in **Box 1**.

The VAP prevention bundles have been revised and reevaluated in recent times. An update on the Strategies to Prevent Ventilator-Associated Pneumonia in Acute-Care Hospitals, published in 2014, was updated in 2022.[10] Some of the most important changes suggested have been as under.

- *Avoid Intubation and reintubation:*
  - Use high-flow nasal oxygen and noninvasive positive pressure ventilation (NIPPV): High-flow nasal oxygen reduces intubation rates in hypoxemic patients and helps prevent reintubation postextubation.[11] NIPPV lowers rates of intubation, VAP, and mortality in patients with respiratory failure. Combining high-flow nasal oxygen with NIPPV after extubation further reduces reintubation risk.[12]

BOX 1: Eight elements of the VAP prevention bundle.

1. Subglottic suction endotracheal/tracheostomy tubes should be used in patients who it is anticipated will be mechanically ventilated for >72 hours
2. Mechanically-ventilated patients should be tracheally intubated with an orotracheal tube and cuff pressure maintained between 20 and 30 cmH_2O (optimally 25 cmH_2O)
3. Cuff pressure measurements should be carried out every 4–6 hours as a minimum and following any significant movement of the patient, i.e., transfer, mobilization.
4. Daily sedation hold (unless contraindicated) or based on targeted RASS
5. Patients should be nursed in a semirecumbent position (>300°) unless contraindicated
6. Ventilator tubing and suction systems should only be changed if specifically indicated, such as by visible soiling, to avoid unnecessary changes (in conjunction with manufacturers' recommendations)
7. SUP should be used judiciously, and only in patients considered to be at high risk of upper GI bleeding. If a patient is prescribed SUP, this should be reviewed regularly and specifically when enteral feeding is established
8. Regular oral hygiene should be maintained; oral care should be assessed and delivered according to identified risk

(GI: gastrointestinal; RASS: Richmond Agitation Sedation Scale; SUP: stress ulcer prophylaxis; VAP: ventilator-associated pneumonia)

    - Prone positioning in coronavirus disease 2019 (COVID-19) patients: Placing nonintubated patients with acute hypoxemic respiratory failure in the prone position may decrease the need for intubation.[13]
- *Minimize sedation:*
    - *Reduce sedation use:* Minimizing sedation in ventilated patients leads to better outcomes, including shorter ventilation duration and ICU stay.
    - *Prefer nonbenzodiazepine medications:* Use Dexmedetomidine or Propofol for agitation instead of benzodiazepines. These alternatives are linked to shorter ICU stays and lower mortality rates.
    - *Implement sedation protocols:* Nurse-driven protocols and daily sedation interruptions (spontaneous awakening trials).
- *Enhance patient recovery and shorten ICU stays:*
    - *Ventilator liberation protocols*: Conduct daily assessments of extubation readiness using spontaneous breathing trials, which can lead to earlier extubation. Promote physical conditioning.
    - *Early mobilization and exercise:* Implementing early exercise and mobility programs shortens mechanical ventilation duration, reduces ICU stays, and improves functional recovery. These programs are also cost-effective.[14]
- *Optimize bed positioning:* Elevate the head of the bed—keeping the patient's head elevated to 30–45° significantly reduces VAP incidence with minimal risk and cost.

- *Oral care and nutrition:*
    - *Daily oral care with tooth brushing:* Regular oral hygiene lowers VAP rates and improves patient outcomes.[15] However, avoid chlorhexidine-based oral care due to the potential increased mortality risk.
    - *Early enteral nutrition*: Enteral feeding reduces pneumonia risk, shortens ICU stays, and enhances patient recovery compared to parenteral nutrition.
- *Ventilator circuit maintenance:*
    - *Change circuits only when necessary:* Replacing ventilator circuits only when visibly soiled or malfunctioning reduces costs without affecting VAP rates.
    - *Follow infection control guidelines:* Adhere to CDC and manufacturer guidelines for sterilization and disinfection of respiratory equipment.
- *Additional strategies for high-risk settings*:
    - Selective decontamination of the oropharynx and digestive tract. This strategy may lower hospital mortality rates in ICUs with low antibiotic resistance but is not advisable in high-resistance settings.[16]
    - *Use of ETTs with subglottic secretion drainage:* These specialized tubes help prevent VAP in patients requiring prolonged intubation (more than 48–72 hours).
    - *Early tracheostomy:* Performing tracheostomy within seven days of intubation may reduce VAP incidence and mechanical ventilation duration but does not significantly affect mortality.
    - *Postpyloric feeding:* For patients at high risk of aspiration, postpyloric feeding decreases pneumonia rates compared to gastric feeding.[17]

CONCLUSION

- Ventilator-associated infections, particularly ventilator-associated pneumonia (VAP), remain a critical concern in intensive care units. Mechanical ventilation, which compromises natural airway defenses due to many reasons, increases the risk of microbial colonization. The diagnosis of VAP is complex, requiring standardized surveillance systems such as the ventilator-associated event (VAE) algorithm to enhance detection accuracy.
- Prevention is key to reducing VAP incidence. Strategies such as minimizing sedation, ensuring proper oral hygiene, maintaining optimal ventilator settings, and implementing spontaneous breathing trials help in reducing infection rates. Additionally, the use of high-flow nasal oxygen and non-invasive ventilation can prevent the need for intubation, thereby lowering VAP risk.
- The role of multidrug-resistant pathogens complicates treatment, highlighting the importance of antimicrobial stewardship. Balancing

immune response is crucial, as excessive inflammation can worsen lung injury. Emerging research on lung microbiota and immune modulation provides new insights into infection control and treatment strategies.

- In conclusion, a multidisciplinary approach incorporating updated guidelines, improved ventilatory management, and strict infection control measures can significantly decrease VAP occurrence. Continued research and innovation are essential to further refine preventive strategies and improve outcomes for mechanically ventilated patients.

REFERENCES

1. Liang J, Li Z, Dong H, Xu C. Prognostic factors associated with mortality in mechanically ventilated patients in the intensive care unit: A single-center, retrospective cohort study of 905 patients. Medicine (Baltimore). 2019;98(42):e17592.
2. Fialkow L, Farenzena M, Wawrzeniak IC, Brauner JS, Vieira SRR, Vigo A, et al. Mechanical ventilation in patients in the intensive care unit of a general university hospital in southern Brazil: an epidemiological study. Clinics. 2016;71(3):145-51.
3. Semet C. The ongoing challenge of ventilator-associated pneumonia: epidemiology, prevention, and risk factors for mortality in a secondary care hospital intensive care unit. Infect Prev Pract. 2023;5(4):100320.
4. Goetz RL, Vijaykumar K, Solomon GM. Mucus Clearance Strategies in Mechanically Ventilated Patients. Front Physiol. 2022;13:834716.
5. Ben Lakhal H, M'Rad A, Naas T, Brahmi N. Antimicrobial Susceptibility among Pathogens Isolated in Early- versus Late-Onset Ventilator-Associated Pneumonia. Infect Dis Rep. 2021;13(2):401-10.
6. Gunalan A, Sastry AS, Ramanathan V, Sistla S. Early- vs Late-onset Ventilator-associated Pneumonia in Critically Ill Adults: Comparison of Risk Factors, Outcome, and Microbial Profile. Indian J Crit Care Med. 2023;27(6):411-5.
7. Huang L, Zhang X, Pang L, Sheng P, Wang Y, Yang F, et al. Viral reactivation in the lungs of patients with severe pneumonia is associated with increased mortality, a multicenter, retrospective study. J Med Virol. 2023;95(1):e28337.
8. Howroyd F, Chacko C, MacDuff A, Gautam N, Pouchet B, Tunnicliffe B, et al. Ventilator-associated pneumonia: pathobiological heterogeneity and diagnostic challenges. Nat Commun. 2024;15(1):6447.
9. Horn KJ, Fulte S, Yang M, Lorenz BP, Clark SE. Neutrophil responsiveness to IL-10 impairs clearance of *Streptococcus pneumoniae* from the lungs. J Leukoc Biol. 2024;115(1):4-15.
10. Klompas M, Branson R, Eichenwald EC, Greene LR, Howell MD, Lee G, et al. Strategies to prevent ventilator-associated pneumonia in acute care hospitals: 2014 update. Infect Control Hosp Epidemiol. 2014;35(8):915-36.
11. Yasuda H, Okano H, Mayumi T, Narita C, Onodera Y, Nakane M, et al. Post-extubation oxygenation strategies in acute respiratory failure: a systematic review and network meta-analysis. Crit Care. 2021;25(1):135.
12. Vaschetto R, Pecere A, Perkins GD, Mistry D, Cammarota G, Longhini F, et al. Effects of early extubation followed by noninvasive ventilation versus standard extubation on the duration of invasive mechanical ventilation in hypoxemic

non-hypercapnic patients: a systematic review and individual patient data meta-analysis of randomized controlled trials. Crit Care. 2021;25(1):189.

13. Ehrmann S, Li J, Ibarra-Estrada M, Perez Y, Pavlov I, McNicholas B, et al. Awake Prone Positioning Meta-Trial Group. Awake prone positioning for COVID-19 acute hypoxaemic respiratory failure: a randomised, controlled, multinational, open-label meta-trial. Lancet Respir Med. 2021;9(12):1387-95.
14. Hsieh SJ, Otusanya O, Gershengorn HB, Hope AA, Dayton C, Levi D, et al. Staged Implementation of Awakening and Breathing, Coordination, Delirium Monitoring and Management, and Early Mobilization Bundle Improves Patient Outcomes and Reduces Hospital Costs. Crit Care Med. 2019;47(7):885-93.
15. Sozkes S, Sozkes S. Use of toothbrushing in conjunction with chlorhexidine for preventing ventilator-associated pneumonia: A random-effect meta-analysis of randomized controlled trials. Int J Dental Hygiene. 2023;21(2):389-97.
16. Minozzi S, Pifferi S, Brazzi L, Pecoraro V, Montrucchio G, D'Amico R. Topical antibiotic prophylaxis to reduce respiratory tract infections and mortality in adults receiving mechanical ventilation. Cochrane Database of Systematic Reviews. 2021;1(1):CD000022.
17. Klompas M, Branson R, Cawcutt K, Crist M, Eichenwald EC, Greene LR, et al. Strategies to prevent ventilator-associated pneumonia, ventilator-associated events, and nonventilator hospital-acquired pneumonia in acute-care hospitals: 2022 Update. Infect Control Hosp Epidemiol. 2022;43(6):687-713.

11

CHAPTER Catheter-associated Infections

Archana Srivastava

LEARNING OBJECTIVES

- To know the definition of central line-associated bloodstream infection (CLABSI) and catheter-associated urinary tract infection (CAUTI).
- To learn the diagnosis and evaluation of CLABSI and CAUTI.
- To understand the pathogenesis of catheter-associated infections.
- To learn evidence-based preventive strategies to reduce the incidence of CLABSI and CAUTI, which include insertion and maintenance bundles.

INTRODUCTION

Catheter-associated infections are common hospital-acquired infections that lead to prolonged hospital stay, an increase in morbidity, mortality, and a substantial financial burden.

As per American data, 80,000 CLABSIs occur in ICUs every year.[1] There is limited Indian data for the incidence of CLABSI. As per one prospective study, the incidence of CLABSI was 9.3/1,000 catheter days and 6.7 per 1,000 inpatient days with a 0.7 device utilization ratio in a tertiary care center in northern India.[2] One more similar study conducted in a trauma ICU in a tertiary care hospital showed the incidence of CLABSI as 16.4/1,000 central line days and 13.2/1,000 inpatient days with a 0.8 device utilization ratio.[3]

>25% of hospitalized patients have a urinary catheter in situ during hospitalization. CAUTI is the most common hospital-acquired infection in the United States and the second most common in Southeast Asia.[4] In developing countries, the incidence is estimated to be 8.8/1,000 catheter days.[5]

In order to reduce the incidence of catheter-associated infections and thereby reduce morbidity and cost burden, it is essential to have a multidisciplinary approach, which includes healthcare providers (who are involved in the insertion and maintenance of catheters), the infection control department, healthcare managers, and senior management.

CENTRAL LINE-ASSOCIATED BLOOD STREAM INFECTIONS

Definition

CLABSI is defined as a laboratory-confirmed bloodstream infection where an eligible bloodstream infection organism is identified and an eligible central line (that has been in place for more than 2 consecutive calendar days) is present on the laboratory confirmed bloodstream infection date of the event or the day before.[6]

Risk Factors

- Prolonged hospital stays before catheterization.
- Central venous catheters inserted in emergencies.
- Catheters needed for extended periods.
- Heavy microbial colonization at the hub and insertion site.
- Catheters having multiple lumens.
- Neutropenic patients, immunosuppression, and chemotherapy patients.
- Compromised nurse–patient ratio.
- Poor infection control practices.
- Total parenteral nutrition.
- Thrombosis of the catheter.
- Increased manipulation of the catheter.

Pathogenesis

- Colonization of intracutaneous and intravascular portions of the catheter by microorganisms present in the patient's skin or due to healthcare worker handling is the most common source.[7] Biofilm formation on the catheter, both externally and internally, significantly contributes to the colonization process.
- Intraluminal or hub contamination is also an important contributor to CLABSI, especially in long-standing (>2 weeks) central venous catheters (CVCs).[8]
- In critically ill patients with long-standing CVCs, hematogenous seeding from another source of infection, commonly from a gastrointestinal source, can occur.[9]
- Infusate contamination can occur due to poor handling, during manufacture, during solution preparation, or retrogradely via a contaminated catheter.

Common Causative Organisms

The most commonly isolated gram-negative bacteria include *Escherichia coli, Klebsiella pneumoniae, Pseudomonas* species, *Enterobacter* species, *Serratia* species, and *Acinetobacter* species.[10] *Stenotrophomonas maltophilia* bacteremia is a particular problem in cancer patients. CLABSI caused by multidrug-resistant gram-negative bacilli has become a major worry, especially in Indian intensive care units (ICUs). *Candida* infections are quite common, especially in patients receiving intravenous hyperalimentation. In hemodialysis patients, gram-positive infections are more common.

Diagnosis and Evaluation

Central line-associated bloodstream infection should be suspected in patients having symptoms of fever, chills, hypotension, in the setting of CVC in situ for at least 48 hours before the development of symptoms. Clinical examination may reveal redness and the presence of purulent discharge at the insertion site. It is important to rule out possible alternative sources of infection during the evaluation of CLABSI.

In cases where CLABSI is suspected, blood cultures should be collected before antibiotic administration. Blood cultures should be collected from a separate peripheral site by fresh prick and also from the existing CVC.[11] While collecting blood through CVC, extra caution should be taken to avoid contamination. Due to low positive predictive value, catheter tip cultures are no longer recommended.[12]

Interpretation of Blood Culture

- Cultures must be interpreted as per clinical context.
- Other alternative sources of infection must be ruled out.
- If there is a positive blood culture from a central line showing organisms such as *coagulase-negative Staphylococcus aureus* and any other possible skin contaminant along with a negative peripheral culture, then this indicates catheter colonization.
- *Differential time to positivity (DTTP)*:[13] It is a tool for diagnosis of CLABSI, though its predictive value is uncertain. If peripheral culture becomes positive 2 hours after the central line blood culture becomes positive, then the DTTP is considered positive and a diagnosis of CLABSI is made. The predictability of this tool is poor in many common enteric gram-negative bacteria, as well as *S. aureus* and *Candida*.
- To label CLABSI due to *Coagulase*-negative *S. aureus*, two or more positive blood cultures drawn from different sites are needed.

Prevention Strategies[14]

Before Insertion

- Minimize unnecessary central venous catheter insertion, to be done only when indicated.
- Regular education and competency checking of healthcare professionals involved in the insertion and maintenance of CVC.
- Daily bathing of ICU patients with chlorhexidine preparation (patient age >2 months).

AT Insertion

- A checklist is preferred to ensure infection control measures during CVC insertion **(Box 1)**.

BOX 1: Checklist for prevention of CLABSI.

At insertion:
- Hand hygiene before procedure
- Maximum sterile barrier precautions
- Adequate skin preparation with an alcoholic solution containing at least 2% chlorhexidine
- Full body sterile drape
- Appropriate site selection as per clinical condition
- Appropriate sterile precautions for ultrasound assistance
- Proper dressing application and wrapping of ports with a sterile towel post procedure

For maintenance:
- Hand hygiene before handling of CVC
- Daily bath of ICU patients (>2 months of age) with chlorhexidine preparation
- Scrub the ports/hubs with antiseptic (chlorhexidine, povidone-iodine, or 70% alcohol) with friction before accessing
- Daily check of dressing, whether changed if soiled, damp, or loose
- Appropriate wrapping of ports with a sterile towel
- Change of administration sets as advised
- Assessment for the need for continuation of CVC

(CVC: central venous catheter; ICU: intensive care unit)

- Hand hygiene is mandatory before catheter insertion or manipulation with an alcohol based waterless product or soap and water.
- The subclavian site is preferred in order to minimize infectious complications.
- The insertion site should be selected on an individual basis depending on clinical condition, risk of infectious and noninfectious complications.
- Availability of a catheter trolley or kit, which contains all the essential components to ensure aseptic technique of insertion.
- Though use of ultrasound assistance may lead to breach in asepsis if due precautions and technique are not followed, it is associated with a lesser risk of noninfectious complications.
- It is mandatory to use maximum barrier precautions by the healthcare professional performing the procedure. Mask, cap, sterile gown, and sterile gloves should be donned by the healthcare worker doing the CVC insertion. The patient should be covered by a full-body sterile drape.
- For skin preparation, an alcoholic solution having at least 2% chlorhexidine gluconate should be used. The solution must be allowed to dry before taking the puncture.

After Insertion

- Adequate nurse-patient ratio should be maintained to reduce the risk of CLABSI. In ICUs, float nurses are not recommended.

- For nontunneled CVCs, change dressing every 7 days, if using a transparent dressing, unless the dressing is visibly soiled, loose, or damp. Gauze dressing should be changed every 2 days or earlier if soiled, loose, or damp.
- Insertion site care should be performed with a chlorhexidine-based antiseptic solution.
- Scrub with catheter ports or hubs with alcoholic chlorhexidine solution or 70% alcohol for a minimum of 5 seconds every time before accessing.
- During ICU rounds, there should be a daily assessment for the need for continuation of CVCs. The catheters no longer needed should be removed.
- Replacements of administration sets can be considered at intervals of up to 7 days unless they are used for administering blood and blood products or lipid formulations.
- Constant surveillance of CLABSI rates should be performed and should be shared and discussed amongst nursing, doctors, and administrators regularly.

Additional Measures

- Antiseptic or antibiotic-impregnated CVCs can be used in certain conditions:
    - Units where CLABSI rates are higher than institutional goals despite optimum compliance with infection control practices.
    - Patients with recurrent CLABSI along with limited vascular access.
    - Patients having recently implanted intravascular prosthetic devices.
- Antimicrobial lock therapy can be considered in certain long-term CVCs. It should be used judiciously as its use poses a risk of antimicrobial resistance. Lock therapy can be used in:
    - Long-term hemodialysis catheters with recurrent CLABSI.
    - Limited vascular access and recurrent CLABSI.
    - Recently transplanted intravascular prosthetic devices.
- Recombinant tissue plasminogen activating factor (rt-PA) once weekly after hemodialysis in patients undergoing hemodialysis through a CVC.
- Apply polysporin "triple" (where available) or povidone iodine ointment to the hemodialysis catheter insertion site if compatible with the catheter material.
- Use an antiseptic-containing hub/connector cap/port protector to cover connectors.

Checklist for Prevention of Central Line-associated Bloodstream Infection

Refer **Box 1**.

BOX 2: Points to remember for prevention of CLABSI.

- Avoid unnecessary CVC placement
- Remove CVC when no longer needed
- Daily bathing of ICU patients with Chlorhexidine preparation
- Checklist to ensure infection control practices for insertion as well as maintenance
- Hand hygiene is a must before insertion and handling of CVC
- Maximum sterile barrier precautions mandatory for insertion of CVC
- Always disinfect CVC hubs/ports before accessing
- Use of chlorhexidine dressing for CVCs
- No antibiotic prophylaxis for CVC insertion or while catheters are in situ
- No routine replacement of CVCs or arterial catheters

(CLABSI: central line-associated bloodstream infection; CVC: central venous catheter)

Points to Remember

Refer **Box 2**.

CATHETER-ASSOCIATED URINARY TRACT INFECTION

Definition

A urinary tract infection where an indwelling urinary catheter was in place for >2 consecutive days in a patient setting on the day of the event or the day before, with day of device placement considered as day 1.[15]

If a urinary catheter was in place for >2 consecutive days in an inpatient location and then removed, the date of the event for the urinary tract infection (UTI) must be the date of discontinuation of the urinary catheter or the next day for the infection to be considered as CAUTI.[15]

Pathogenesis

Pathogenesis of CAUTI includes both extra- and intraluminal routes.[16] Extraluminal inoculation occurs by direct contamination during catheter insertion, while intraluminal inoculation occurs by upward movement of bacteria from a contaminated urinary catheter, drainage tube, or urine bag due to poor handling.

Risk Factors

- Catheterization and duration of catheterization.
- Catheterization is done outside the operating room.
- Female sex
- Old age
- Underlying illness
- Colonization of the catheter, drainage bag, and periurethral segment.

Common Causative Organisms

Escherichia coli is the commonest causative organism for CAUTI. Other pathogens are *Proteus, Pseudomonas, Klebsiella, Enterobacter, Enterococci,*

Candida, and Serratia. Out of these, *Enterobacter cloacae* exhibit the highest biofilm production.

Diagnosis and Evaluation

Refer **Box 3**.

The urine sample collection should be done absolutely by aseptic technique. In case of long-standing catheters, the preferred method is to change the catheter and obtain a sample from the freshly placed catheter. Alternatively, samples can be collected from the catheter port in the drainage system after thorough disinfection with an appropriate disinfectant.

Prevention Strategies[17]

- Catheterization only when indicated.
- Daily assessment for the need for continuation of urinary catheter.
- Only trained healthcare providers should be allowed to do urinary catheterization along with routine competency assessment.
- To have a kit available with all the necessary supplies so as to ensure aseptic technique.
- Perform surveillance for CAUTI rates in ICU as well as non-ICU settings.
- To have a standardized institutional protocol for urine culture.
- Concerned, healthcare providers should be regularly trained regarding insertion, maintenance of urinary catheters, and the importance of urine culture stewardship.

BOX 3: Catheter-associated urinary tract infection (CAUTI) in any age.

Patients must meet the following criteria:

Patient had an indwelling urinary catheter that had been in place for >2 consecutive days in an inpatient location on the date of the event AND was either:
- Present for any portion of the calendar day on the date of the event

Or

- Removed the day before the date of the event

Patient has *at least one* of the following signs or symptoms:
- Fever (>38.0°C)
- Suprapubic tenderness
- Costovertebral angle pain or tenderness
- Urinary urgency
- Urinary frequency
- Dysuria

Patients have a urine culture with no more than two species of organisms identified, at least one of which is a bacterium of $\geq 10^5$ CFU/m.

The following excluded organisms cannot be used to meet the UTI definition:
- Any yeast
- Mould
- Dimorphic fungi
- Parasites

Indications for Sending Urine Culture

Refer **Box 4**.

Inappropriate Indications for Sending Urine Culture

Refer **Box 5**.

At Insertion

- Hand hygiene is necessary before the procedure or handling of a catheter or a drainage system.
- Aseptic techniques should be followed.
- Use sterile gloves, drape, and sponges, a sterile antiseptic solution for cleaning the urethral meatus, and a sterile single-use packet of lubricant jelly for insertion.

Maintenance of Indwelling Urinary Catheters

- Urinary catheters should always be secured after insertion to avoid movement and urethral traction.
- A closed drainage system is recommended.
- For sending a urine sample for examination, the collection is to be done by aspirating urine from the needleless sampling port with a sterile syringe after thorough cleansing of the port with disinfectant.
- Timely transport (within an hour) of the urine sample to the laboratory should be ensured. If not feasible, then the sample should be refrigerated.
- The collecting bag should always be below the bladder level and should never touch the floor.
- The catheter should be kept free from kinking to ensure unobstructed flow.

BOX 4: The following are appropriate indications for sending urine culture:[17]

- Presence of symptoms indicating UTI, such as acute hematuria and flank pain
- New onset or worsening of sepsis without any evidence of an alternative source of infection
- Fever or altered sensorium without any evidence of an alternative source
- Increased spasticity, autonomic dysreflexia in patients with spinal cord injury, >40% burns, postkidney transplant recipient with graft failure

BOX 5: Inappropriate indications for sending urine culture.[17]

- To diagnose response to therapy unless there is no resolution of symptoms
- Pyuria during routine analysis without any indications
- Presence of cloudy, smelly, or discolored urine with absence of any relevant signs and symptoms

TABLE 1: Checklist for prevention measures for catheter-associated urinary tract infection (CAUTI).

Insertion bundle:	
Presence of appropriate indication for urinary catheterization	☐
Availability of a catheterization kit containing a disposable urinary catheterization set, sterile gloves, disinfectant, and single-use lubricant jelly	☐
Surgical hand hygiene before the procedure	☐
Aseptic technique during insertion	☐
Proper cleansing of the genitalia	☐
Maintenance bundle:	
Daily review of the need for catheter continuity	☐
Hand hygiene before and after handling the catheter system	☐
Maintenance of the closed drainage system	☐
Unobstructed urine flow, no kinks	☐
Urine collecting bag below the level of the bladder	☐
Urine collecting bag not touching the floor	☐
Collection bag emptied when half full or before any procedures/activities	☐
Drainage port cleaned with 70% alcohol before and after draining the urine	☐
Catheter secured to the lateral aspect of the patient's thigh	☐

- The collecting bag should be emptied regularly using a separate container for each patient. The draining port of the collecting bag should not touch the container while doing the same.
- Regular catheter care and cleaning of the meatal area with antiseptic solution.

Checklist to Ensure Prevention Measures for Catheter-associated Urinary Tract Infection

Refer **Table 1**.

POINTS TO REMEMBER

Refer **Box 6**.

BOX 6: Points to remember for prevention measures for catheter-associated urinary tract infection (CAUTI).

- Urinary catheterization only when indicated
- Daily review for the need of catheter continuity
- Hand hygiene is a must before insertion and before/after catheter handling
- Checklist should be followed during insertion and management of a urinary catheter
- Do not treat asymptomatic bacteriuria in order to prevent CAUTI
- Continuous bladder irrigation with antimicrobials is not recommended as a prevention strategy
- No routine changing of urinary catheters
- In case of a catheter of >7 days duration, the catheter can be changed to obtain a fresh urine sample
- Alcohol based products should be avoided over the genital mucosa

CONCLUSION

- Catheter-related infections are very common in ICU settings.
- It is important to understand their pathogenesis and risk factors.
- Catheters should be inserted only when indicated.
- There has to be a daily assessment for the need for continuation of existing catheters.
- Checklists and prevention bundles are important tools in the prevention of catheter-related infections.
- Regular audits should be conducted to check adherence to infection control practices.
- Surveillance for CLABSI and CAUTI is essential in ICU and non-ICU settings.

REFERENCES

1. Mermel LA. Prevention of intravascular catheter-related infections. Ann Intern Med. 2000 Mar 7;132(5):391-402. Erratum in: Ann Intern Med 2000; 133(5):395.
2. Maqbool S, Sharma R. Incidence of Central Line-Associated Bloodstream Infection in a Tertiary Care Hospital in Northern India: A Prospective Study. Cureus. 2023;15(8):e44501.
3. Maqbool S, Sharma R. A Two-Year Surveillance of Central Line-Associated Bloodstream Infections in the Trauma ICU of a Tertiary Care Hospital in India. Cureus. 2023;15(9):e45325.

4. Ling ML, Apisarnthanarak A, Madriaga G. The Burden of Healthcare-Associated Infections in Southeast Asia: A Systematic Literature Review and Meta-analysis. Clin Infect Dis. 2015;60(11):1690-9.
5. Allegranzi A. (2011). Report on the Burden of Endemic Health Care-Associated Infection: Worldwide World Health Organization. [online] Available from https://iris.who.int/bitstream/handle/10665/80135/9789241501507_eng.pdf [Last accessed August, 2025].
6. National Healthcare Safety Network. (2025). Bloodstream Infection Event (Central Line-Associated Bloodstream Infection and Non-central Line Associated Bloodstream Infection). [online] Available from https://www.cdc.gov/nhsn/pdfs/pscmanual/4psc_clabscurrent.pdf.
7. Snydman DR, Gorbea HF, Pober BR, Majka JA, Murray SA, Perry LK. Predictive value of surveillance skin cultures in total-parenteral-nutrition-related infection. Lancet. 1982 Dec 18;2(8312):1385-8.
8. Salzman MB, Isenberg HD, Shapiro JF, Lipsitz PJ, Rubin LG. A prospective study of the catheter hub as the portal of entry for microorganisms causing catheter-related sepsis in neonates. J Infect Dis. 1993;167(2):487-90.
9. Mermel LA, McCormick RD, Springman SR, Maki DG. The pathogenesis and epidemiology of catheter-related infection with pulmonary artery Swan-Ganz catheters: a prospective study utilizing molecular subtyping. Am J Med. 1991;91(3B):197S-205S.
10. Weiner LM, Webb AK, Limbago B, Dudeck MA, Patel J, Kallen AJ, et al. Antimicrobial-Resistant Pathogens Associated With Healthcare-Associated Infections: Summary of Data Reported to the National Healthcare Safety Network at the Centers for Disease Control and Prevention, 2011-2014. Infect Control Hosp Epidemiol. 2016;37(11):1288-1301.
11. Chatzinikolaou I, Hanna H, Hachem R, Alakech B, Tarrand J, Raad I. Differential quantitative blood cultures for the diagnosis of catheter-related bloodstream infections associated with short- and long-term catheters: a prospective study. Diagn Microbiol Infect Dis. 2004;50(3):167-72.
12. Ulrich P, Lepak AJ, Chen DJ. Diagnostic and Therapeutic Utility of Positive Intravascular Catheter Tip Cultures. Microbiol Spectr. 2022;10(6):e0402222.
13. Tomlinson D, Mermel LA, Ethier MC, Matlow A, Gillmeister B, Sung L. Defining bloodstream infections related to central venous catheters in patients with cancer: a systematic review. Clin Infect Dis. 2011;53(7):697-710.
14. Buetti N, Marschall J, Drees M, Fakih MG, Hadaway L, Maragakis LL, et al. Strategies to prevent central line-associated bloodstream infections in acute-care hospitals: 2022 Update. Infect Control Hosp Epidemiol. 2022;43(5):553-69.
15. National Healthcare Safety Network. (2025). Urinary Tract Infection (Catheter-Associated Urinary Tract Infection [CAUTI] and Non-Catheter-Associated Urinary Tract Infection [UTI]) Events. [online] Available from: https://www.cdc.gov/nhsn/pdfs/pscmanual/7psccauticurrent.pdf [Last accessed August, 2025].
16. Kass EH, Schneiderman LJ. Entry of bacteria into the urinary tracts of patients with inlying catheters. N Engl J Med. 1957;256(12):556-7.
17. Patel PK, Advani SD, Kofman AD, Lo E, Maragakis LL, Pegues DA, Pettis AM, Saint S, Trautner B, Yokoe DS, Meddings J. Strategies to prevent catheter-associated urinary tract infections in acute-care hospitals: 2022 Update. Infect Control Hosp Epidemiol. 2023;44(8):1209-31.

12

CHAPTER **Surgical Site and Wound Infections**

Susovan Mitra

LEARNING OBJECTIVES

- *Understand the pathophysiology of surgical site infections (SSIs):* Comprehend the biological mechanisms and factors contributing to SSIs in the critical care setting.
- *Implement preventive strategies effectively:* Implement preventive measures and evidence-based prophylactic antibiotic protocols to reduce the incidence of SSIs.
- *Optimize postoperative wound care in the intensive care unit (ICU):* Utilize best practices for wound management to enhance healing and minimize infection risks.
- *Utilize practical tools for clinical application*: Employ checklists, guidelines to standardize and improve SSI prevention and management in the ICU.

INTRODUCTION

Surgical site infections (SSIs) are one of the most common and serious complications in the healthcare facility, especially in the intensive care unit (ICU). SSIs occur within 30 days postoperatively along the incision site of a surgical procedure and are further categorized as superficial or deep tissue infections.[1,5] The importance of SSIs is derived from their contribution to increased morbidity of patients, extended stay in the hospital, added costs of care, and even mortality rates.[6-8] The patients in the ICU are more prone to SSIs due to various reasons, which include compromised immune system, the presence of invasive devices, and the severity of the underlying conditions.[5,11,17]

The pathogenesis of SSI essentially represents an interaction between the microbial pathogens on one hand and the immune defense of the host on the other. Understanding this would obviously be pivotal to the evolution of effective prophylaxis or therapy. Besides these, prophylaxis via judiciously used antibiotics, optimization of surgical techniques, and stringent asepsis are measures which are cardinal for keeping the rate of SSIs at a minimum.[2-4,18,19] Moreover, postoperative wound care in the ICU requires greater attention to detail because active management of a wound accelerates the course of healing and also acts as an important barrier against potential pathogens.[34-36]

In essence, this chapter covers the pathophysiology of SSI, various methods of prevention, and best practices in providing postoperative ICU care for infected wounds, and integrates relevant recent guidelines with high-borough evidence-based approach for clinicians to work safely and effectively within their scope through improving patient outcomes and promoting affordable treatment.

PATHOPHYSIOLOGY OF SURGICAL SITE INFECTIONS

Microbial Etiology

A vast majority of SSIs are caused by bacterial pathogens, and the most common causative agents belong to the *Staphylococcus* genus: *Staphylococcus aureus*, including methicillin-resistant strains, and *Staphylococcus epidermidis*.[5,9,10] Gram-negative bacteria such as *Escherichia coli, Pseudomonas aeruginosa*, and *Klebsiella pneumoniae* are also common causes of SSIs, especially following abdominal and thoracic surgeries.[5,11] The emergence of multidrug-resistant organisms (MDOs) complicates treatment, making targeted antimicrobial therapy necessary.[8-11]

Host Factors

It is, therefore, important to consider a variety of predisposing factors relating to the patient that predispose an individual to SSIs. Comorbidities such as diabetes mellitus, obesity, malnutrition, and immunosuppression weaken the host response to infection.[5,14] Advanced age and prolonged hospitalization increase the risk of SSIs among patients.[5,7] Other risk factors include smoking and poor glycemic control, which not only impede the process of wound healing but also are reported to have a depressive effect on the immune system, thereby further increasing the risk of development of SSI.[14-16]

The risk of SSI is greatly affected by the nature and complexity of the surgical procedure. Surgical procedures classified as "clean", like orthopedic implants, tend to have much lower infection rates compared to clean-contaminated or contaminated surgeries, like gastrointestinal operations, which inherently involve much higher microbial load.[1,3,5]

PREVENTIVE STRATEGIES

- *Preoperative skin cleansing*: Emphasize proper cleansing of the skin with povidone-iodine or chlorhexidine in preparation for surgery in an attempt to minimize microbial burden at the site of incision. [2-4,18]
- The maintenance of normothermia involves keeping the patient warm while an anesthetic is being administered, as hypothermia is linked to an increased risk of SSIs. [2,3,18]
- *Maintenance of normothermia*: Ensure normothermic maintenance of the patient during surgery, with hypothermia being a causative factor for SSI increased risk.[2,3,18]
- *Glycemic control*: Emphasize how important it is to maintain optimal blood sugar levels, especially in diabetics, in order to mitigate the threat of infection.[14,16,30,31]

- Encourage patients to stop smoking at least a few weeks before surgery to promote wound healing and reduce the chance of complications from SSI.[15]
- *Minimizing invasive devices*: Have recommendations for minimizing use of invasive devices such as catheters and for timely removal to mitigate infection risk.[17,44]
- *Postoperative wound care*: Educate patient and caregiver in proper care for a wound to prevent infection.[34-37]

PROPHYLACTIC ANTIBIOTICS

Prophylactic antibiotics prevent SSIs, and the judicious use of prophylactic antibiotics is crucial. The prophylaxis should be given 1 hour prior to surgical incision for attaining optimal tissue concentration at the time of potential microbial contamination of the wound site.[3,18-20] The antibiotic should be appropriately selected by the surgical site, history of patient allergy, and local microbial flora. Usual agents that can be employed are cefazolin and cefoxitin. The choice would also be vancomycin in settings where the prevalence of methicillin-resistant *Staphylococcus aureus* (MRSA) is very high.[3,10,19]

Antibiotic Stewardship

Antibiotic stewardship programs are very much significant for the optimization of prophylactic antibiotics and reducing the risk of resistance. In general, these programs advocate judicious selection, dosing, and duration of antibiotic therapy, so that optimum efficacy may be achieved with least adverse events and resistance.[21,22] Stewardship protocols, when applied in the ICUs, have immense potential to bring about drastic reduction of SSIs, eventually bringing MDOs down too.[8,9,21,22]

Current Guidelines and Key Studies

The current guidelines and key studies regarding the use of prophylactic antibiotics to prevent SSIs are summarized in **Table 1**.

USE OF ANTIMICROBIAL-IMPREGNATED DEVICES

Antimicrobial-impregnated sutures and implants are among the most significant advancements toward SSI prevention, particularly during high-risk surgeries.[23,46,47] These devices elute antimicrobial agents locally from the surgical site, thus allowing a prolonged action of antimicrobials in reducing the chance of bacterial colonization.[23,46] These devices prevent the pathogenic growth successfully by maintaining optimal local concentrations of antimicrobials throughout their action time and hence ensure lower SSI rates, with most important events during the sensitive postoperative period.[23,46,47]

TABLE 1: Current guidelines and key studies regarding the use of prophylactic antibiotics to prevent SSIs.

Guideline/study	*Key recommendations/findings*	*Year*	*Reference*
World Health Organization (WHO) global guidelines on SSI prevention	Emphasize timely prophylactic antibiotic administration and procedure-appropriate drug selection as part of a broader SSI prevention bundle	2016 (2nd ed. 2018)	2
CDC guideline for the prevention of surgical site infection	Recommends giving prophylactic antibiotics within 1 hour before incision (2 hours for vancomycin/fluoroquinolones) and redosing in prolonged procedures	2017	3
Clinical practice guidelines for antimicrobial prophylaxis in surgery	Provide detailed advice on drug choice, dose, timing, and duration; adherence is linked with reduced SSI rates	2013	19
Strategies to prevent surgical site infections in acute care hospitals	Stresses evidence-based prophylaxis, normothermia, glycaemic control, and care bundles for SSI prevention in hospitals and ICUs	2023	18
Meta-analysis of timing of antimicrobial prophylaxis	Shows that antibiotics given within 60 minutes before incision are associated with lower SSI rates compared with earlier or later administration	2017	20
IDSA/SHEA guideline on antibiotic stewardship	Highlights stewardship as central to optimizing perioperative prophylaxis and limiting resistance	2016	21

(CDC: Centers for Disease Control and Prevention; MRSA: methicillin-resistant *Staphylococcus aureus*; SSIs: surgical site infections; WHO: World Health Organization)

Antimicrobial-impregnated devices, such as sutures coated with triclosan or implants treated with silver nanoparticles, have shown to decrease the rates of SSI in several surgical disciplines, including orthopedic and cardiac surgery.[23,46,47] For example, triclosan-coated sutures have been shown to decrease SSIs in clean and clean-contaminated procedures through mechanisms that inhibit bacterial adherence and biofilm formation.[46] Similarly, the implantation of joint replacements with antimicrobial coating has been associated with a decrease in the number of infected wounds, hence increasing patient satisfaction while minimizing the incidence of revision surgeries.[23]

Moreover, local delivery of antimicrobials with the use of such devices minimizes systemic antibiotic exposure, hence reducing the occurrences of adverse effects and development of antibiotic resistance.[23] This approach not only improves the prophylactic efficacy but also follows the principles of antibiotic stewardship through avoiding unnecessary systemic use of antibiotics.[21-23]

However, despite the advantages, evidence-based guidelines are still required to assist in their appropriate use and maximize their effectiveness.[2,3,18,23] Such devices should be selected by healthcare facilities based on the type of surgery, risk profile of patients, and pattern of local resistance to antimicrobials.[2,3,18,23] Basic research and clinical trials continue to evaluate optimal configurations and combinations of antimicrobial agents to further enhance SSI prevention.[23,46,47]

Current Guidelines and Key Studies

Table 2 summarizes the current guidelines and key studies using antimicrobial-impregnated devices for the prevention of SSIs.

TABLE 2: Current guidelines and key studies using antimicrobial-impregnated devices for the prevention of surgical site infections (SSIs).

Guideline/study	*Key recommendations/findings*	*Year*	*Reference*
World Health Organization (WHO) SSI prevention guidelines	Recognize antimicrobial sutures and implants as optional components of comprehensive SSI prevention strategies, particularly in high-risk surgery	2016 /2018	2
Centers for Disease Control and Prevention (CDC) guidelines—SSI prevention	Notes that antimicrobial-impregnated sutures may be used in selected procedures as part of multimodal SSI prevention efforts	2017	3
Triclosan-coated sutures reduce the risk of SSI (meta-analysis)	Triclosan-coated sutures significantly lower SSI risk compared with standard sutures	2015	46
Abdominal surgery meta-analysis	Triclosan-coated sutures for fascial closure in abdominal surgery reduce SSIs compared with uncoated sutures	2024	47
Local antimicrobial strategies and implants	Reviews local antimicrobial strategies and antimicrobial-coated implants for fracture-related infection; supports selective use in high-risk orthopedic procedures	2020	23
SSI prevention update	Suggests considering antimicrobial-impregnated devices for specific high-risk patients and procedures within broader SSI prevention bundles	2023	18

GLYCEMIC CONTROL STRATEGIES

Preoperative Assessment

Before any surgery, the blood glucose of a patient needs to be investigated and optimized. The glycemic condition of the patient should be maintained within a stable level of glucose over a given range for that specific disease to prevent further complications before and after surgery.[14,16,30,31]

Insulin Management

The main factor that maintains blood glucose within the target range, normally between 80 and 180 mg/dL, is insulin therapy. This should be titrated according to the individual's needs to avoid hyperglycemia and hypoglycemia.[30,31]

Continuous Glucose Monitoring

Since the level of blood glucose is monitored in real time throughout the perioperative period, spikes and dips in levels are quickly ascertained, allowing immediate action to be instituted.[30,31]

Collaborative Care

Management of diabetes in surgical patients should be a collaborative effort. It is crucial to involve an endocrinologist, surgeon, and nursing staff for total and coordinated care regarding the condition of the patient.[16,30,31]

NUTRITIONAL SUPPORT

Adequate nutrition is important to ensure healthy tissue repair and good immune function to prevent SSIs.[26-29] Malnutrition adversely affects the body's tissue repair system and its infection-fighting capabilities, putting the patient at risk for SSI.[26,27] Conversely, good nutritional status promotes anabolic processes and enhances the immune response, accelerating wound healing.[26-29]

Nutritional Support Strategies

Preoperative Nutrition Assessment

It should include a comprehensive nutrition assessment for identifying deficiencies and malnutrition.[26-29]

Nutritional Supplementation

Ingestion of nutritional supplements according to the specific needs, such as proteins, vitamins (for example, vitamin C, vitamin D), and minerals (for example, zinc) in order to provide specific nutrient deficiencies.[26-29]

Enteral Nutrition

Provide early enteral nutrition in the perioperative period, when possible, to maintain gut integrity and immune function.[26-29] Enhanced Recovery After Surgery (ERAS) protocols specifically endorse early oral or enteral feeding as part of multimodal perioperative care.[28,29] The links between glycemic control, nutrition, and SSI prevention are summarized in **Table 3**.

PROPER WOUND CARE IN THE INTENSIVE CARE UNIT

Good care of the wound is essential in the ICU to avoid infections and promote wound healing. Attention should be given to several aspects.[34-39]

Hand Hygiene and Infection Control Practices

All health professionals should strictly follow the protocols of hand hygiene as a part of good wound care and the prevention of contamination and SSIs.[2,40-42] These include:

- *Alcohol-based hand sanitizers*: They are effective in reducing microbial load on hands.[40,41]
- *Glove use*: Changing gloves between patient contacts and after contact with contaminated surfaces to prevent cross contamination.[40,42]

Wound Assessment

The principle of early detection of SSI is based on the regular and detailed assessment of the wound. Careful observation will reveal warning signs such as the following:

- *Redness and swelling*: These are indicative of inflammation or onset of an infection.[34,35]
- *Localized heat and pain*: The most common sign of infection is warmth and tenderness around the wound.[34,35]
- *Discharge*: The purulent or serous discharge will then indicate infection and requires attention as soon as possible.[34-36]

Choice of Dressing

Selection of appropriate dressing is very important to ensure a healing process with minimal chance of infection. The type of wound, the amount of exudate, and the infection risk all play a role in making a decision on dressing. Options available include:

- *Antimicrobial dressings:* These are treated with agents such as silver or iodine and should be utilized with infected wounds or those at high risk to provide local antimicrobial protection.[35,39]
- *Hydrocolloid dressings:* These are recommended for lesions with moderate exudate. They foster autolytic debridement, which is the

TABLE 3: Year wise guidelines and key recommendations for glycemic control and enteral nutrition.

Guideline/study	*Key recommendations/findings*	*Year*	*Reference*
Meta-analysis of glycemic regimens	Structured perioperative glycemic protocols reduce SSI rates in surgical patients with diabetes	2022	16
American Diabetes Association (ADA) Standards of Care	Keep perioperative blood glucose generally 100–180 mg/dL (ICU often 140–180 mg/dL) to reduce complications including SSI	2024	30
Endocrine Society guideline	Detailed guidance on inpatient hyperglycaemia management, including perioperative insulin strategies	2012	31
WHO SSI prevention guidelines	Identify glycemic control and adequate nutrition as important components of SSI prevention bundles	2016/ 2018	2
ESPEN guideline on clinical nutrition in surgery	Appropriate nutrition improves wound healing and reduces infectious complications	2017	27
ESPEN guideline on clinical nutrition in the ICU	Individualized nutrition supports immunity and tissue repair in critical illness	2019	26
ERAS Society guidelines & Ljungqvist et al. review	Emphasize nutritional assessment, carbohydrate loading, and early postoperative feeding within ERAS pathways	2017–2021	28,29
Meta-analysis of smoking cessation	Perioperative smoking cessation programmes lower wound complication and SSI rates	2012	15
Supplemental oxygen trial	Higher perioperative oxygen fractions can reduce SSI in some high-risk patients	2000	32
Strategies to prevent SSIs	Advocates for integrated bundles that include glycaemic control, nutrition, and other risk factor modification	2023	18

natural sloughing off of dead tissue by the body, and establish a moist environment in the wound.[38]

- *Transparent film dressings*: These dressings ensure that the healing process is not disrupted by frequent alterations, allowing for continuous visualization of the wound.[35,36]

The ICU team must be proficient in the provision of optimal postoperative care to reduce morbidity through the systematic evaluation of wounds and the deliberate selection of dressings.[34-39]

Negative Pressure Wound Therapy

Negative pressure wound therapy (NPWT) has also become an evidence-based modality in ICU complex wound care by applying intermittent and continuous-controlled negative pressure to the wound bed in efforts to increase the formation of granulation tissue and reduce the levels of edema along with promoting removal of excess exudates.[24,25] Research demonstrates NPWT not only increases healing rates but significantly lowers SSI complications in high-risk surgical populations.[24,25]

Early Mobilization and Physical Therapy

Early mobilization and mobilization through physical rehabilitative support allow for improvement in wound healing by providing better aeration and reducing the tendency to develop lesions such as pressure ulcers caused by poor circulation. Mobilization promotes respiratory function, minimizing the chances of SSIs through improving circulation and enhancing recovery of the patient overall.[45]

Monitoring and Documentation

Precise documentation of assessment and the changes in wounds and infection signs is relevant to the ongoing management of the patient and to the control of infection in general. Correct record maintenance ensures timely intervention but also enables monitoring of the SSI trends within the ICU to inform quality improvement efforts.[17,18,43]

Multidisciplinary Approach

Full care and early intervention, when necessary, require collaboration in the ICU among surgeons, intensivists, nurses, and infection control specialists for the proper management of wounds. This multidisciplinary collaboration significantly enhances strategies for the prevention of SSI and nurtures a culture of safety and continuous improvement in healthcare institutions.[18,26-29,44,45]

PRACTICAL TOOLS

Surgical Site Infection Prevention Checklist

- *Preoperative*:
    - Appropriate prophylactic antibiotics to be administered within 1 hour before incision.[3,19,20]

  - Ensure patient optimization measures, such as glycemic control and smoking cessation.[14-16,26-30]
- *Intraoperative:*
  - Adhere to sterile techniques and aseptic practices intraoperatively.[2-4,18]
  - Maintain normothermia and proper oxygenation intraoperatively.[18,32,33]
- *Postoperative:*
  - Conduct regular wound assessments and document findings.[34,35,43]
  - Implement appropriate wound dressing protocols.[35-39]
  - Monitor for signs of infection and intervene promptly, including culture-directed antibiotics when indicated.[3,11,17]

Algorithm for the Management of Suspected Surgical Site Infection

- *Assess clinical signs*:
  - Redness, swelling, heat, pain, and discharge
- *Obtain wound cultures:*
  - Swab or biopsy for microbiological analysis[11,17]
- *Initiate empirical antibiotic therapy:*
  - Based on likely pathogens and local antibiogram[3,10,11,19]
- *Adjust therapy based on culture results:*
  - Tailor antibiotics to specific pathogens and sensitivities.[8,9,21,22]
- *Implement wound management strategies:*
  - Debridement, dressing changes, and NPWT as indicated[23-25,35-39]
- *Monitor patient response:*
  - Evaluate clinical improvement and adjust management as necessary.

IMPORTANT POINTS TO REMEMBER

- *Timely administration of prophylactic antibiotics*: It ensures optimal tissue concentration during the critical period of microbial contamination.[3,18-20]
- *Strict adherence to aseptic techniques*: It minimizes the risk of introducing pathogens during surgery.[2-4,18]
- *Regular wound monitoring*: This facilitates early detection and management of SSIs, improving patient outcomes.[34,35,43]
- *Multidisciplinary collaboration*: This enhances the effectiveness of SSI prevention and management strategies.[18,26-29,44,45]
- *Antibiotic stewardship*: It balances effective infection control with the prevention of antimicrobial resistance.[8,9,21,22]

CONCLUSION

Surgical site infections are one of the major yet preventable complications in the ICU, which require multimodal and comprehensive approaches to both prevention and management. Understanding the pathophysiology involved in SSIs is important for the development of effective strategies to combat infection.[5,12,13] Preventive measures of importance include the proper use of prophylactic antibiotics, adherence to sterile surgical technique, and patient optimization.[2-4,14-16,18-21,26-31] Wound care in the postoperative period in the ICU involves very close monitoring, proper selection of dressings, and a multidisciplinary approach for timely intervention and promotion of healing, including selective use of NPWT.[23-25,34-39,44,45] Evidence-based protocols and some practical tools will enable the practitioner in the ICU to go a long way in reducing the risk of SSIs and improving patient outcomes while reducing the burden on healthcare systems.

REFERENCES

1. Centers for Disease Control and Prevention. National Healthcare Safety Network (NHSN) Patient Safety Component Manual: Surgical Site Infection (SSI) Event. Atlanta (GA): CDC; 2024.
2. World Health Organization. Global guidelines for the prevention of surgical site infection. 2nd ed. Geneva: World Health Organization; 2018.
3. Berríos-Torres SI, Umscheid CA, Bratzler DW, Leas B, Stone EC, Kelz RR, et al. Centers for Disease Control and Prevention guideline for the prevention of surgical site infection, 2017. JAMA Surg. 2017;152(8):784-91.
4. National Institute for Health and Care Excellence (NICE). Surgical site infections: prevention and treatment. NICE Guideline NG125. London: NICE; 2019.
5. Anderson DJ. Surgical site infections. Infect Dis Clin North Am. 2011;25(1): 135-53.
6. Gillespie BM, Harbeck E, Rattray M, Liang R, Walker R, Latimer S, et al. Worldwide incidence of surgical site infections in general surgical patients: a systematic review and meta-analysis of 488,594 patients. Int J Surg.2021;95:106136.
7. Tola HH, Mekonnen ZA, Bisetegn TA, Gebreagziabher SB. Global incidence of surgical site infection among patients: systematic review and meta-analysis. Inquiry. 2023;60:00469580231162549.
8. Badia JM, Casey AL, Petrosillo N, Hudson PM, Mitchell SA, Crosby C. Impact of surgical site infection on healthcare costs and patient outcomes: a systematic review in six European countries. J Hosp Infect.2017;96(1):1-15.
9. Tacconelli E, Carrara E, Savoldi A, Harbarth S, Mendelson M, Monnet DL, et al. Discovery, research, and development of new antibiotics: the WHO priority list of antibiotic-resistant bacteria and tuberculosis. Lancet Infect Dis. 2018;18(3):318-27.
10. Klevens RM, Morrison MA, Nadle J, Petit S, Gershman K, Ray S, et al. Invasive methicillin-resistant *Staphylococcus aureus* infections in the United States. JAMA. 2007;298(15):1763-71.
11. Solomkin JS, Mazuski JE, Bradley JS, Rodvold KA, Goldstein EJ, Baron EJ, et al. Diagnosis and management of complicated intra-abdominal infection in adults and children: guidelines by the Surgical Infection Society and the Infectious Diseases Society of America. Clin Infect Dis. 2010;50(2):133-64.
12. Medzhitov R. Origin and physiological roles of inflammation. Nature. 2008;454(7203):428-35.

13. Costerton JW, Stewart PS, Greenberg EP. Bacterial biofilms: a common cause of persistent infections. Science.1999;284(5418):1318-22.
14. Martin ET, Kaye KS, Knott C, Nguyen H, Santarossa M, Evans R, et al. Diabetes and risk of surgical site infection: a systematic review and meta-analysis. Infect Control Hosp Epidemiol. 2016;37(1):88-99.
15. Sørensen LT. Wound healing and infection in surgery: the clinical impact of smoking and smoking cessation: a systematic review and meta-analysis. Arch Surg. 2012;147(4):373-83.
16. Lai F, Wang J, He Y, Luo Y, Ye Y, Deng G, et al. Intensive versus conventional glucose control in surgical patients: a systematic review and meta-analysis. Front Surg. 2022;9:836218.
17. Centers for Disease Control and Prevention. Identifying healthcare-associated infections (HAI) for NHSN surveillance. In: NHSN Patient Safety Component Manual. Atlanta (GA): CDC; 2024.
18. Calderwood MS, Anderson DJ, Bratzler DW, Dellinger EP, Garcia Houchins S, Maragakis LL, et al. Strategies to prevent surgical site infections in acute-care hospitals: 2022 update. Infect Control Hosp Epidemiol.2023;44(5):695-720.
19. Bratzler DW, Dellinger EP, Olsen KM, Perl TM, Auwaerter PG, Bolon MK, et al. Clinical practice guidelines for antimicrobial prophylaxis in surgery. Am J Health Syst Pharm. 2013;70(3):195-283.
20. de Oliveira GS Jr, Chang R, Kendall MC, Fitzgerald PC, McCarthy RJ. Timing of antimicrobial prophylaxis and the risk of surgical site infections: a systematic review. Ann Surg. 2017;265(5):893-901.
21. Barlam TF, Cosgrove SE, Abbo LM, MacDougall C, Schuetz AN, Septimus EJ, et al. Implementing an antibiotic stewardship program: guidelines by the Infectious Diseases Society of America and the Society for Healthcare Epidemiology of America. Clin Infect Dis. 2016;62(10):e51-77.
22. Dyar OJ, Huttner B, Schouten J, Pulcini C. What is antimicrobial stewardship? Clin Microbiol Infect.2017;23(11):793-8.
23. Metsemakers WJ, Emanuel N, Cohen O, Serra Torres J, Chadayammuri V, Egol KA, et al. Evidence-based recommendations for local antimicrobial strategies and dead space management in fracture-related infection. J Orthop Trauma. 2020;34(1):18-29.
24. Willy C, Agarwal A, Andersen CA, Santis G, Gabriel A, Hudson DA, et al. Closed incision negative pressure therapy: international multidisciplinary consensus recommendations. Int Wound J. 2017;14(2):385-98.
25. Hyldig N, Vinter CA, Kruse M, Mogensen O, Bille C, Sorensen JA, et al. Prophylactic incisional negative pressure wound therapy reduces the risk of surgical site infection after caesarean section in obese women: a pragmatic randomised clinical trial. BJOG. 2019;126(5):628-35.
26. Singer P, Blaser AR, Berger MM, Alhazzani W, Calder PC, Casaer MP, et al. ESPEN guideline on clinical nutrition in the intensive care unit. Clin Nutr. 2019;38(1):48-79.
27. Weimann A, Braga M, Carli F, Higashiguchi T, Hübner M, Klek S, et al. ESPEN guideline: clinical nutrition in surgery. Clin Nutr. 2017;36(3):623-50.
28. Ljungqvist O, Scott M, Fearon KC. Enhanced Recovery After Surgery: a review. JAMA Surg. 2017;152(3):292-8.

29. Enhanced Recovery after Surgery (ERAS) Society. ERAS Society guidelines [Internet]. Stockholm: ERAS Society; c2017–2025 [cited 2025 Aug 20]. Available from: https://erassociety.org/guidelines/
30. American Diabetes Association Professional Practice Committee. 16. Diabetes care in the hospital: Standards of Medical Care in Diabetes—2024. Diabetes Care. 2024;47(Suppl 1):S266-78.
31. Umpierrez GE, Hellman R, Korytkowski MT, Kosiborod M, Maynard GA, Montori VM, et al. Management of hyperglycemia in hospitalized patients in non-critical care setting: an Endocrine Society clinical practice guideline. J Clin Endocrinol Metab. 2012;97(1):16-38.
32. Greif R, Akça O, Horn EP, Kurz A, Sessler DI; Outcomes Research Group. Supplemental perioperative oxygen to reduce the incidence of surgical wound infection. N Engl J Med. 2000;342(3):161-7.
33. Apfel CC, Kranke P, Eberhart LHJ, Roewer N. High-concentration perioperative oxygen to reduce surgical site infection: is it the right solution? Anesthesiology. 2010;113(2):340-7.
34. Ayello EA, Sibbald RG. TIME heals all wounds. Nurs Manage. 2003;34(4):36-43.
35. Sibbald RG, Goodman L, Woo KY, Krasner DL, Smart H, Tariq G, et al. Special considerations in wound bed preparation 2011: an update. Adv Skin Wound Care. 2011;24(9):415-36.
36. Harding K, Dowsett C, Fias L, Leaper D, Mayer D, Romanelli M, et al. Simplifying venous leg ulcer management: consensus recommendations. Wounds Int. 2015;6(1):1-10.
37. Malone M, Bjarnsholt T, McBain AJ, James GA, Stoodley P, Leaper D, et al. The prevalence of biofilms in chronic wounds: a systematic review and meta-analysis of published data. J Wound Care. 2017;26(1):20-5.
38. Vermeulen H, Westerbos SJ, Ubbink DT. Benefit and harm of silver-containing dressings in infected and noninfected chronic wounds: a systematic review and meta-analysis. J Wound Care. 2007;16(6):245-52.
39. Leaper D, Drake R, Assadian O, Edmiston CE Jr, Goves J, Lang S, et al. Appropriate use of silver dressings in wounds: international consensus document. Int Wound J. 2012;9(1 Suppl):1-21.
40. Pittet D, Allegranzi B, Boyce J; World Health Organization World Alliance for Patient Safety First Global Patient Safety Challenge Core Group of Experts. The World Health Organization guidelines on hand hygiene in health care and their consensus recommendations. Infect Control Hosp Epidemiol. 2009;30(7): 611-22.
41. Larson EL. A patient safety challenge: hand hygiene. J Nurs Care Qual. 2005;20(1):24-8.
42. Boyce JM, Pittet D; Healthcare Infection Control Practices Advisory Committee; HICPAC/SHEA/APIC/IDSA Hand Hygiene Task Force. Guideline for hand hygiene in health-care settings. MMWR Recomm Rep.2002;51(RR-16):1-45.
43. Kalisch BJ, Tschannen D, Lee KH. Missed nursing care, staffing, and patient falls. J Nurs Care Qual.2012;27(1):6-12.
44. Pronovost P, Needham D, Berenholtz S, Sinopoli D, Chu H, Cosgrove S, et al. An intervention to decrease catheter-related bloodstream infections in the ICU. N Engl J Med. 2006;355(26):2725-32.

45. Needham DM, Korupolu R, Zanni JM, Pradhan P, Colantuoni E, Palmer JB, et al. Early physical medicine and rehabilitation for patients with acute respiratory failure: a quality improvement project. Arch Phys Med Rehabil. 2010;91(4):536-42.
46. Apisarnthanarak A, Thongphubeth K, Sirinvaravong S, Kitkhuandee A, Apisarnthanarak P, Warren DK, et al. Triclosan-coated sutures reduce the risk of surgical site infections: a meta-analysis. Infect Control Hosp Epidemiol. 2015;36(2):169-79.
47. Depuydt M, Van Egmond S, Petersen SM, Muysoms F, Henriksen NA, Deerenberg EB. Surgical site infection in abdominal surgery: a systematic review and meta-analysis comparing triclosan-coated and uncoated sutures. Hernia. 2024;28(3):1-13. Epub ahead of print.

13

CHAPTER Biofilm-related Infections

Saswati Sinha

LEARNING OBJECTIVES

- Biofilm-related infections—their importance in clinical practice.
- The stages of biofilm formation, structure, composition, and mechanisms of tolerance to standard therapies.
- Common device-associated infections related to biofilms with challenges in diagnosis and treatment.
- Newer insights in biofilm diagnostic and therapeutic strategies.
- Future prospects with regard to antibiofilm strategies.

INTRODUCTION

Device-associated infections are dreaded complications in clinical practice and pose challenges with respect to diagnosis and treatment and are notorious in terms of recurrence.[1] The predominant reason is the formation of biofilms which are complex microbial communities encased in extracellular polymeric substances (EPS) which behave differently from planktonic microorganisms in terms of structural properties, growth rate, and microenvironments.[2] The unique challenges of biofilm-related infections include decreased susceptibility to antimicrobials as well as resistance to innate and adaptive immune host immune response. With the advancement of medical technology, and the advent of an array of medical devices, biofilm-related infections have become increasingly common, making the understanding of these infections vital for clinicians and microbiologists.

Biofilms may be formed by a single microorganism, or there may be a mix of bacteria, fungi, and protozoa. They are usually characterized by adhesion to surfaces of devices, but free-floating microorganisms can also aggregate to form biofilms on body tissues causing chronic or persistent infections that are difficult to treat and eradicate.[3] Once a biofilm matures and is >7 days old, the embedded microorganisms become 500–5,000-fold less susceptible to antimicrobials compared to their planktonic counterparts.[4] The concept of biofilms was demonstrated 80–90 years ago in environmental and technical microbiology on the surface of submerged structures such ships, but relevance of biofilms in medicine was highlighted by identification of heaps of *Pseudomonas aeruginosa* in sputum and lung tissue of patients with cystic fibrosis by Hoiby and acquired dental pellicles by Jendresen.[5]

The term "biofilm" was introduced in the medical field by Costerton in 1985 and thereafter, the importance of these infections is now widely understood and appreciated.[6] Apart from being resistant to antimicrobials and disinfectants, the microorganisms in the biofilm are difficult to identify from routine clinical samples. The treatment based on the susceptibility pattern of planktonic organisms may be ineffective against biofilms leading to treatment failure and recurrence.

DEFINITION

A biofilm is defined as "an aggregate of microorganisms adherent to a biotic or abiotic surface, embedded within a matrix of EPS".[7]

STRUCTURE OF BIOFILMS

A biofilm is a "structured consortium of microbial cells surrounded by a self-produced polymer matrix". In addition to microorganisms such as bacteria and/or fungi, host components such as fibrin, platelets, and immunoglobulins also form a part of the matrix. The biofilms have physiological and biochemical gradients from the surface to the deeper layers including nutrients, oxygen, genetics, and rate of growth. They could be monomicrobial and polymicrobial depending on the type of device and the length of time, it is in situ and their characteristics differ from nonaggregated (planktonic) organisms.[8] The structure is a three-dimensional matrix which adheres to the medical device and is formed when the free-floating bacteria come in contact with the device surface and secrete polymers. When the biofilms reach a critical level, they trigger an inflammatory response in the host and may even lead to implant failure. The most common microorganisms which cause medical device-associated infections include *Staphylococcus aureus* and *Staphylococcus epidermidis*. Multidrug-resistant gram-negative organisms such as *Escherichia coli, Klebsiella pneumoniae, P. aeruginosa,* and *Acinetobacter baumannii* can also form biofilms.[9]

STAGES OF BIOFILM FORMATION

The stages in biofilm formation include initial attachment, growth, maturation, and dispersal/detachment **(Fig. 1)**.

Initial Attachment

The attachment of the microorganisms to the surface of a device or tissue is the first stage. Microbes are transported by convection, Brownian motion, and sedimentation.[10] Furthermore, chemotaxis allows the bacterial cells to traverse the gradient toward chemically induced nutrient substrates such as sugars and amino acids. The ability to adhere to the surface depends on the device surface characteristics such as roughness, hydrophobicity,

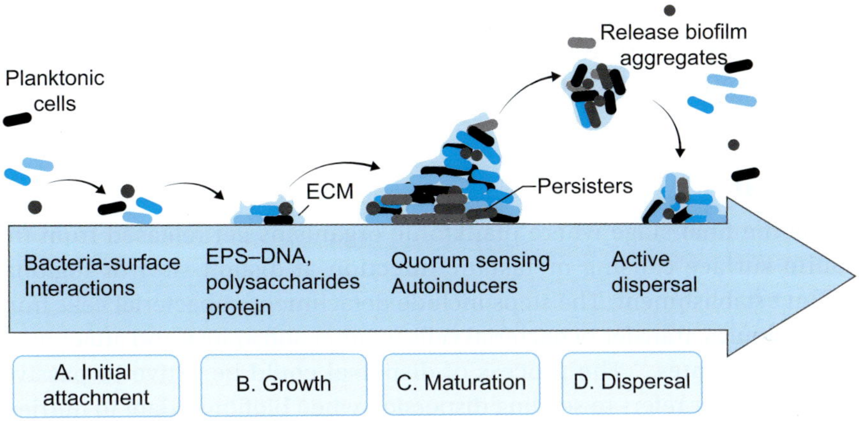

Fig. 1: Stages of biofilm formation.

surface charge, and film modulation.[11] In addition, the structural and physicochemical properties of the bacterial cells determine the adhesive properties which depend on the species, age, environmental pH, ionic strength, and culture medium.[12] Microorganisms adhere to medical devices via cell surface proteins such as biofilm associated protein—a fimbria-like polymer, the protein autolysin of *S. epidermidis*, and other coagulase-negative Staphylococci. In addition, host-derived proteins such as fibrinogen, fibronectin, and vitronectin get absorbed on the surface of medical devices, producing a conditioning film which enhances the interaction between the microbial and host proteins thereby promoting microbial colonization.[13]

Growth

During this stage, the bacterial cells begin to proliferate, the individual cells adhere to each other and become surrounded by EPS. EPS plays a crucial role in biofilm formation which includes surface adhesion, formation of the internal structure, mutual recognition between cells, signal transduction, acquisition of nutrients, cell maintenance, etc.[14] Among the components of EPS, extracellular polysaccharides play the key role in forming and promoting development of the biofilm. In addition, EPS also contains proteins in form of enzymes, protein structures such as fimbriae as well as extracellular DNA (eDNA) which helps in connecting the bacterial cells as well as lipids.[2]

Maturation

As bacteria multiply and replicate, they form small microbial colonies and a three-dimensional matrix leading to biofilm maturation. A multicellular structural community is formed, water channels are generated whereby available nutrients can be delivered to the cellular community and extraneous products can be rejected. It also helps in protecting the organisms in the biofilm from host defense mechanisms as well as antimicrobials. Microorganisms also release autoregulators and alter gene expression thereby stimulate production of virulence factors thereby enhancing their own survival.[15]

Dispersal

This is the final stage where planktonic organisms get released from the biofilm surface causing metastatic infection at distant sites or regional biofilm establishment. The steps include detachment of bacterial cells from small colonies, transfer of bacterial cells to other substrates, and attachment to new substrates.[16] The process of dispersal could be active or passive. Active behavior refers to seeding dispersion when biofilms adapt to nutrient deprivation, matrix degrading enzymes, or antimicrobials. Passive behavior refers to dispersion triggered by external forces such as shear leading to shedding or erosion. Changes in factors such as temperature, pH, nutritional inadequacy, or oxygen can also contribute to dispersal.[17]

UNIQUE CHARACTERISTICS OF BIOFILMS

Biofilms form a stable environment with excellent homeostatic mechanisms whereby they protect the microorganisms from the effects of blood pH, osmotic pressure and nutrient deficiencies as well as prevent the entry of antimicrobial agents and host immune cells.

They create a unique communication system by which the bacteria can communicate and coexist with each other even in adverse situations. This is known as quorum sensing (QS), which comprises chemical signals through which they sense bacterial population density as well as regulate biofilm formation and maturation as well as antimicrobial resistance and bacterial-host interactions.[18] In addition, some signaling molecules such as cyclic-di-guanosine monophosphate (GMP) present in microorganisms modulate several aspects of biofilm process including cell cycle, cell movement, pili formation, stress response, and bacterial virulence. Cells use c-di-GMP as a checkpoint to proceed across stages of biofilm development until they fully commit to the biofilm lifestyle, although they have the choice to revert at any time.[19] Biofilms also have a variety of immune escape mechanisms such as mechanical protection, altered gene expression, impaired immune recognition as well as functional impairment of immune cells.[20]

MECHANISMS OF RESISTANCE IN BIOFILMS

Biofilm-associated infections are difficult to treat with antimicrobials due to innate and acquired mechanisms of resistance, physiological gradients, and matrix diffusion limit all of which make treatment challenging. The main mechanisms are as follows:

Delayed Penetration of Antimicrobials

Transport of nutrients and antimicrobials are hampered as they must diffuse through the EPS matrix. This could be due to physical difficulty in diffusion or inactivation of the antimicrobials by enzymes within the polymeric matrix.[21]

Altered Cellular Growth Rate

The growth rate of biofilm-associated microorganisms (sessile cells) is significantly lower as compared to their planktonic counterparts, thereby diminishing the uptake of antimicrobial agents. This phenomenon can be amplified by phenotypic variants called "persister cells" who display tolerance to antimicrobial agents owing to them being in a dormant state.[22] However, once planktonic microorganisms are dispersed from the biofilm, they may regain the susceptibility to antimicrobial agents thereby making targeted dispersal a potential adjuvant strategy while treating biofilm associated infections.[23]

Other Mechanisms

Certain other mechanisms include increased expression of gene-coded efflux pumps, acquisition of genetic changes such as gene transfer and mutations. Plasmid conjugation has been shown to be 700-fold more efficient in biofilms as compared with free-floating organisms increasing resistance risk. Finally, the altered microenvironment within the biofilm including nutrient and oxygen deficiency can compromise the efficacy of antimicrobials.[22,24]

BIOFILM-ASSOCIATED INFECTIONS

Biofilms can cause device-related and nondevice-related infections. Almost 65% of all bacterial infections are reportedly caused by biofilms which are highly recalcitrant and associated with morbidity and mortality.[25] With the advancement of medical science, there is an increasing utilization of medical devices for acute and chronic medical ailments. Among patients with indwelling intravenous catheters in the intensive care unit, catheter-related bloodstream infections (CRBSI) can occur in 5 per 1,000 catheter days. Biofilms on endotracheal tubes can lead to ventilator associated pneumonia which may occur in up to 9–27% of ventilated patients.[26] The rates of urinary catheter-related infections are even higher as 50% of the catheters get colonized within 10–14 days post insertion.[27] Apart from these, 0.5–2% of patients with orthopedic implants may develop infections within 2 years postoperatively.[28] Practically, all kinds of devices implanted are susceptible to develop biofilms and infections therefrom. A majority of nondevice related infections which are difficult to treat and become chronic and resistant could also be related to biofilms which are depicted in **Figure 2**.

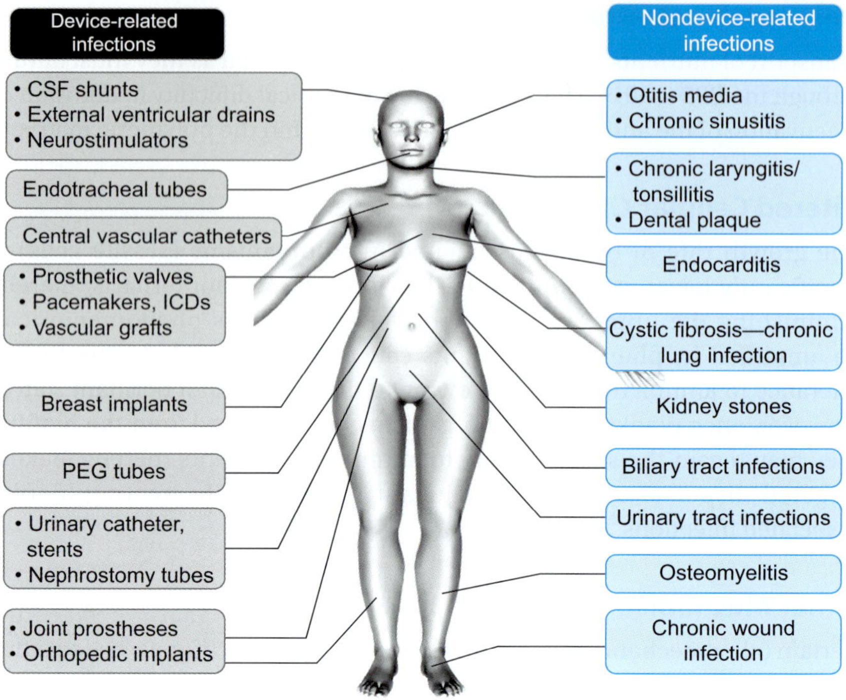

Fig. 2: Biofilm-related infection sites and devices. (CSF: cerebrospinal fluid; ICDs: implantable cardioverter defibrillators; PEG: percutaneous endoscopic gastrostomy)

CHALLENGES IN DIAGNOSIS

The diagnosis of biofilms is challenging as standard diagnostic modalities may be insufficient and there is no established protocol. The search for biofilms in conventional clinical specimens may not be representative of the focus of infection and yield false positive results.

As per the ESCMID guidelines (2015), certain clinical and laboratory features indicative of biofilm-related infections have been put forward **(Box 1)**.[29]

SAMPLING AND PROCESSING MICROBIOLOGICAL SAMPLES IN DETECTING BIOFILM INFECTIONS

Most device-related infections are associated with biofilms on the surface of devices. However, appropriate sampling might be difficult. At times, the device may need to be removed but, cultures may still be negative as the biofilm may have organisms which are slow growing which are "viable but not culturable (VBNC)" which renders it undetectable on standard culture media.[30] Sonication might improve the culture yield in large prosthetic infections and when combined with nucleic acid amplification can enhance

BOX 1: Clinical and laboratory features indicative of biofilm-related infections.

Clinical features and history:
- *Signs of infection* such as fever (usually low grade), rubor, dolor, tumor and loss of function
- *History of predisposing condition*—medical device implanted, cystic fibrosis, etc.
- *Persistent infection* >7 days
- *Failure of antibiotic treatment* and infection *recurrence* (especially if the same pathogen is identified on multiple occasions)
- Documented history/evidence of antibiotic failure
- Systemic *signs and symptoms of infection* which *resolve but recur* after cessation of antibiotic therapy

Microbiological diagnostics:
- *Microscopic evidence from fluid or tissue samples from infection site*:
  - Microscopic presence of microbial aggregates/biofilm structure from fluid or smear, preferably tissue
  - Microbial aggregates colocalized with inflammatory cells
  - Microbiological evidence of microbial aggregates of infectious etiology
- *Positive culture/nonculture-based techniques (PCR) from fluid/tissue samples*:
  - Culture-based identification of pathogens (MALDI-TOF)
  - Presence of mucoid colonies or small colony variants of *P. aeruginosa* in culture–positive samples
  - PCR, quantitative or multiplex PCR positive for pathogen associated with infection (*Staphylococcus aureus* in implant and *Pseudomonas aeruginosa* in cystic fibrosis)
  - Fluorescence in situ hybridization (FISH) for known pathogen showing aggregates of microorganisms
  - Nonculture-based identification of microbial pathogen (pyrosequencing, next generation sequencing)

(MALDI-TOF: matrix-assisted laser desorption/ionization time-of-flight; PCR: polymerase chain reaction)

the sensitivity for infection diagnosis.[31,32] Molecular diagnostic techniques may identify bacteria in culture-negative cases or additional organisms which may help in pathogen identification from tissues in infections such as culture-negative infective endocarditis or arthroplasty failure.[33] Advanced methods such as scanning electron microscopy or confocal laser scanning microscopy can detect biofilms from resected samples but are more for research purposes and not available for clinical use at present.[34]

Table 1 shows the diagnostic sampling and interpretation of common device-related biofilm infections.

PREVENTION OF BIOFILM-RELATED INFECTIONS

The basic tenet of infection prevention is to avoid microbial contamination of implanted devices which is the first step in biofilm formation. This can be achieved by adhering to strict asepsis and guidelines during device insertion,

TABLE 1: The diagnostic sampling and interpretation of common device-related biofilm infections.[26,35-41]

Type of infection	*Samples to be sent*	*Method of processing*	*Inference*
Vascular catheters/ Implantable venous ports	• If catheter removed, 3–4 cm of the distal tip to be sent for semiquantitative or quantitative cultures • If catheter in situ, simultaneous paired blood cultures from catheter and peripheral blood for qualitative and quantitative cultures • In case of implantable vascular access port, the port and reservoir to be sent	• *Semiquantitative*: Catheter tip is rolled on an agar plate (Maki method) • *Quantitative*: Tip is sonicated in 1 mL solution (Brun–Buisson method) • For port infections—catheter tip, port sonication fluid, and culture from internal surface	• *Semiquantitative:* Differential time to positivity—growth >2 hours earlier in blood drawn from CVC • *Quantitative*: Colony counts threefold greater in blood drawn from CVC than periphery
Endotracheal tube (ETT) biofilm (VAP)	• Lower respiratory secretions from endotracheal aspirate, bronchoalveolar lavage, or protected specimen brush as per situation • Mucus shaver—a device to remove the biofilm from inside the ETT to identify the etiology of VAP	• Matching pathogens have been discovered from biofilms and ETT samples in 56–70% of patients with VAP • Mucus and biofilm from the ETT as well as the inner surface of the ETT can be microscopically examined for biofilm	• Appropriately, collected lower respiratory samples are sufficient to diagnose VAP in addition to clinical and radiological features • Demonstration of biofilm not mandatory for VAP diagnosis
Urinary catheters or ureteral stents	• Urine sample from the catheter for culture • Removed catheters may be subjected to microscopy or culture-independent techniques to depict biofilm	• Urinary samples from catheter sent for culture might be false negative in 50–64% cases in case of biofilms • Examination of removed catheter or stents may reveal biofilm	• Negative cultures do not rule out a biofilm-related urinary tract infection • Routine examination of removed catheter or stents are not recommended

Contd...

Contd...

Type of infection	*Samples to be sent*	*Method of processing*	*Inference*
Orthopedic devices and implants	• Synovial fluid for cell counts and microbiological work up • If infection confirmed and surgery indicated, biopsies from peri-implant tissues and device/prosthesis or modular parts of it (3–6 biopsies recommended)	• The foreign material should be subjected to sonication before culture • Crushing or tissue homogenization in case of foreign body	• Biopsies should be paired with culture specimens to differentiate contamination from infection • At least 2 specimens culture positive with same organism confirms periprosthetic infection
Tissue fillers, breast implants	Removed material and contiguous tissue	Like other prosthesis	

(CVC: Central venous catheter; VAP: ventilator-associated pneumonia)

appropriate perioperative prophylaxis in case of surgical implants and daily assessment of the need of the indwelling device.

Current approaches include:

- Modification of surface (coating/elution)
- Physical, mechanical, electrical, and biological

Topical Antimicrobials or Surface Coating

- *Patients with central venous catheter (CVC):* Chlorhexidine impregnated sponges can cost effectively reduce CRBSI incidence.[42] Antiseptic/antibiotic impregnated catheters should be considered if the incidence of CRBSI remains high despite adherence to standard measures. Minocycline-rifampin-coated catheters are better than chlorhexidine-silver sulphadiazine-coated catheters in reducing CRBSI and should be considered if the catheter is likely to be in situ for >8 days.[43,44]
    - *Preventive antibiotic lock technique (ALT):* Small volume of a concentrated antimicrobial allowed to dwell inside lumen for 12–24 hours. It is recommended in patients who get repeated CRBSI despite standard precautions. Minocycline-ethylenediaminetetraacetic acid (EDTA), mix of taurolidine/citrate/heparin, or ethanol locks have been found to be effective. For prevention of fungal infections, the most effective antifungal lock therapy (ALT) includes amphotericin B, ethanol, or echinocandins.[45-48]

- *Endotracheal tube (ETT) biofilm and ventilator-associated pneumonia (VAP):* Surface coating of ETT with silver can hinder biofilm formation and has been shown to reduce incidence of VAP and mortality with maximal effect in first 10 days and is recommended if the patient is at a risk and is likely to be ventilated for more than a week.[29,49,50] The "Mucus shaver" is a device with an inflatable balloon with two or more silicon rings which keeps the ETT lumen free of mucus and mechanically removes the biofilm. It has been shown to reduce biofilm formation and incidence of VAP.[51]
- *Indwelling urinary catheters:* Coating with antimicrobials can postpone but not prevent biofilm-related infections.[52,53]
- *Orthopedic alloplastics/implants:* Antibiotic impregnated materials particularly gentamicin, tobramycin, and vancomycin are effective in reducing prosthesis-associated biofilm infections.[54,55]

Hygiene and Sterilization

Proper sterilization protocol of medical devices and cleaning and disinfection plays a major role.

Vaccination and Immunotherapies

Targeting biofilms through vaccines is under evaluation and conjugate vaccines targeting *S. aureus, P. aeruginosa* and certain other organisms are under evaluation. Better molecular identification of biofilm-associated genes holds a promise for vaccine development in future.[56,57]

Recent advances in surface technologies have ushered in novel methods to prevent biofilms. Materials such as electropolished stainless steel and zirconium oxide reduce bacterial adhesion and an engineered micropattern on central venous devices (Sharklet pattern) may reduce microbial colonization and biofilm formation. In addition, surface modification with antifouling polyurethane and hydrogels reduce bacterial colonization.[58,59]

TREATMENT

Biofilm-related infections may need prolonged treatment ranging from few weeks to lifelong and might resurface when antibiotics are stopped. The EPS in biofilms keeps getting dynamically modified rendering it impervious to many antibiotics. Although difficult to treat, these infections can be treated with the correct dosing of appropriate agents in conjunction with adjuvant therapies, topical agents, and sometimes device removal.

Conventional Therapies

- *Patients with CVCs:* In CRBSI, systemic antimicrobials should always be combined with ALT. In case of CRBSI caused by *S. aureus*, the catheter should always be removed to prevent hematogenous complications, endocarditis and treatment failure.[60] Similarly in case of *Candida species*, nonremoval of catheter prolongs candidemia and increases mortality.[61]

The ALT may be used in uncomplicated CRBSI due to coagulase negative *staphylococci, Enterobacteriaceae,* and *P. aeruginosa* but if catheter retention is chosen, close monitoring of clinical status and cultures is needed to detect treatment failure which mandates catheter removal.[62]

- *Patients with ETT and VAP:* Systemic antibiotics as per culture reports can treat VAP but does not help in clearing biofilms. Duration of treatment depends on the clinical response which can range from 7 days in most patients up to 14–21 days in case of *Methicillin-resistant S. aureus (MRSA)* or *P. aeruginosa*. Treatment may need to be modified in case of lack of appropriate response in 48–72 hours.[26]
- *Patients with indwelling catheters or ureteral stents:* Use of appropriate renally excreted antibiotics combined with change of catheter or stent is recommended. The duration is 7 days for rapid responders in case of catheter-associated UTI and 10–14 days for patients who are slow responders.[63]
- *Patients with orthopedic implants/joint prostheses:* In case of therapeutic difficulties, implant removal serves as definitive therapy but may not be desirable or feasible and associated with increased cost and complications. There is a critical time dependent success rate for implant retention—3 weeks from onset of symptoms (hematogenous infections) or 4 weeks (perioperative). If implant is stable, no sinus tract present and microorganisms are susceptible to biofilm-validated antibiotics, debridement, implant retention, and prolonged antibiotics can have a success rate of 85%. In case of chronic infections (>3 weeks symptoms or 4 weeks perioperative), implant removal and thorough debridement is recommended.[64] In case of two-stage exchange, antibiotic containing spacer is used in the intervening period. Duration of antibiotic therapy is 6–12 weeks with biofilm-validated antibiotics such as rifampin against staphylococci or quinolones against gram negatives.[65] Combination therapy using glycopeptides or linezolid with rifampin is recommended to prevent rifampin resistance. Newer molecules such as dalbavancin and oritavancin are effective against staphylococcal and enterococcal biofilms.[66,67]

RECENT ADVANCES

Deeper understanding of the biofilm structure and biology and its complexities have brought forward novel antibiofilm strategies directed against each stage of biofilm formation until dispersal. Most of these are under investigation but some hold promise in combating biofilm-related infections in years to come.

Biofilm disrupting agents—EPS degrading enzymes such as deoxyribonuclease1 (DNAase1) and Dispersin B (DspB) may enhance the activity of antimicrobials by improving penetration. They can act as adjuvants and are being investigated as biomedical coatings on devices. These enzymes act on the matrix proteins and degrade eDNA thereby reducing the stability and rigidity of the biofilm.[68,69]

Physical Disruption

- *Ultrasound-assisted therapy:* Low-frequency ultrasound in combination of antibiotics increases the penetration across the biofilm known as a bioacoustic effect. Studies have shown the efficacy of these noninvasive techniques to improve antibiotic efficacy and thereby have an antibiofilm effect in treating device-associated infections.[70,71]
- *Electrical and electromagnetic methods:* The stress caused by electric and electromagnetic field can break down membranes and are under investigation in combination with antibiotics or host immunity against biofilms called a bioelectric effect. They have been tested in animal studies and need further investigation.[70,72]
- *Photodynamic therapy:* Reactive oxygen species are produced when light absorbing compounds react with light and oxygen. This technique has been used to eradicate bacterial cells in vitro and in vivo using yttrium aluminum garnet (YAG), potassium yttrium tungstate (KYW), femtosecond, and near-infrared lasers against biofilms. Although effective, they need further investigation regarding their cytotoxicity.[73-75]

Emerging Therapies

- *Phage therapy:* Bacteriophages are viruses which propagate in the bacterial host and can kill the host or produce antibiofilm substances. Experimental and clinical studies have shown an effect of phage therapy which depolarizes the EPS and leads to biofilm disruption. Limitations include resistance by mature biofilms, clearance by host immune system, ineffectiveness against certain strains, and rapid development of phage resistant subpopulations.[76,77]
- *Nanoparticles:* They are an exciting novel method of targeting biofilms through their own antibacterial activity as well as strong antibiofilm potential. They can also act as carriers for targeted delivery of antimicrobial and antibiofilm agents. Antimicrobial catheters, implants, and wound dressings using silver nanoparticles are available but there is still need for further studies to establish their therapeutic applications.[78,79]
- *Quorum sensing inhibitors (QSIs):* The use of QS systems play a major role in driving the virulence and biofilm formation and can serve as a novel

target for antibiofilm strategies. QS requires the binding of a signaling molecule to a corresponding transcriptional regulator to activate a downstream transcription of selected targets. This signaling of QS can be disrupted by a process called "quorum quenching" by modifying, mimicking, or degrading signaling molecules by molecules called QSIs. Several molecules including plant extracts, oils, and traditional medicinal plants have been evaluated as QSIs but need further evaluation including toxicity.[80-82]

- *Gener-editing techniques:* Gene-editing tools such as short palindromic repeats CRISPR-associated (CRISPR Cas) systems can make the biofilm pathogens less virulent through genetic alterations. These techniques are being studied in isolation or combination with phage or conjugative delivery to inhibit or eliminate biofilms in vivo and may emerge as options in future.[83-85]

CONCLUSION

- Treatment of biofilm-related infections on medical devices are challenging due to their unique mechanism of tolerance to standard antimicrobial agents.
- The sessile biofilm organisms remaining in their "viable but non-culturable" state renders diagnostic difficulties. Hence, appropriate sampling, sonication techniques, and use of molecular diagnostics can improve pathogen identification and microbial diversity.
- Standard therapeutics include high-dose antibiotics with a potential for biofilm penetration for a prolonged duration and device removal if necessary.
- Inhibition of initial microbial attachment using surface-coating and eluting and biofilm removal using physical/chemical/biological/ mechanical and electrical methods has been the focus of emerging antibiofilm strategies and research.
- Novel therapies such as EPS degrading enzymes, Phage therapy, nanoparticles, QSIs, and Gene editing are likely to improve upon the current armamentarium in overcoming current treatment hurdles in the years to come.

REFERENCES

1. Percival SL, Suleman L, Vuotto C, Donelli G. Healthcare-associated infections, medical devices and biofilms: risk, tolerance and control. J Med Microbiol. 2015;64(Pt 4):323–334.
2. Flemming HC, Wingender J, Szewzyk U, Steinberg P, Rice SA, Kjelleberg S. Biofilms: an emergent form of bacterial life. Nat Rev Microbiol. 2016;14(9):563-75.
3. Wi YM, Patel R. Understanding Biofilms and Novel Approaches to the Diagnosis, Prevention, and Treatment of Medical Device-Associated Infections. Infect Dis Clin North Am. 2018;32(4):915-29.

4. Khoury AE, Lam K, Ellis B, Costerton JW. Prevention and control of bacterial infections associated with medical devices. ASAIO J. 1992;38(3):M174-8.
5. Høiby N. A personal history of research on microbial biofilms and biofilm infections. Pathog Dis. 2014;70(3):205-11.
6. Høiby N, Bjarnsholt T, Givskov M, Molin S, Ciofu O. Antibiotic resistance of bacterial biofilms. Int J Antimicrob Agents. 2010;35(4):322-32.
7. Hall-Stoodley L, Stoodley P, Kathju S, Høiby N, Moser C, Costerton JW, et al. Towards diagnostic guidelines for biofilm-associated infections. FEMS Immunol Med Microbiol. 2012;65(2):127-45.
8. Bjarnsholt T, Ciofu O, Molin S, Givskov M, Høiby N. Applying insights from biofilm biology to drug development - can a new approach be developed? Nat Rev Drug Discov. 2013;12(10):791-808.
9. Palmer J, Flint S, Brooks J. Bacterial cell attachment, the beginning of a biofilm. J Ind Microbiol Biotechnol. 2007;34(9):577-88.
10. Yu P, Wang C, Zhou J, Jiang L, Xue J, Li W. (2016). Influence of surface properties on adhesion forces and attachment of streptococcus mutans to zirconia in vitro. BioMed Res Int. 2016;2016:8901253.
11. Rochford ET, Richards RG, Moriarty TF. Influence of material on the development of device-associated infections. Clin Microbiol Infect. 2012;18(12):1162-7.
12. Tuson HH, Weibel DB. Bacteria-surface interactions. Soft Matter. 2013;9(18):4368-80.
13. Heilmann C, Hussain M, Peters G, Götz F. Evidence for autolysin-mediated primary attachment of Staphylococcus epidermidis to a polystyrene surface. Mol Microbiol. 1997;24(5):1013-24.
14. Costa OYA, Raaijmakers JM, Kuramae EE. Microbial Extracellular Polymeric Substances: Ecological Function and Impact on Soil Aggregation. Front Microbiol. 2018;9:1636.
15. Mangwani N, Dash HR, Chauhan A, Das S. Bacterial quorum sensing: functional features and potential applications in biotechnology. J Mol Microbiol Biotechnol. 2012;22(4):215-27.
16. Shen D, Langenheder S, Jürgens K. Dispersal Modifies the Diversity and Composition of Active Bacterial Communities in Response to a Salinity Disturbance. Front Microbiol. 2018;9:2188.
17. Lee K, Yoon SS. *Pseudomonas aeruginosa* Biofilm, a Programmed Bacterial Life for Fitness. J Microbiol Biotechnol. 2017;27(6):1053-64.
18. Whiteley M, Diggle SP, Greenberg EP. Progress in and promise of bacterial quorum sensing research. Nature. 2017;551(7680):313-20.
19. Loera-Muro A, Guerrero-Barrera A, Tremblay DNY, Hathroubi S, Angulo C. Bacterial biofilm-derived antigens: a new strategy for vaccine development against infectious diseases. Expert Rev Vaccines. 2021;20(4):385-96.
20. Campoccia D, Mirzaei R, Montanaro L, Arciola CR. Hijacking of immune defences by biofilms: a multifront strategy. Biofouling. 2019;35(10):1055-74.
21. Donlan RM. Role of biofilms in antimicrobial resistance. ASAIO J. 2000; 46(6):S47-52.
22. Conlon BP, Rowe SE, Lewis K. Persister cells in biofilm associated infections. Adv Exp Med Biol. 2015;831:1-9.
23. Thuptimdang P, Limpiyakorn T, McEvoy J, Prüß BM, Khan E. Effect of silver nanoparticles on Pseudomonas putida biofilms at different stages of maturity. J Hazard Mater. 2015;290:127-33.

24. Hausner M, Wuertz S. High rates of conjugation in bacterial biofilms as determined by quantitative in situ analysis. Appl Environ Microbiol. 1999; 65(8):3710-3.
25. Fleming D, Rumbaugh KP. Approaches to Dispersing Medical Biofilms. Microorganisms. 2017;5(2):15.
26. American Thoracic Society; Infectious Diseases Society of America. Guidelines for the management of adults with hospital-acquired, ventilator-associated, and healthcare-associated pneumonia. Am J Respir Crit Care Med. 2005; 171(4):388-416.
27. Stickler DJ. Bacterial biofilms in patients with indwelling urinary catheters. Nat Clin Pract Urol. 2008;5(11):598-608.
28. Cataldo MA, Petrosillo N, Cipriani M, Cauda R, Tacconelli E. Prosthetic joint infection: recent developments in diagnosis and management. J Infect. 2010;61(6):443-8.
29. Høiby N, Bjarnsholt T, Moser C, Bassi GL, Coenye T, Donelli G, et al. ESCMID Study Group for Biofilms and Consulting External Expert Werner Zimmerli. ESCMID guideline for the diagnosis and treatment of biofilm infections 2014. Clin Microbiol Infect. 2015;21 Suppl 1:S1-25.
30. Li L, Mendis N, Trigui H, Oliver JD, Faucher SP. The importance of the viable but non-culturable state in human bacterial pathogens. Front Microbiol. 2014;5:258.
31. Trampuz A, Piper KE, Jacobson MJ, Hanssen AD, Unni KK, Osmon DR, et al. Sonication of removed hip and knee prostheses for diagnosis of infection. N Engl J Med. 2007;357(7):654-63.
32. Bereza PL, Ekiel A, Auguściak-Duma A, Aptekorz M, Wilk I, Kusz DJ, et al. Identification of silent prosthetic joint infection: preliminary report of a prospective controlled study. Int Orthop. 2013;37(10):2037-43.
33. Liesman RM, Pritt BS, Maleszewski JJ, Patel R. Laboratory Diagnosis of Infective Endocarditis. J Clin Microbiol. 2017;55(9):2599-608.
34. Stoodley P, Nistico L, Johnson S, Lasko LA, Baratz M, Gahlot V, et al. Direct demonstration of viable Staphylococcus aureus biofilms in an infected total joint arthroplasty. A case report. J Bone Joint Surg Am. 2008;90(8):1751-8.
35. Brun-Buisson C, Abrouk F, Legrand P, Huet Y, Larabi S, Rapin M. Diagnosis of central venous catheter-related sepsis. Critical level of quantitative tip cultures. Arch Intern Med. 1987;147(5):873-7.
36. Maki DG, Weise CE, Sarafin HW. A semiquantitative culture method for identifying intravenous-catheter-related infection. N Engl J Med. 1977;296(23):1305-9.
37. Longuet P, Douard MC, Arlet G, Molina JM, Benoit C, Leport C. Venous access port—related bacteremia in patients with acquired immunodeficiency syndrome or cancer: the reservoir as a diagnostic and therapeutic tool. Clin Infect Dis. 2001;32(12):1776-83.
38. Raad I, Hanna HA, Alakech B, Chatzinikolaou I, Johnson MM, Tarrand J. Differential time to positivity: a useful method for diagnosing catheter-related bloodstream infections. Ann Intern Med. 2004;140(1):18-25.
39. Mietto C, Foley K, Salerno L, Oleksak J, Pinciroli R, Goverman J, et al. Removal of endotracheal tube obstruction with a secretion clearance device. Respir Care. 2014;59(9):e122-6.
40. Holá V, Ruzicka F, Horka M. Microbial diversity in biofilm infections of the urinary tract with the use of sonication techniques. FEMS Immunol Med Microbiol. 2010;59(3):525-8.

41. Xu Y, Moser C, Al-Soud WA, Sørensen S, Høiby N, Nielsen PH, et al. Culture-dependent and independent investigations of microbial diversity on urinary catheters. J Clin Microbiol. 2012;50:3901- 8.
42. Loveday HP, Wilson JA, Pratt RJ, Golsorkhi M, Tingle A, Bak A, et al. UK Department of Health. epic3: national evidence-based guidelines for preventing healthcare-associated infections in NHS hospitals in England. J Hosp Infect. 2014;86 Suppl 1:S1-70.
43. Darouiche RO, Raad II, Heard SO, Thornby JI, Wenker OC, Gabrielli A, et al. A comparison of two antimicrobial-impregnated central venous catheters. Catheter Study Group. N Engl J Med. 1999;340(1):1-8.
44. Marciante KD, Veenstra DL, Lipsky BA, Saint S. Which antimicrobial impregnated central venous catheter should we use? Modeling the costs and outcomes of antimicrobial catheter use. Am J Infect Control. 2003;31(1):1-8.
45. Campos RP, do Nascimento MM, Chula DC, Riella MC. Minocycline-EDTA lock solution prevents catheter-related bacteremia in hemodialysis. J Am Soc Nephrol. 2011;22(10):1939-45.
46. Betjes MG, van Agteren M. Prevention of dialysis catheter-related sepsis with a citrate-taurolidine-containing lock solution. Nephrol Dial Transplant. 2004;19(6):1546-51.
47. Slobbe L, Doorduijn JK, Lugtenburg PJ, El Barzouhi A, Boersma E, van Leeuwen WB, et al. Prevention of catheter-related bacteremia with a daily ethanol lock in patients with tunnelled catheters: a randomized, placebo-controlled trial. PLoS One. 2010;5(5):e10840.
48. Walraven CJ, Lee SA. Antifungal lock therapy. Antimicrob Agents Chemother. 2013;57(1):1-8.
49. Berra L, Kolobow T, Laquerriere P, Pitts B, Bramati S, Pohlmann J, et al. Internally coated endotracheal tubes with silver sulfadiazine in polyurethane to prevent bacterial colonization: a clinical trial. Intensive Care Med. 2008;34(6):1030-7.
50. Afessa B, Shorr AF, Anzueto AR, Craven DE, Schinner R, Kollef MH. Association between a silver-coated endotracheal tube and reduced mortality in patients with ventilator-associated pneumonia. Chest. 2010;137(5):1015-21.
51. Berra L, Coppadoro A, Bittner EA, Kolobow T, Laquerriere P, Pohlmann JR, et al. A clinical assessment of the Mucus Shaver: a device to keep the endotracheal tube free from secretions. Crit Care Med. 2012;40(1):119-24.
52. Lai KK, Fontecchio SA. Use of silver-hydrogel urinary catheters on the incidence of catheter-associated urinary tract infections in hospitalized patients. Am J Infect Control. 2002;30(4):221-5.
53. Srinivasan A, Karchmer T, Richards A, Song X, Perl TM. A prospective trial of a novel, silicone-based, silver-coated foley catheter for the prevention of nosocomial urinary tract infections. Infect Control Hosp Epidemiol. 2006;27(1):38-43.
54. Parvizi J, Saleh KJ, Ragland PS, Pour AE, Mont MA. Efficacy of antibiotic-impregnated cement in total hip replacement. Acta Orthop. 2008;79(3):335-41.
55. Marschall J, Lane MA, Beekmann SE, Polgreen PM, Babcock HM. Current management of prosthetic joint infections in adults: results of an Emerging Infections Network survey. Int J Antimicrob Agents. 2013;41(3):272-7.
56. Freire MO, Devaraj A, Young A, Navarro JB, Downey JS, Chen C, et al. A bacterial-biofilm-induced oral osteolytic infection can be successfully treated by

immuno-targeting an extracellular nucleoid-associated protein. Mol Oral Microbiol. 2017;32(1):74-88.
57. Estellés A, Woischnig AK, Liu K, Stephenson R, Lomongsod E, Nguyen D, et al. A High-Affinity Native Human Antibody Disrupts Biofilm from Staphylococcus aureus Bacteria and Potentiates Antibiotic Efficacy in a Mouse Implant Infection Model. Antimicrob Agents Chemother. 2016;60(4):2292-301.
58. Lebeaux D, Ghigo JM, Beloin C. Biofilm-related infections: bridging the gap between clinical management and fundamental aspects of recalcitrance toward antibiotics. Microbiol Mol Biol Rev. 2014;78(3):510-43.
59. May RM, Magin CM, Mann EE, Drinker MC, Fraser JC, Siedlecki CA, et al. An engineered micropattern to reduce bacterial colonization, platelet adhesion and fibrin sheath formation for improved biocompatibility of central venous catheters. Clin Transl Med. 2015;4:9.
60. Fowler VG Jr, Justice A, Moore C, Benjamin DK Jr, Woods CW, Campbell S, et al. Risk factors for hematogenous complications of intravascular catheter-associated *Staphylococcus aureus* bacteremia. Clin Infect Dis. 2005;40(5): 695-703.
61. Andes DR, Safdar N, Baddley JW, Playford G, Reboli AC, Rex JH, et al; Mycoses Study Group. Impact of treatment strategy on outcomes in patients with candidemia and other forms of invasive candidiasis: a patient-level quantitative review of randomized trials. Clin Infect Dis. 2012;54(8):1110-22.
62. Funalleras G, Fernández-Hidalgo N, Borrego A, Almirante B, Planes AM, Rodríguez D, et al. Effectiveness of antibiotic-lock therapy for long-term catheter-related bacteremia due to Gram-negative bacilli: a prospective observational study. Clin Infect Dis. 2011;53(9):e129-32.
63. Hooton TM, Bradley SF, Cardenas DD, Colgan R, Geerlings SE, Rice JC, et al.; Infectious Diseases Society of America. Diagnosis, prevention, and treatment of catheter-associated urinary tract infection in adults: 2009 International Clinical Practice Guidelines from the Infectious Diseases Society of America. Clin Infect Dis. 2010;50(5):625-63.
64. Osmon DR, Berbari EF, Berendt AR, Lew D, Zimmerli W, Steckelberg JM, et al; Infectious Diseases Society of America. Diagnosis and management of prosthetic joint infection: clinical practice guidelines by the Infectious Diseases Society of America. Clin Infect Dis. 2013;56(1):e1-e25.
65. Penterman J, Nguyen D, Anderson E, Staudinger BJ, Greenberg EP, Lam JS, et al. Rapid evolution of culture-impaired bacteria during adaptation to biofilm growth. Cell Rep. 2014;6(2):293-300.
66. Fernández J, Greenwood-Quaintance KE, Patel R. In vitro activity of dalbavancin against biofilms of staphylococci isolated from prosthetic joint infections. Diagn Microbiol Infect Dis. 2016;85(4):449-51.
67. Yan Q, Karau MJ, Patel R. In vitro activity of oritavancin against biofilms of staphylococci isolated from prosthetic joint infection. Diagn Microbiol Infect Dis. 2018;92(2):155-7.
68. Okshevsky M, Regina VR, Meyer RL. Extracellular DNA as a target for biofilm control. Curr Opin Biotechnol. 2015;33:73-80.
69. Darouiche RO, Mansouri MD, Gawande PV, Madhyastha S. Antimicrobial and antibiofilm efficacy of triclosan and DispersinB combination. J Antimicrob Chemother. 2009;64(1):88-93.

70. Freebairn D, Linton D, Harkin-Jones E, Jones DS, Gilmore BF, Gorman SP. Electrical methods of controlling bacterial adhesion and biofilm on device surfaces. Expert Rev Med Devices. 2013;10(1):85-103.
71. Cai Y, Wang J, Liu X, Wang R, Xia L. A Review of the Combination Therapy of Low Frequency Ultrasound with Antibiotics. Biomed Res Int. 2017;2017:2317846.
72. Bordi C, de Bentzmann S. Hacking into bacterial biofilms: a new therapeutic challenge. *Ann. Intensive Care.* 2011;1:19.
73. Eick S, Meier I, Spoerlé F, Bender P, Aoki A, Izumi Y, et al. In Vitro-Activity of Er:YAG Laser in Comparison with other Treatment Modalities on Biofilm Ablation from Implant and Tooth Surfaces. PLoS One. 2017;12(1):e0171086.
74. Schnell G, Staehlke S, Duenow U, Nebe JB, Seitz H. Femtosecond Laser Nano/Micro Textured Ti6Al4V Surfaces-Effect on Wetting and MG-63 Cell Adhesion. Materials (Basel). 2019;12(13):2210.
75. Damestani Y, De Howitt N, Halaney DL, Garay JE, Aguilar G. Evaluation of laser bacterial anti-fouling of transparent nanocrystalline yttria-stabilized-zirconia cranial implant. Lasers Surg Med. 2016;48(8):782-9.
76. Furfaro LL, Payne MS, Chang BJ. Bacteriophage Therapy: Clinical Trials and Regulatory Hurdles. Front Cell Infect Microbiol. 2018;8:376.
77. Fu W, Forster T, Mayer O, Curtin JJ, Lehman SM, Donlan RM. Bacteriophage cocktail for the prevention of biofilm formation by Pseudomonas aeruginosa on catheters in an in vitro model system. Antimicrob Agents Chemother. 2010;54(1):397-404.
78. Gallo J, Panacek A, Prucek R, Kriegova E, Hradilova S, Hobza M, et al. Silver Nanocoating Technology in the Prevention of Prosthetic Joint Infection. Materials (Basel). 2016;9(5):337.
79. Schütz CA, Juillerat-Jeanneret L, Mueller H, Lynch I, Riediker M; NanoImpactNet Consortium. Therapeutic nanoparticles in clinics and under clinical evaluation. Nanomedicine (Lond). 2013;8(3):449-67.
80. Bjarnsholt T, Givskov M. Quorum sensing inhibitory drugs as next generation antimicrobials: worth the effort? Curr Infect Dis Rep. 2008;10(1):22-8.
81. Koo H, Allan RN, Howlin RP, Stoodley P, Hall-Stoodley L. Targeting microbial biofilms: current and prospective therapeutic strategies. Nat Rev Microbiol. 2017;15(12):740-55.
82. Brackman G, Cos P, Maes L, Nelis HJ, Coenye T. Quorum sensing inhibitors increase the susceptibility of bacterial biofilms to antibiotics in vitro and in vivo. Antimicrob Agents Chemother. 2011;55(6):2655-61.
83. Gholizadeh P, Aghazadeh M, Asgharzadeh M, Kafil HS. Suppressing the CRISPR/Cas adaptive immune system in bacterial infections. Eur J Clin Microbiol Infect Dis. 2017;36(11):2043-51.
84. Zuberi A, Misba L, Khan AU. CRISPR Interference (CRISPRi) Inhibition of luxS Gene Expression in *E. coli*: An Approach to Inhibit Biofilm. Front Cell Infect Microbiol. 2017;7:214.
85. Garrido V, Piñero-Lambea C, Rodriguez-Arce I, Paetzold B, Ferrar T, Weber M, et al. Engineering a genome-reduced bacterium to eliminate *Staphylococcus aureus* biofilms in vivo. Mol Syst Biol. 2021;17(10):e10145.

4

SECTION

Multidrug-resistant Organisms and Antibiotic Stewardship

Section Editor: *Nishant Kumar*

14

CHAPTER Multidrug-resistant Organisms

Suresh Ramasubbaman, Dipanjan Hojai

LEARNING OBJECTIVES

- Understand the growing prevalence of infections caused by multidrug-resistant organisms (MDROs).
- Comprehend the ways in which organisms develop resistance mechanisms.
- Understand management of infections with MDROs.
- Discuss the role of isolation and cohorting to prevent the spread of infections due to MDROs.

INTRODUCTION

Antimicrobials are medicines used to treat infectious diseases caused by bacteria, viruses, fungi, and parasites. Resistance to antimicrobials emerged very soon after the discovery and therapeutic use of antimicrobials. Since the discovery of penicillin, numerous classes of antibiotics have been discovered; however, microbes have kept up with the progress in the pharmaceutical industry, and resistance has also grown across classes of antibiotics. Resistance is not only something restricted to bacteria, but viruses, parasites, and fungi all have the propensity to develop resistance. Antimicrobial resistance (AMR) refers to this situation wherein bacteria, viruses, fungi, and parasites do not respond to treatment with antimicrobials. AMR is almost a natural phenomenon as microbes slowly develop genetic changes to the new challenge in their environment. Adaptation is the key to survival, and the fittest organism passes its genes to its progeny. And microorganisms follow this Darwinian principle to the hilt. The culmination of the process of acquiring resistance by microbes is to be pan-drug resistant (PDR). Multidrug-resistance (MDR) is an important intermediary in this evolution. There has been a sustained increase in the prevalence of multidrug-resistance organisms (MDRO) over the last two decades, and this problem is compounded by the parching of the new antibiotic manufacturing pipeline. This problem of growing resistance and dearth of new drugs to combat resistance has raised alarms in various quarters. The World Health Organization (WHO) has flagged this as the top public health and development issue in the world. WHO estimates that in the year 2019, bacterial AMR directly resulted in 1.27 million deaths and had an indirect contribution in 4.95 million deaths.[1] The increase in AMR is not only the genetic ability of microbes but is largely driven by human and societal issues. Overuse and misuse of antimicrobials in animals and humans are one of the biggest drivers of this epidemic. The mortality consequence is easily observable by practicing intensivists, but the financial burden is generally not easily appreciated. The World Bank estimates that by 2050, AMR would lead to an increase of 1 trillion $ in health care costs, and there will be a loss of 3.4 trillion $ in Gross Domestic Product per year by 2030.[2] Critical care medicine, where sepsis, infections, and use of antimicrobials are highly prevalent, is itself at the verge of annihilation due to the specter of AMR. All the good that science has achieved in health care will be undone if the spiral of AMR continues to gallop.

DEFINITIONS

There are a lot of terms in the literature, like MDR, extremely drug-resistant (XDR), and PDR, in the context of AMR. Multidrug-resistance, as the name implies, means resistance to more than one antimicrobial agent. Standardized definitions have been in place since 2011 following a consensus meeting of the Centers for Disease Control and Prevention of the USA and Europe.[3] The method advocated is based on in vitro antimicrobial susceptibility testing. The definition used for gram-positive and gram-negative bacteria is "resistant to more than or equal to one agent in three or more antimicrobial classes." The term XDR originated from the tubercular resistance nomenclatures, wherein XDR TB is defined as resistance to first-line medicines such as isoniazid and rifampicin, to fluoroquinolones, and to at least one of the three second-line medications. A similar approach is used in bacteria and is defined as "resistant to more than or equal to one agent in all but two or fewer categories." PDR implies that an organism is resistant to all the antimicrobials. The categories of antibiotic classes tested differ for various organisms; a few examples are shown in **Tables 1 to 3**. The more commonly used method to define MDR is, however, based on "resistance to one key antimicrobial agent." A common example is Methicillin-resistant *Staphylococcus aureus* (MRSA). With MRSA, resistance to one agent, i.e., methicillin, implies public health importance and cross- or coresistance to other classes of antimicrobial agents.

EPIDEMIOLOGY OF ANTIMICROBIAL RESISTANCE

Resistance to antimicrobials is increasing in a prolific fashion. Gram-negative bacteria lead this brigade of resistant pathogens. However, resistance is widespread across the microbial world. Gram-positive bacteria are not far behind *Staphylococcus* and *Enterococcus,* being the prime culprits. Other microorganisms concerned are *Mycobacterium tuberculosis,* parasites, such as *Plasmodium* species, and fungi. In this review, we will restrict ourselves to the epidemiology, management, and infection control of MDR bacteria and *Candida*.

TABLE 1: To define MDR, XDR, and PDR for *Staphylococcus aureus* isolates.

Antimicrobial class	*Antimicrobial drugs*	*Antimicrobial susceptibility result*
Ansamycins	Rifampicin	
Aminoglycosides	Gentamicin	
Antistaphylococcal β-lactam	Oxacillin or cefoxitin*	
Anti-MRSA cephalosporins	Ceftaroline	
Folate pathway inhibitors	Trimethoprim–sulfamethoxazole	
Fucoidanes	Fusidic acid	
Fluoroquinolones	Moxifloxacin, ofloxacin	
Glycylcyclines	Tigecycline	
Glycopeptides	Teicoplanin, vancomycin	
Lipopeptides	Daptomycin	
Lincosamides	Clindamycin	
Macrolides	Azithromycin	
Oxazolidinones	Linezolid	
Phosphonic acid	Fosfomycin	
Tetracyclines	Doxycycline, minocycline	
Streptogramins	Quinupristin–dalfopristin	

Note: Criteria for defining:

- *MDR*: (1) An MRSA is considered MDR and (2) Non susceptible to more than or equal to one drug in more than or equal to three antimicrobial classes.
- *XDR*: Nonsusceptible to more than one drug in all but less than or equal to two antimicrobial classes.
- *PDR*: Nonsusceptible to all the antimicrobial classes listed.

*Oxacillin resistance predicts resistance to all other β-lactams with the exception of anti-MRSA cephalosporins, which include all categories of penicillins, cephalosporins, β-lactamase inhibitors, and carbapenems.

(MDR: multidrug-resistant; MRSA: methicillin-resistant *Staphylococcus aureus*; PDR: pandrug-resistant; XDR: extensively drug-resistant)

Drug Resistance in Bacteria

Epidemiology of MDR bacteria is obtained from the WHO global antimicrobial resistance and use surveillance system (GLASS) report of 2022.[4] MDR *Escherichia coli,* i.e., extended spectrum β-lactamase (ESBL) production rates are as high as 41.8% and ESBL *K. pneumoniae* rates range from 59 to 64.7% and carbapenem resistance in *Acinetobacter* species (CRAB) ranges from 69 to 73.4%. Data regarding the epidemiology of MDRO in India is obtained from the annual report of the National Antimicrobial Surveillance Network

TABLE 2: To define MDR, XDR, and PDR for Enterobacteriaceae isolates.

Antimicrobial class	*Antimicrobial drugs*	*Antimicrobial susceptibility result*	*Intrinsic resistance to antimicrobials*
Aminoglycosides	• Gentamycin • Tobramycin • Netilmicin • Amikacin		*Providencia rettgeri, Providencia stuarti* *P. rettgeri, P. stuarti,* *P. rettgeri, P. stuarti*
Antipseudomonal penicillins + β-lactamase inhibitors	• Ticarcillin-clavulanic acid • Piperacillin-tazobactam		*Escherichia hermannii* *E. hermannii*
Anti-MRSA cephalosporin	• Ceftaroline		
Carbapenem	• Meropenem • Imipenem • Ertapenem • Doripenem		
First and second generation cephalosporins	• Cefazolin • Cefuroxime		*Morganella morganii, Proteus penneri, Proteus Vulgaris, P. rettgeri, P. stuarti, Serratia marcescens, Citrobacter freundii, Enterobacter aerogenes, and Enterobacter cloacae* *M. morganii, P. penneri, P. vulgaris, S. marcescens*
Third and fourth generation cephalosporins	• Cefotaxime or ceftriaxone • Ceftazidime and cefepime		
Cephamycins	• Cefoxitin		*C. freundi, E. aerogenes, E. cloacae, H. alvei*
Folate pathway inhibitors	• Trimethoprim–sulfamethoxazole		
Fluoroquinolones	• Ofloxacin		
Glycylcyclines	• Tigecyclines		*Proteus mirabilis, M. morganii, P. penneri, P. vulgaris, P. rettgeri, P. stuarti*
Monobactams	• Aztreonam		
Phenicols	• Chloramphenicol		
Phosphonic acid	• Fosfomycin		

Contd...

Contd...

Antimicrobial class	*Antimicrobial drugs*	*Antimicrobial susceptibility result*	*Intrinsic resistance to antimicrobials*
Penicillins	• Ampicillin		*C.freundii, E. aerogenes, E. cloacae, M. morgani, klebsiellae spp, P. vulgaris, P. penneri, P. rettgeri, P. stuarti*
Penicillins + β-lactamase inhibitor	• Amoxicillin clavulanic acid • Ampicillin-sulbactam		*C. freundii, E. aerogenes, E. cloacae, M. morgani, P. vulgaris, P. penneri, P. rettgeri, P. stuarti*
Polymyxins	Colistin		
Tetracyclines	• Tetracycline • Doxycycline/ Minocycline		*M. morganii, P. mirabilis, P. penneri, P. vulgaris, P. rettgeri, P. stuarti* *M. morganii, P. penneri, P. vulgaris, P. rettgeri, P. stuarti*

Note: Criteria for defining:

- *MDR*: Nonsusceptible to more than or equal to one drug in more than or equal to three antimicrobial classes.
- *XDR*: Nonsusceptibility to more than or equal to one drug in all but less than or equal to two antimicrobial classes.
- *PDR*: Nonsusceptible to all antimicrobial drugs listed.

(MDR: multidrug-resistant; MRSA: methicillin-resistant *Staphylococcus aureus*; PDR: pandrug-resistant; XDR: extensively drug-resistant)

(NARS-Net), a part of the government of India's National Programme on AMR containment.[5] The last published report is from 2023, which includes data up to December 2022. The NARS-Net has identified seven pathogens, which pose a significant risk for AMR, and they include *S. aureus, Enterococcus species, E. coli, Klebsiella* species, *Pseudomonas species, Acinetobacter species, and Salmonella enterica* serotype *Typhi* and *Paratyphi*. The report noted consistency with previous years as *E. coli* remains the most commonly isolated pathogen (33% of all pathogens), the most common source being urine (43%). Most of the priority pathogens are isolated from in-patient wards (56%), with the remaining from the out-patient sites. ESBL *E. coli* rates have decreased from 86% in 2018 to 76% in the year 2022. This decreased trend in ESBL rates in *E. coli* may be attributed to more stringent microbiologic criteria and better-quality control on antibiotic discs for testing. The rates of carbapenem-resistant *Enterobacterales* (CRE) are static, and about 35% of

TABLE 3: To define MDR, PDR, and XDR for *Acinetobacter* spp. Isolates.

Antimicrobial class	*Antimicrobial drug*	*Antimicrobial susceptibility result*
Antipseudomonal carbapenem	• Imipenem • Meropenem • Doripenem	
Antipseudomonal fluoroquinolones	• Ciprofloxacin • Levofloxacin	
Antipseudomonal penicillin + β-lactamase inhibitors	• Piperacillin–tazobactam • Ticarcillin–clavulanic acid	
Aminoglycosides	• Amikacin • Gentamicin • Tobramycin • Netilmicin	
Extended-spectrum cephalosporin	• Ceftriaxone • Ceftazidime • Cefotaxime • Cefepime	
Folate pathway inhibitors	• Trimethoprim–sulfamethoxazole	
Polymixins	• Colistin • Polymyxin B	
Tetracyclines	• Tetracycline • Minocycline • Doxycycline	
Penicillins + β-lactamase inhibitors	Ampicillin–sulbactam	

Note: Criteria for defining:
- *MDR:* Nonsusceptibility to more than or equal to 1 drug in more than or equal to 3 antimicrobial class.
- *XDR:* Nonsusceptibility to more than or equal to 1 drug in all but less than or equal to 2 antimicrobial class.
- *PDR:* Nonsusceptible to all antimicrobial drug listed.

(MDR: multidrug-resistant; PDR: pandrug-resistant; XDR: extensively drug-resistant)

E. coli and 47% of *Klebsiella* species are CRE. Amongst the nonfermenting gram-negative bacilli, *Pseudomonas* had MDR rates of 50% and carbapenem resistance of 27%, while amongst *Acinetobacter*, carbapenem resistance was 65–69%. *Staphylococcus* species were predominantly seen in pus cultures, and MRSA rates of 59% and vancomycin-resistant *Enterococcus* rates were at 13%. Unfortunately, these resistance rates were reported by government hospitals, mostly medical colleges providing tertiary care. If private hospitals were to be involved, the rates would be far more than those reported in this data. This data is still reflective of the burden of MDRO in India.

Drug Resistance in *Candida*

Antifungal resistance in *Candida* is the non-susceptibility to an antifungal agent based on in vitro susceptibility testing, when comparing with isolates of the same *Candida* species. Resistance in *Candida* is intrinsic or acquired. Many *Candida* species are intrinsically resistant to antifungal agents. There has been an uptick in the prevalence of invasive *Candida* infections across the world, and now *Candida* is the fourth most common cause of bloodstream infections (BSI), especially in the ICU.[6] There has been a steady shift in the species of *Candida* causing invasive infections over the last two decades, and non-albicans *Candida* species are the predominant pathogens in many ICUs.[7] Fungal susceptibility testing across *Candida* species in the US revealed a rate of 7% fluconazole resistance.[8] In India, MDR rates in *Candida* species are 1.9%. A significant proportion of the non-albicans *Candida* have reduced susceptibility to antifungal drugs and are MDR. There is now a plethora of MDR *Candida* species, including *Candida glabrata, Candida guilliermondii, Candida krusei, Candida lusitaniae,* and the most prominent amongst these being *Candida auris*. *Candida auris* was initially misidentified as *Candida haemulonii* species, but was identified as a separate species from 2015 onward. It has become a notifiable disease because of its MDR nature, and worldwide, there is an increasing number of infections due to *Candida auris*. *Candida auris* is a critical priority organism as per the WHO.[9] One of the main reasons for this is the almost 100% resistance to fluconazole and 43% resistance to polyene antifungals, making it very difficult to treat MDRO.

MECHANISM OF RESISTANCE

Antimicrobial resistance can be either intrinsic resistance or acquired resistance. Intrinsic resistance is the ability of bacteria to deny the activity of an antimicrobial agent via its inherent functional and structural properties, which will allow resistance to that antimicrobial class of drug. It can be due to drug inaccessibility into the cell wall, presence of gene-encoded active export channels or pumps, production of antimicrobial-degrading enzymes, and lack of affinity for the target site. For example, aerobic bacteria have innate resistance to metronidazole due to the inability of the drug to reduce to its active form in aerobic conditions.[10]

Acquired resistance happens when a particular organism acquires the ability to resist the activity of a particular antimicrobial agent to which it was previously susceptible to. This may happen from gene mutation and transfer across species via vertical or horizontal gene transfer by transformation, transduction, or conjugation.[11]

There are various ways by which gram-negative bacteria become resistant to antibiotics[12] **(Fig. 1)**. They include the following mechanisms:

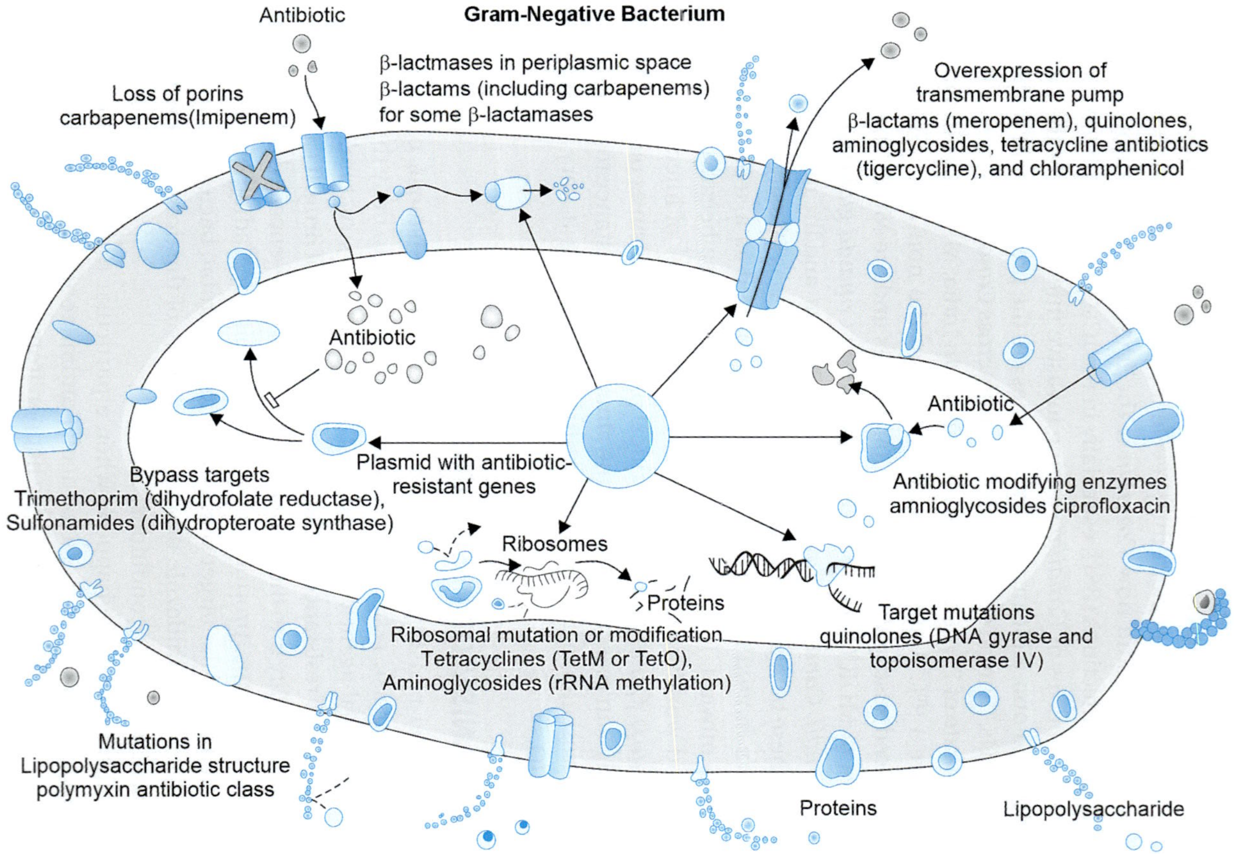

Fig. 1: Gram-negative bacteria. (DNA: deoxyribonucleic acid)

- *Loss of porin channels:* Gram-negative bacilli have an outer cell membrane, which confers protection and a barrier to penetration of antibiotics to target the penicillin-binding proteins (PBPs) in the peptidoglycan layers. As a result, the antibiotic molecules need to pass through the hydrophilic porin channels situated in the outer membrane of the bacterial cell wall to reach the inner cell membrane. Mutations that result in decreased amounts of porin channels confer resistance to antibiotics like carbapenems.
- *β-lactamases:* The presence of enzymes like β-lactamases in the periplasmic space results in degradation of β lactam antibiotics and prevents them from exerting their action on the PBPs in the inner cell membrane. These enzymes are classified based on their structure into four molecular classes (A to D), may be classified based on their substrate, and lastly based on their response to inhibitors **(Flowchart 1)**. This is the major defense mechanism of gram-negative organisms against β-lactam antibiotics. These enzymes have evolved alongside the development of β-lactam antibiotics. Ever since the discovery of penicillin, there has been an increase in the prevalence of β-lactamases in organisms that naturally possess these enzymes, like *S. aureus*. Subsequently, these enzymes spread to organisms that did not naturally possess these enzymes, such as *Hemophilus influenzae* and *Neisseria gonorrhoeae,* to become broad-spectrum β-lactamases. Introduction of a multitude of cephalosporins about 30 years ago resulted in an explosion of β-lactamases, such as extended-spectrum β-lactamases (ESBL) and carbapenem-hydrolyzing β-lactamases (carbapenemase) **(Table 4)**.
- *Efflux pump overexpression:* Overexpression of the transmembrane efflux pump in bacteria can result in expulsion of the drug from the bacterium

Flowchart 1: Classification of β-lactamases.

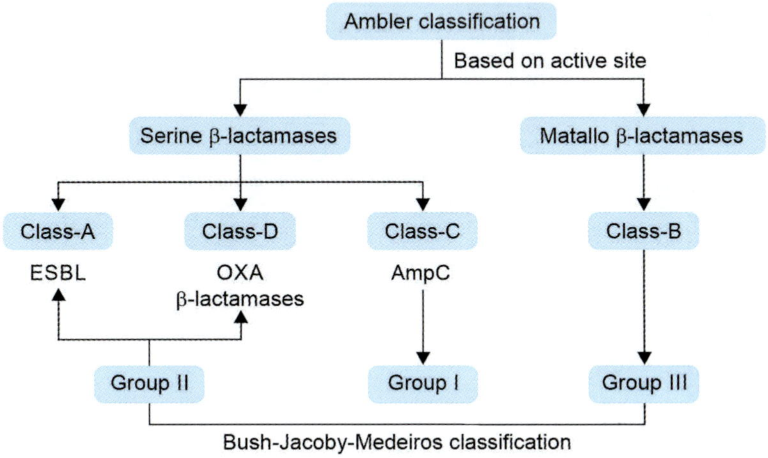

TABLE 4: Description of selected β-lactamases of gram-negative bacteria.

β-lactamases	*Examples*	*Substrates*	*Inhibition by clavulanic acid*	*Molecular class*
Broad spectrum	TEM-1, TEM-2, SHV-1	• Benzylpenicillin, aminopenicillins, carboxypenicillins, piperacillin, narrow-spectrum cephalosporins, such as cefuroxime, cefazolin, and other	+++	A
	OXA family	• Substrates of the broad-spectrum group, plus cloxacillin, methicillin, and oxacillin	+	D
Expanded spectrum	TEM family and SHV family	• Substrates of the broad-spectrum group PLU oxyimino cephalosporins (ceftazidime, cefpodoxime, cefotaxime, and ceftriaxone) and monobactams (aztreonam)	++++	A
	Others(BES-1, GES/IBC family, PER-1, PER-2, SFO-1, TLA-1, VEB-1 and VEB-2)	• Same as for the TEM family and the SHV family	++++	A
	CTX-M family	• Substrates of the expanded spectrum group, plus, for some enzymes, cefepime	++++	A
	OXA family	• Same as for the CTX-M family	+	D
Amp c	ACC-1, ACT-1, CFE-1, CMY family,DHA-1, DHA-2, FOX family, LAT family, MIR-1, MOX-1, and MOX-2	Substrates of expanded-spectrum group plus cephamycins (cefotetan, cefoxitin, and others)	0	C
Carbapenemase	IMP family, VIM family, GIM-1, and SPM-1	• Substrates of the expanded-spectrum group plus cephamycins and carbapenems	0	B
	KPC-1, KPC-2, and KPC-3	• Same as for IMP family, VIM family, GIM-1, and SPM-1	+++	A
	OXA-23,OXA-24, OXA-25, OXA-26, OXA-27, OXA-40, and OXA-48	• Same as for IMP family, VIM family, GIM-1, and SPM-1	+	D

Note: Table above showing the type of β-lactamases produced by the gram-negative bacteria with examples and the substrates it acts on, along with the degree of inhibition by β-lactamase inhibitor such as clavulanic acid, with a plus(+) sign denoting the relative sensitivity to inhibition.

before it can have an effect. This is an important mechanism for resistance against carbapenems, quinolones, aminoglycosides, tetracyclines, and chloramphenicol.

- *Antibiotic-modifying enzymes:* Certain gram-negative organisms possess enzymes in the cytoplasm that can modify the antibiotics, making them incapable of interacting with their target. This mechanism is important to prevent the actions of aminoglycosides and quinolones.
- *Target site mutations:* Mutations in certain targets, like deoxyribonucleic acid (DNA) gyrase and topoisomerase intravenous (IV) in certain gram-negative bacteria, can lead to resistance to quinolone antibiotics.
- *Ribosomal mutations:* Antibiotics that act on ribosomes, like aminoglycosides and tetracyclines, are affected by mutations or modifications of the ribosomes, leading to the antibiotic not being able to bind to the ribosome and inhibiting protein synthesis.
- *Metabolic bypass mechanisms:* Certain gram-negative bacteria develop an alternative resistant enzyme to bypass the inhibitory effect of antibiotics like trimethoprim and sulfonamides.
- *Lipopolysaccharide mutation:* A mutation in the lipopolysaccharide structure in certain gram-negative organisms results in resistance to the polymyxin class of antibiotics.

Mechanism of Resistance in Gram-positive Organisms

National Antimicrobial Resistance Surveillance Network (NARS-Net): NARS-Net has identified two gram-positive pathogens, which pose a significant risk for AMR, and they include *S. aureus* and *Enterococcus* species and the discussion of the mechanism of resistance will be restricted to these two gram-positive organisms.

Staphylococcus aureus: Ever since the introduction of penicillin, *S. aureus* has been quick to develop resistance and has been the quintessential smart organism that develops resistance to any introduced antibiotic. Resistance to penicillin is due to β-lactamase production. Resistance to methicillin, which epitomizes MDR status, is due to production of PBP2a, a homologue of PBP, which is resistant to β-lactams.[13] Vancomycin resistance in *S. aureus* (VRSA) is due to the acquisition of the vanA operon from *enterococci*, which allows *S. aureus* to alter the structure of peptidoglycan precursors, leading to reduced affinity to vancomycin.

Enterococcus species: Enterococcus species are intrinsically resistant to β-lactams because their PBP has low affinity for β-lactams. Vancomycin-resistant *enterococci* (VRE) are the MDR of concern, and the mechanism of resistance is the same as that of VRSA, i.e., possession of vanA operons.

Mechanism of Antifungal Resistance

Like bacteria, some species of *Candida* are intrinsically resistant to certain antifungals. This is due to the ineffective binding to drug targets and/or efflux activities in all members of a given species. For instance, *C. krusei* and *C. auris* are intrinsically resistant to fluconazole; similarly, environmental molds are resistant to fluconazole. The problem, however, is acquired resistance, i.e., the ability of the fungal cells to grow at a higher concentration of antifungal drugs as compared to the fungal cells of the wild type of population. Another characteristic observed in fungal cells, like bacteria, is tolerance, also called heteroresistance. This is the ability of a susceptible isolate to grow slowly in the presence of drug concentrations above the minimum inhibitory concentrations (MICs). Acquired resistance results in changes in the interaction between the drug and the target[14] **(Fig. 2)**. This may arise due to:

- Genetic changes to the binding site of the antifungal agent. For example, mutation of the genes encoding the synthesis of lanosterol demethylase results in azole resistance, and mutation of genes encoding for β-glucan synthase results in echinocandin resistance.
- *Increased abundance of target:* Overexpression of ERG11 can lead to azole resistance to *C. albicans*, by increasing target abundance, which would require more drug to be available for effectiveness.
- Altering the effective drug concentration acts by increasing drug efflux pumps, leading to decreased intracellular concentration of drugs like azoles or inhibition of prodrugs like flucytosine.

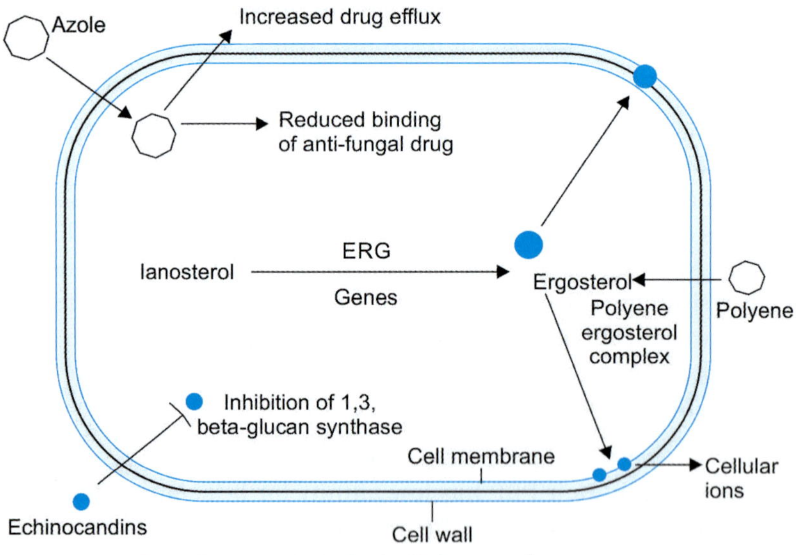

Fig. 2: Resistance results in changes in the interaction between the drug and the target.

MANAGEMENT OF INFECTIONS WITH MULTIDRUG-RESISTANT ORGANISMS

The management of infections caused by MDR gram-negative infections is based on the recommendations of the European Society of Clinical Microbiology and Infectious Diseases (ESCMID) and European Society of Intensive Care Medicine (ESICM).[15]

- *Infections caused by third-generation resistant Enterobacterales (ESBL):* In patients with BSI and sepsis/septic shock, the MERINO trial has clearly demonstrated the superiority of meropenem as compared to piperacillin–tazobactam and is the drug of choice.[16] In patients with low-risk infections (this Classification into low-risk and high-risk infections is based on the INCREMENT score), that is originating from a urinary tract source or biliary infections after source control, use of piperacillin–tazobactam, amoxicillin–clavulanic acid, or quinolones can be used with close monitoring. For a nonsevere complicated urinary tract infection, which is in the absence of sepsis or septic shock, cotrimoxazole can also be considered. In case of complicated UTI without septic shock, use of a short-duration course of aminoglycosides or IV fosfomycin may be useful. In the management of infections caused by third-generation resistant *enterobacterales*, it is considered good practice to step down therapy to a targeted drug following the use of carbapenem and patient stabilization.
- *Carbapenem-resistant enterobacterales (CRE): The recommendation for treatment of severe CRE infections is the use of meropenem-vabor*bactam or ceftazidime-avibactam; this may not be useful in critical care practice in countries like India, where there is a high prevalence of metallo-β-lactamase (MBL) producing organisms. In such situations, a combination of ceftazidime-avibactam with aztreonam or treatment with cefiderocol may be considered. For the treatment of non-severe CRE infections, use of an antibiotic from among the in vitro active drugs on a case-by-case basis is a good practice. In case of complicated UTI, aminoglycosides, including plazomicin, are preferred. Tigecycline should be avoided in cases of complicated UTI and bloodstream infection. In patients with pneumonia, tigecycline can be used at high doses. The practice of using a combination of polymyxins, tigecycline, aminoglycosides, or fosfomycin in combination is recommended in the absence of new beta-lactamase inhibitor (BLBLI) agents. Monotherapy with these agents can be used in nonsevere and low-risk carbapenem-resistant Enterobacterales (CRE) infections based on in vitro susceptibility and source of infection.
- *Carbapenem-resistant Pseudomonas aeruginosa (CRPA):* In severe infections due to CRPA, ceftolozane–tazobactam is recommended if active in vitro. If this agent is not available, then a combination of polymyxins,

aminoglycosides, or fosfomycin can be used. While in non-severe, low-risk infections, monotherapy with these agents can be considered.

- *Carbapenem-resistant Acinetobacter baumanii (CRAB):* In patients with CRAB infections susceptible to sulbactam, using high-dose sulbactam is preferred. If strains are not susceptible to sulbactam, then polymyxin or high-dose tigecycline can be used if there is in vitro susceptibility. For severe and high-risk infections with CRAB, A combination of two in vitro active antibiotics among the following drugs, i.e., polymyxin, aminoglycoside, tigecycline, and sulbactam, is preferred.
- *MRSA:* The initial treatment recommended for management of MRSA BSI consists of monotherapy with glycopeptides, such as vancomycin and teicoplanin. Daptomycin is an alternative for the treatment of BSI with MRSA. Other alternative agents include ceftaroline, ceftobiprole, telavancin, linezolid, tedizolid, dalbavancin, and oritavancin.
- *VRE:* The preferred treatment of enterococcal infections with resistance to vancomycin (VRE) includes daptomycin and linezolid. In the setting of BSI with VRE and possible endocarditis, daptomycin is the preferred agent.
- *Fluconazole-resistant Candida:* The initial therapy in critically ill patients with BSI with *Candida species* is with echinocandins as per the recommendation of the Infectious Disease Society of America guidelines (IDSA).[17] However, treatment depends on the species identified and in vitro susceptibility. In patients with infections due to *Candida auris*, initial treatment is with echinocandins, but if there is no response or there is persistent candidemia, then a switch to the lipid formulation of amphotericin B is suggested.

PREVENTION AND CONTROL OF INFECTIONS WITH MULTIDRUG-RESISTANT ORGANISMS

Multidrug-resistant organisms control can be discussed under the following six headings:[18]

1. *Improve hand hygiene compliance:* MDR organisms are transmitted through direct or indirect contact from health care workers, environmental surfaces, as well as medical equipment. WHO, in its 2009 guidelines on improving hand hygiene, promulgated the "five moments of hand hygiene." Despite the obvious importance of hand hygiene, results from the 2019 WHO "hand hygiene self-assessment" global survey showed a poor implementation of hand hygiene practices. Focusing on education and training, improving the infrastructure to promote hand hygiene, having reminder tools, providing feedback on hand hygiene techniques, and conducting audits are the mainstay to improve compliance. Newer technologies like the automated hand hygiene monitoring systems are

in place in certain countries and have shown substantial improvement in hand hygiene compliance. Such innovations need to be brought in to control the menace of MDRO.

2. *Environmental cleanliness:* It is well known that CRAB, CRE, MRSA, and VRE can persist in the environment for extended periods of time. To prevent their spread having thorough surface cleaning and equipment are essential. Regular surface cleaning followed by disinfection is the standard care practice as advocated by CDC.[19] Low-level disinfectants like quaternary ammonium compounds and intermediate-level disinfectants, either alcohol based or chlorine-based based are suggested based on the nature of the surface and equipment. Recent research is pointing towards using hydrogen peroxide devices (intermediate level disinfectants) and the use of ultraviolet light for disinfecting patient rooms, a process known as automated whole room disinfection (WRD).
3. *Contact isolation:* CDC also advocates contact isolation for all patients infected or colonized with MDRO. These precautions entail a single room, donning isolation gowns and gloves before encountering the patient or his surroundings, and doffing personal protective equipment before exiting the isolation room. Implementing such guidelines in open plan ICUs is a challenge, and most of the ICUs in India are open plan, making contact isolation methods non-compliant with guidelines.
4. *Decolonization:* Decolonization involves treating colonized patients to eliminate their carriage. This is well documented for treating MRSA carriage in hospitalized patients. Chlorhexidine bathing and nasal mupirocin have been used for eliminating the carriage of MRSA. However, no data exists for eliminating the problem of MDRO that plagues our country.
5. *Cluster intervention:* Clustering or bundling means doing a set of evidence-based interventions together to improve outcomes. Bundling hand hygiene practices and disinfection of the hospital environment is an example of clustering.
6. *Early screening for pathogens:* Early detection of pathogenic microorganisms can lead to appropriate antibiotic use and thereby result in decreasing the emergence of MDRO infections. Pneumonia diagnosis with polymerase chain reaction (PCR) testing, as compared to conventional cultures, shortens the duration of inappropriate antimicrobial use; whether this will lead to a reduction in the emergence of MDRO is uncertain as of now.

CONCLUSION

Multidrug-resistance is a growing epidemic, and prevalence is increasing leaps and bounds in both gram-positive and gram-negative organisms, parasites, mycobacterium species, and in yeasts. CRE is the main Gram-negative threat in our ICUs. Rising fluconazole-resistant *Candida species* is also an emerging threat. Production of β-lactamases is the main mechanism driving gram-negative MDR, and this may happen from gene mutation and transfer across species via vertical or horizontal gene transfer. The mechanism of drug resistance is complex and involves multiple mechanisms, which differ in various organisms. A clear understanding of the mechanism of resistance is necessary for targeting therapy with antimicrobial agents. Treatment regimens for CRE, CRAB, and MRSA are evolving, and some new molecules are being introduced. Prevention remains the cornerstone for management of MDRO, and decreasing the emergence of MDRO focuses primarily on hand hygiene and environmental sanitation.

REFERENCES

1. World Health Organization. (2025). News. [Online]. Available from https://www.who.int/news [Last accessed August, 2025].
2. World Bank Group. (2017). Drug-resistant infections: A threat to our economic future (Vol. 2): final report. [Online]. Available from http://documents.worldbank.org/curated/en/323311493396993758/final-report [Last accessed August, 2025].
3. Magiorakos A-P, Srinivasan A, Carey RB, Carmeli Y, Falagas ME, Giske CG, et al. Multidrug-resistant, extensively drug-resistant and pandrug-resistant bacteria: an international expert proposal for interim standard definitions for acquired resistance. Clin Microbiol Infect. 2012;18(3):268-81.
4. World Health Organization. (2022). Global Antimicrobial Resistance and Use Surveillance System (GLASS) report: 2022. [Online]. Available from https://www.who.int/publications/i/item/9789240062702 [Last accessed August, 2025].
5. National Centre for Disease Control. (2024). Antimicrobial Resistance (AMR) Containment. [Online] Available from https://ncdc.mohfw.gov.in/antimicrobial-resistance-amr-containment/ [Last accessed August, 2025].
6. Timsit JF, Ruppé E, Barbier F, Tabah A, Bassetti M. Bloodstream infections in critically ill patients: an expert statement. Intensive Care Med. 2020;46(2):266-84.
7. Chakrabarti A, Sood P, Rudramurthy S, Chen S, Kaur H, Capoor M, et al. Incidence, characteristics and outcome of ICU-acquired candidemia in India. Intensive Care Med. 2015;41(2):285-95.
8. Toda M, Williams SR, Berkow EL, Farley MM, Harrison LH, Bonner L, et al. Population-Based Active Surveillance for Culture-Confirmed Candidemia - Four Sites, United States, 2012-2016. MMWR Surveill Summ. 2019;68(8):1-15.
9. World Health Organization. WHO fungal priority pathogens list to guide research, development and public health action. [Online]. Available from https://www.who.int/publications/i/item/9789240060241 [Last accessed August, 2025].
10. Devi NS, Mythili R, Cherian T, Dineshkumar R, Sivaraman GK, Jayakumar R, et al. Overview of antimicrobial resistance and mechanisms: The relative status of the past and current. Microbe. 2024;3(3):100083.
11. Devi NS, Mythili R, Cherian T, Dineshkumar R, Sivaraman GK, Jayakumar R, et al. Overview of antimicrobial resistance and mechanisms: The relative status

of the past and current. The Microbe [Internet]. 2024 Jun 1;3:100083. Available from: https://www.sciencedirect.com/science/article/pii/S2950194624000505

12. Peleg AY, Hooper DC. Hospital-Acquired Infections Due to Gram-Negative Bacteria. N Engl J Med. 2010;362(19):1804-13.
13. Kakoullis L, Papachristodoulou E, Chra P, Panos G. Mechanisms of Antibiotic Resistance in Important Gram-Positive and Gram-Negative Pathogens and Novel Antibiotic Solutions. Antibiotics. 2021;10(4):415.
14. Fisher MC, Izquierdo AA, Berman J, Bicanic T, Bignell EM, Bowyer P, et al. Tackling the emerging threat of antifungal resistance to human health. Nat Rev Microbiol. 2022;20(9):557-71.
15. Paul M, Carrara E, Retamar P, Tängdén T, Bitterman R, Bonomo RA, et al. European Society of Clinical Microbiology and Infectious Diseases (ESCMID) guidelines for the treatment of infections caused by multidrug-resistant Gram-negative bacilli (endorsed by European society of intensive care medicine). Clin Microbiol Infect. 2022;28(4):521-47.
16. Harris PNA, Tambyah PA, Lye DC, Mo Y, Lee TH, Yilmaz M, et al. Effect of Piperacillin-Tazobactam vs Meropenem on 30-Day Mortality for Patients With E coli or Klebsiella pneumoniae Bloodstream Infection and Ceftriaxone Resistance. JAMA. 2018;320(10):984-94.
17. Pappas PG, Kauffman, CA, Andes DR, Clancy CJ, Marr KA, Ostrosky-Zeichner L, et al. Clinical Practice Guideline for the Management of Candidiasis: 2016 Update by the Infectious Diseases Society of America. 2016;62(4):e1-50.
18. Ji B, Ye W. Prevention and control of hospital-acquired infections with multidrug-resistant organism: A review. PubMed. 2024;103(4):e37018-8.
19. Siegel JD, Rhinehart E, Jackson M, Chiarello L; Healthcare Infection Control Practices Advisory Committee. Management of multidrug-resistant organisms in healthcare settings, 2006. Atlanta (GA): Centers for Disease Control and Prevention; 2006. Available from: https://www.cdc.gov/infection-control/hcp/mdro-management/prevention-control.html.

15 CHAPTER

Antimicrobial Stewardship in Intensive Care Unit

Swapna Khanzode

LEARNING OBJECTIVES

- Understand the burden of antibiotic resistance.
- Antibiotic resistance in intensive care unit (ICU).
- Concept of "antimicrobial stewardship (AMS)" also know as antibiotic stewardship.
- Current available guidelines on AMS.
- Strategies to implement AMS in ICU.

INTRODUCTION

The global burden of antimicrobial resistance is on the rise. The prevalence of drug-resistant bacteria has increased in hospital settings. The limited reserve of antibiotics and paucity in development of new antibiotics are adding insult to injury. Antimicrobial resistance also leads to increased length of hospital stay and increased cost of healthcare. Healthcare-associated infections (HCAIs) are infections which develop in patients while receiving treatment for any illness.[1] Patients who are inadvertently exposed to antibiotics in either hospitals, nursing homes, or other healthcare facilities are at risk of developing resistance from them.[2] HCAIs are one of the important adverse events affecting hospitalized patients.[3] As a consequence, there is an increasing incidence of antibiotic resistance among patients getting admitted to the intensive care unit (ICU). The current classification of antibiotic-resistant bacteria divides pathogens into three classes:[4] (1) Multidrug-resistant (MDR), indicating nonsusceptibility to at least one antibiotic within three or more antibiotic categories; (2) extensively drug-resistant (XDR), indicating nonsusceptibility to at least one antibiotic in all but two or fewer antibiotic categories; and (3) pandrug-resistant (PDR), indicating nonsusceptibility to all antibiotics in all antibiotic categories. The antibiotic classes are penicillin, cephalosporins, monobactams, carbapenems, aminoglycosides, fluoroquinolones, folate pathway inhibitors, glycylcyclines, phosphonic acids, polymyxins, phenicols, and tetracyclines. Correcting the inappropriate usage of antibiotics and developing a tailor-made approach for individual patients are the need of the hour.

ANTIMICROBIAL RESISTANCE IN INTENSIVE CARE UNIT

As far as ICU is concerned, the prescription of antibiotics at times becomes a mandatory part of the treatment, which is not always required. As per evidence and records, up to 50% of antibiotic prescriptions are unnecessary.[5] Hence, a watchful practice is needed in order to segregate the patients who really need antibiotics. Antibiotic resistance in ICU is a difficult situation as it is governed by multiple factors such as advanced age, immunosuppression, previous antibiotic treatment, invasive procedures, and prolonged hospitalization.[6]

One of the most crucial steps in preventing colonization and infection by MDR bacteria is to implement infection control procedures in the ICU.[7] Along with infection control, misuse of antibiotics also needs to be curtailed. The concept of "antimicrobial stewardship (AMS)" also known as antibiotic stewardship came into force due to WHO adversity. The World Health Organization (WHO) has been working on antibiotic resistance and strategies to prevent it for a decade now. AMS is directed toward developing an approach to use of the antibiotics with proper indications and justifications along with adequate duration. It is also helpful in avoiding unnecessary and misguided use of the same.

ANTIMICROBIAL STEWARDSHIP: DEFINITION AND CONCEPT

Antimicrobial stewardship is defined as the optimal selection, dosage, and duration of antimicrobial treatment that results in the best clinical outcome for the treatment or prevention of infection with low harm to the patient and minimal impact on eventual resistance.[3] The purpose is to develop a stringent discipline in the usage of antibiotics in patients.[8] John McGowan and Dale Gerding were the first to use the term antimicrobial stewardship, where they suggested a causal association between antimicrobial agent usage and resistance.[9] Stewardship in simple terms means careful and responsible management of something that is entrusted to one's care.[10] Initially, it was used only in context with antimicrobials, but now the term has expanded to the health sector as a whole. Healthcare system can remain strong based on three main aspects: (1) AMS, (2) infection prevention and control (IPC), and (3) patient and medicine safety. According to WHO guidelines, AMS helps to control antimicrobial resistance when used aptly in conjunction with antimicrobial use surveillance and the WHO essential medicine list (EML), AWaRe [three groups of antibiotics: (1) Access, (2) Watch, and (3) Reserve].[11,12] In a systematic review and meta-analysis of 52 studies with more than 1.7 million patients conducted in different healthcare and income settings, AMS programs were associated with reduced consumption of overall antibiotics as well as decreased use of antibiotics in the WHO Watch group.[13]

STRUCTURE OF ANTIMICROBIAL STEWARDSHIP PROGRAM

The Centers for Disease Control and Prevention (CDC), along with Society for Healthcare Epidemiology of America (SHEA) and others, has formulated

AMS recommendations for hospitals. The AMS program mainly comprises two components: (1) Goals and (2) core elements.

Goals of AMS include:[8]

- To work with healthcare practitioners to prescribe "five Ds" of antimicrobial therapy, which are: (1) The right Drug, (2) correct Dose, (3) right Drug route, (4) suitable Duration, and (5) timely De-escalation to pathogen-directed therapy.
- To prevent antimicrobial overuse, misuse, and abuse in inpatient, outpatient, and community settings, including the agriculture industry
- To reduce antibiotic-related adverse effects, for example, *Clostridioides difficile* infection
- To minimize resistance
- To reduce healthcare-associated costs

The core elements of AMS include:[14]

- Leadership commitment
- Accountability and responsibility
- Actions
- Tracking and surveillance
- Reporting and feedback
- Education.

Each component is important and needs to be modified depending upon the healthcare facility where AMS needs to be implemented. *Leadership commitment* forms an important step in the AMS structure. A stand-alone or multidisciplinary leadership can be implemented. Physicians with formal training in infectious disease and AMS have been found to be effective in the stewardship program. Similarly, appointing a single pharmacist leader as a coleader has shown better implementation and outcomes.[15] They can initiate policies and certain directives made for monitoring antibiotic use (AU). The leader should ensure that every team member is giving enough time and involvement for the stewardship. *Accountability* and *responsibility* are built on the basis of regular activities pertaining to AMS. *AMS action* includes proper implementation of the policies. For example, whenever any antibiotic is prescribed, specifying dose, duration, and indication should be mandatory. This kind of accountability also helps to keep a check on misguided indications and prompt and appropriate de-escalation of the antibiotics.[16] Information on local organisms and antibiogram-based susceptibility patterns should be updated regularly. Physicians can use "time-out" after 48 hours of initiation of antibiotics in order to reassess the clinical situation. This can help in revising the choice of antibiotics based on diagnostic tests and early de-escalation, if indicated.[17] The dose adjustments based on organ parameters can also be done. Unnecessary use of antibiotics based only on laboratory results needs to be avoided (e.g., asymptomatic bacteriuria).

Tracking involves keeping a track of clinical condition of the patient and surveillance of implementation of policies. *Reporting* is documenting the data for further record. Development of proper medical charts and records which can store all the patient- and treatment-related information in one place is very useful. Proper clinical and investigational criteria used for diagnosis, monitoring, and indication of antibiotics also can be recorded in the same chart. AU developed by the CDC is very helpful in doing this. It automatically records and keeps a track of the abovementioned points. The AU module is available for facilities capable of submitting electronic medication administration records.[18] Most importantly, tracking helps in knowing the potential impact that AMS policies have made on clinical outcomes of the patients. It also gives us feedback about areas which need improvement in terms of infection control and antibiotic usage. *Education and training* are an indispensable part of AMS programs. Training sessions should include modules on antibiotic resistance, importance of antibiotic stewardship, and infection control measures. Educational sessions and lectures for physicians and staff about local flora, how to read an antibiogram, and information about "reserved or protected" antibiotics should be regularly imparted. Small reminders through messages, charts, or even announcements can help in spreading the right message about AMS. Education has been found to be a very effective tool along with interventions and outcome measurements.

ANTIMICROBIAL STEWARDSHIP IMPLEMENTATION IN INTENSIVE CARE UNIT

In the ICU, the density of MDR pathogens is on the rise and hence AMS policies need to be strengthened.[14]

Salient parameters of AMS specific to ICU include:[19]

- National guidelines and local microbiology of the ICU
- Patient-centric factors, e.g., history of prolonged hospitalization, immunosuppression, and indwelling catheters
- Only fever: *Not* an indication for the use of antibiotics
- Only high C-reactive protein (CRP) and white blood cell (WBC) (without clinical symptoms): *Not* an indication for AU
- Prompt evaluation and diagnosis to avoid unnecessary use of medications
- After initiating treatment, consider pharmacology (PK/PD) of antibiotics.
- Daily monitoring of patients, clinical as well as microbiological (cultures, laboratory tests, etc.)
- Controlling the source of infection
- Appropriate timing of de-escalation of antibiotics
- Documentation of initiation, duration, and de-escalation time of antibiotics along with proper indication

Antimicrobial stewardship and its implementation has been on the forefront since 2015, with WHO taking the lead.[20] Since the emergence of drug-resistant pathogens has been alarming, national surveillance in every country needs to be done so as to know the incidence of these pathogens and morbidity and mortality due to them. According to a report published by the CDC in 2019, more than 2.8 million antibiotic-resistant infections occur each year, and the risk of *Clostridium difficile* infections is also increasing due to overuse of antibiotics.[21]

Important organisms have been classified into four groups according to the threat imposed by them **(Table 1)**.[21]

TABLE 1: Classification of life-threatening organisms.

Urgent threats	*Serious threats*	*Concerning threats*	*Watch list*
Carbapenem-resistant *Acinetobacter baumannii*	Drug-resistant *Campylobacter*	Erythromycin-resistant group A *Streptococcus*	Azole-resistant *Aspergillus fumigatus*
Candida auris	Drug-resistant *Candida*	Clindamycin-resistant group B *Streptococcus*	Drug-resistant *Mycoplasma genitalium*
Clostridioides difficile	Extended spectrum beta-lactamases (ESBL) producing *Enterobacteriaceae*		Drug-resistant *Bordetella pertussis*
Carbapenem-resistant *Enterobacteriaceae*	Vancomycin-resistant *Enterococci* (VRE)		
Drug-resistant *Neisseria gonorrhoeae*	Multidrug-resistant *Pseudomonas aeruginosa*		
	Drug-resistant nontyphoidal *Salmonella*		
	Drug-resistant *Salmonella typhi*		
	Drug-resistant *Shigella*		
	Methicillin-resistant *Staphylococcus aureus* (MRSA)		
	Drug-resistant *Streptococcus pneumoniae*		
	Drug-resistant tuberculosis		

Antimicrobial stewardship in ICU needs a wholesome approach which includes steps taken prior to treatment, during treatment, and after treatment.[19] One needs to be cautious and aware about above organisms while working in ICU. Critically ill patients are prone to infections, more so if they have associated comorbidities. Common high risks of acquiring MDR pathogens are:

- Prolonged hospital stay
- Previous ICU admission
- Immunosuppression: Chemotherapy or corticosteroid use
- Indwelling catheter (central venous catheter, urinary catheter, etc.)
- Mechanical ventilation
- Tracheotomy
- Renal replacement therapy
- Any major surgery
- Previous exposure to higher antibiotics

Careful history taking and detailed clinical examination, keeping in mind the risk factors, help in planning the management of the patient better.

Clinically, symptoms in ICU patients can be deceptive, e.g., fever in ICU patients has multiple reasons. Infection alone need not be the cause of fever in ICU and hence the cause needs to be evaluated before starting the antibiotics. Up to 52% patients can have noninfectious causes of fever in ICU.[22] Common noninfectious causes of fever include: Deep vein thrombosis or pulmonary embolism, viral infections, autoimmune disorders, heat stroke, malignancy, etc. Drug fever is also an important factor to be ruled out. A patient should be thoroughly examined for the focus or source of infection, and appropriate cultures need to be sent. Rapid diagnostic tests such as polymerase chain reaction, microarray technology, fluorescent in situ hybridization (FISH), or matrix-assisted laser desorption/ionization–time-of-flight mass spectrometry (MALDI-TOF MS) can help in faster detection of organisms.[23] Colonization with resistant microorganisms and *Candida* is very common in ICUs. Isolation of *Candida* in a urine culture usually does not require antifungal therapy.[24] Similarly, antibiotics should not be prescribed based on only culture reports without any clinical evidence. Again, it has to be paired with clinical symptoms of the patient. Stand-alone CRP and procalcitonin values have no accuracy.[25]

After the patient is initiated on antimicrobials in ICU, monitoring, especially pharmacodynamics and pharmacokinetics of the drug is essential. The AMS team including clinical pharmacist and ICU staff need to take daily rounds of the patients. Proper dose adjustments based on clinical and laboratory parameters help in prevention of adverse effects and interactions with other drugs. Therapeutic drug monitoring may be indicated in selected patients. An appropriate way of drug administration is also important (intermittent dosing vs. prolonged infusions). In a recent meta-analysis of randomized controlled trials (RCTs), prolonged infusions of antipseudomonal beta-lactams showed better outcomes than intermittent dosing in patients with sepsis.[26] Daily clinical monitoring and subsequent culture reports are helpful. Regular procalcitonin monitoring may aid in decision-making of continuation and de-escalation of antibiotics in ICU.[27] Source control is an important step in controlling infection in patients and decreasing the duration of antibiotic administration. Appropriate intervention is required. Once the focus of infection is identified, appropriate intervention should follow; including surgical procedures when indicated, such as abscess drainage, wound debridement, or insertion of intercostal drains. When organ failure persists or occurs despite resuscitation and the provision of appropriate antimicrobial therapy, the failure of source control should be taken into consideration. In such situations, reevaluation and reassessment of the patient are required including clinical, laboratory, and imaging modalities.[19]

De-escalation of the antibiotics is done based on clinical improvement and taking help from acute-phase reactants as mentioned above. Evidence suggests that short duration of antibiotics is equally effective as long duration of antibiotics. For pneumonia specifically, eight RCTs have shown that 3–5-day courses of antibiotic therapy are as effective as 7–14-day courses for community-acquired pneumonia, and two RCTs demonstrated that 8 days is as effective as 15 days for nosocomial ventilator-associated pneumonia.[28,29]

After the treatment, important points to be noted and practiced are detailed documentation of antibiotic usage, communication, and reporting of any adverse reactions. Antibiotic time-out after 48 hours of treatment with antibiotics is advisable in ICU patients with diagnostic dilemmas. Automatic early warning systems have been found to be beneficial. A detailed reevaluation of the clinical situation is done, and studies have shown to decrease unnecessary antibiotic exposure by doing so, especially in neonates.[30] The AMS team needs to have clear communication regarding escalation, continuation, and de-escalation of antibiotics along with questioning the need and effectiveness of the same. Feedback forms can be given to primary prescribers and real-time feedback can be taken on ICU rounds. This audit helps in filling the lacunae in practice and improving the quality of antibiotic prescription.

An ideal AMS team in an ICU comprises:

- Intensive care physician
- Intensive care nurse
- Infectious disease physician
- Infection control nurse
- Clinical pharmacist
- Clinical microbiologist
- Hospital epidemiologist
- Information system specialist[31]

Infection control in ICU is of prime importance, and the AMS team has to be proactive in implementing infection control strategies. This requires periodic surveillance and consistent efforts toward improving them. A successful AMS in ICU is the one that brings down antibiotic resistance. Infection control is the foundation of AMS. An active epidemiologic survey can help in identifying MDR pathogens and their sources promptly. Various AMS protocols such as tracking of antibiotic consumption, adherence to clinical guidelines, and crude mortality have shown significant improvement in antimicrobial utilization. IPC and AMS go hand in hand for better clinical outcomes and prevention of antibiotic resistance.[14]

WORLD HEALTH ORGANIZATION INITIATIVES

In 2017, the WHO expert committee on selection and use of essential medicines developed the *AWaRe* classification of antibiotics, as a step forward in antibiotic stewardship, which was further revised in 2019 **(Table 2)**.[32] The antibiotics are divided into three categories: (1) Access, (2) Watch, and (3) Reserve. This is to emphasize the importance and impact of correct AU.

TABLE 2: AWaRe classification of common antibiotics.

Access antibiotics list	*Watch antibiotics list*	*Reserve antibiotics list*
Amikacin	Azithromycin	Ceftazidime + avibactam
Amoxicillin	Cefixime	Colistin
Amoxicillin plus clavulanic acid	Cefotaxime	Fosfomycin (intravenous)
Ampicillin	Ceftazidime	Linezolid
Benzyl penicillin	Ceftriaxone	Meropenem + vaborbactam
Cephalexin	Cefuroxime	Plazomicin
Cefazolin	Ciprofloxacin	Polymyxin B
Chloramphenicol	Clarithromycin	
Clindamycin	Meropenem	
Cloxacillin	Piperacillin/tazobactam	
Doxycycline	Vancomycin	
Gentamicin		
Metronidazole		
Nitrofurantoin		
Spectinomycin		
Sulfamethoxazole + trimethoprim		

Access: This group of antibiotics includes antibiotics which are active against commonly encountered pathogens. They have low resistance potential. 60% of these drugs are oral formulations. They should be widely available and affordable.

Watch: This group of antibiotics includes drugs with high resistance potential. They need to be prioritized in AMS programs. They are the first or second choice of treatment in limited clinical conditions and need to be used with word of caution. 40% of these antibiotics are oral formulations and rest are intravenous.

Reserve: This group of antibiotics includes drugs which have to be kept reserved for treatment of infections from suspected or confirmed MDR pathogens. They are to be used in extremely selected cases where all other options have failed.

An ICU physician should be distinctly aware of all these groups while writing a prescription of antibiotics for critically ill patients.

CONCLUSION

Antibiotic resistance is an immediate threat to humans. Judicious and tailor-made use of antibiotics for patients is warranted, especially in ICU. AMS has come into picture to streamline the treatment protocols and reduce antibiotic exposure and thereby reduce antibiotic resistance. Careful evaluation of the patient before initiating antibiotics is necessary. After initiation, regular surveillance, monitoring, and appropriate de-escalation of antibiotics need to be done under supervision of the AMS team. After completion of the treatment, documentation and audit help in measuring outcomes and effectiveness of AMS. Implementation of AMS has demonstrated significant decrease in antibiotic resistance and better clinical outcomes. Adherence to protocols of AMS is the key.

REFERENCES

1. Collins AS. Preventing health care-associated infections. In: Hughes RG (Ed). Patient Safety and Quality: An Evidence-Based Handbook for Nurses. Rockville (MD): Agency for Healthcare Research and Quality (US); 2008.
2. Tamma PD, Avdic E, Li DX, Dzintars K, Cosgrove SE. Association of Adverse Events With Antibiotic Use in Hospitalized Patients. JAMA Intern Med. 2017;177(9):1308-15.
3. Gerding DN. The search for good antimicrobial stewardship. Jt Comm J Qual Improv. 2001;27(8):403-4.
4. Magiorakos AP, Srinivasan A, Carey RB, Carmeli Y, Falagas ME, Giske CG, et al. Multidrug-resistant, extensively drug-resistant and pandrug-resistant bacteria: An international expert proposal for interim standard definitions for acquired resistance. Clin. Microbiol. Infect. 2012;18(3):268-81.

5. Dellit TH, Owens RC, McGowan JE Jr, Gerding DN, Weinstein RA, Burke JP; Infectious Diseases Society of America; Society for Healthcare Epidemiology of America, et al. Infectious Diseases Society of America and the Society for Healthcare Epidemiology of America guidelines for developing an institutional program to enhance antimicrobial stewardship. Clin Infect Dis. 2007;44(2):159-77.
6. Timsit JF, Bassetti M, Cremer O, Daikos G, de Waele J, Kallil A, et al. Rationalizing antimicrobial therapy in the ICU: a narrative review. Intensive Care Med. 2019;45(2):172-89.
7. Türe Yüce Z, Alp E. Infection control bundles for the prevention of hospital infections. Mediterr J Infect Microb Antimicrob. 2016;5(5):8-8.
8. Doron S, Davidson LE. Antimicrobial stewardship. Mayo Clin Proc. 2011;86(11):1113-23.
9. McGowan JE Jr, Gerding DN. Does antibiotic restriction prevent resistance? New Horiz. 1996;4(3):370-6.
10. World Health Organization. (2017). Global framework for development and stewardship to combat antimicrobial resistance: draft roadmap. Geneva; World Health Organization. [online] Available from https://www.who.int/publications/m/item/global-framework-for-development-stewardship-to-combat-antimicrobial-resistance-draft-roadmap [Last accessed August, 2025].
11. Travis P, Egger D, Davies P, Mechbal A. (2002). Towards better stewardship: concepts and critical issues. Geneva; World Health Organization. [online] Available from https://iris.who.int/bitstream/handle/10665/339291/WHO-EIP-DP-02.48-eng.pdf?sequence=1&isAllowed=y [Last accessed August, 2025].
12. World Health Organization. (2017). WHO Model list of essential medicines, 20th List. Geneva; WHO. 2017:8-15.
13. Zay Ya K, Win PTN, Bielicki J, Lambiris M, Fink G. Association Between Antimicrobial Stewardship Programs and Antibiotic Use Globally: A Systematic Review and Meta-Analysis. JAMA Netw Open. 2023;6(2):e2253806.
14. World Health Organization. (2019). Antimicrobial stewardship programmes in health-care facilities in low- and middle-income countries: a WHO practical toolkit. [online] Available from https://www.who.int/publications/i/item/9789241515481 [Last accessed August, 2025].
15. Patel D, Lawson W, Guglielmo BJ. Antimicrobial stewardship programs: interventions and associated outcomes. Expert Rev Anti Infect Ther. 2008;6(2):209-22.
16. Braxton CC, Gerstenberger PA, Cox GG. Improving antibiotic stewardship: order set implementation to improve prophylactic antimicrobial prescribing in the outpatient surgical setting. J Ambul Care Manage. 2010;33(2):131-40.
17. Wolfe JR, Bryant AM, Khoury JA. Impact of an automated antibiotic time-out alert on the de-escalation of broad-spectrum antibiotics at a large community teaching hospital. Infect Control Hosp Epidemiol. 2019;40(11):1287-9.
18. Barlam TF, Cosgrove SE, Abbo LM, MacDougall C, Schuetz AN, Septimus EJ, et al. Implementing an Antibiotic Stewardship Program: Guidelines by the Infectious Diseases Society of America and the Society for Healthcare Epidemiology of America. Clin Infect Dis. 2016;62(10):e51-77.
19. Ture Z, Güner R, Alp E. Antimicrobial stewardship in the intensive care unit. J Intensive Med. 2022;3(3):244-53.

20. World Health Organization.. (2015) Global action plan on antimicrobial resistance. WHO Report. [online] Available from https://www.who.int/publications/i/item/9789241509763 [Last accessed August, 2025].
21. Kadri SS. Key Takeaways From the U.S. CDC's 2019 Antibiotic Resistance Threats Report for Frontline Providers. Crit Care Med. 2020;48(7):939-45.
22. Liu P, Li X, Luo M, Xu X, Su K, Chen S et al. Risk factors for carbapenem-resistant Klebsiella pneumoniae infection: a meta-analysis. Microb Drug Resist. 2018;24(2):190-8.
23. Chiotos K, Tamma PD, Gerber JS. Antibiotic stewardship in the intensive care unit: challenges and opportunities. Infect Control Hosp Epidemiol. 2019;40(6):693-8.
24. Pappas PG, Kauffman CA, Andes DR, Clancy CJ, Marr KA, Ostrosky-Zeichner L et al. Clinical practice guideline for the management of candidiasis: 2016 update by the Infectious Diseases Society of America. Clin Infect Dis. 2016;62(4):e1-50.
25. Peng F, Chang W, Xie JF, Sun Q, Qiu HB, Yang Y. Ineffectiveness of procalcitonin-guided antibiotic therapy in severely critically ill patients: a meta-analysis. Int J Infect Dis. 2019;85:158-66.
26. Hao JJ, Chen H, Zhou JX. Continuous versus intermittent infusion of vancomycin in adult patients: a systematic review and meta-analysis. Int J Antimicrob Agents. 2016;47(1):28-35.
27. Evans L, Rhodes A, Alhazzani W, Antonelli M, Coopersmith CM, French C, et al. Surviving sepsis campaign: international guidelines for management of sepsis and septic shock 2021. Intensive Care Med. 2021;47(11):1181-247.
28. Wald-Dickler N, Spellberg B. Short-course antibiotic therapy–replacing Constantine units with "shorter is better". Clin Infect Dis. 2019;69(9):1476-9.
29. Spellberg B, Rice LB. Duration of Antibiotic Therapy: Shorter Is Better. Ann Intern Med. 2019;171(3):210-1.
30. Tolia VN, Desai S, Qin H, Rayburn PD, Poon G, Murthy K, et al. Implementation of an automatic stop order and initial antibiotic exposure in very low birth weight infants. Am J Perinatol. 2017;34(2):105-10.
31. Quirós RE, Bardossy AC, Angeleri P, Zurita J, Aleman Espinoza WR, Carneiro M; PROA-LATAM Project Group, et al. Antimicrobial stewardship programs in adult intensive care units in Latin America: implementation, assessments, and impact on outcomes. Infect Control Hosp Epidemiol. 2022;43(2):181-90.
32. World Health Organization.. (2019). Executive summary: the selection and use of essential medicines 2019: report of the 22nd WHO Expert Committee on the selection and use of essential medicines. Geneva: World Health Organization. [online] Available from https://www.who.int/publications/i/item/WHO-MVP-EMP-IAU-2019.05 [Last accessed August, 2025].

5 SECTION

Special Considerations in Infection Control

***Section Editor:** Nishant Kumar*

16

CHAPTER

Infection Prevention in Immunocompromised Patients

Priyanka H Chhabra, Sahil Diwan

LEARNING OBJECTIVES

- To understand the immunocompromised states and describe common causes such as transplant recipients, cancer chemotherapy, HIV (human immunodeficiency virus), and tuberculosis (TB).
- To identify common infections occurring in different timelines in immunocompromised patients.
- To understand the factors leading to increased susceptibility to these infections.
- To understand the guiding principles behind infection prevention practices.
- Tailored approach for infection prevention strategies.
- To monitor early signs of infections in immunocompromised patients.
- Counseling of patients in prophylactic measures.

INTRODUCTION

Immunocompromised patients have weakened or impaired immune systems that make them highly susceptible to opportunistic and severe infections. These infections may be caused by bacteria, viruses, fungi, or parasites that rarely affect healthy individuals. The clinical presentation is often atypical, leading to delays in diagnosis and management. Several conditions contribute to immunosuppression, including HIV infection, malignancies, cancer chemotherapy, diabetes, tuberculosis, autoimmune disorders, malnutrition, organ transplantation, and congenital immune defects. Understanding the specific vulnerabilities of each subgroup, the timeline of infections, and the principles of prevention is essential for reducing morbidity and mortality in this high-risk population.

IMMUNOCOMPROMISED PATIENTS

Immunocompromised patient is a person with condition which affects body's immune system and predisposes to unusual [opportunistic infections (OIs)], which do not occur otherwise. Several subgroups of patients are classified as immunocompromised such as transplant recipients, cancer chemotherapy, diabetes, malnutrition, radiation therapy, HIV (human immunodeficiency virus), TB, autoimmune disorders, neutropenic patients, genetic disorders (B-cell or T-cell defect), blood dyscrasias, and hematological malignancies.

Immunodeficiency can be primary, acquired, and iatrogenic.

- Primary immune deficiency occurs due to heredity and is usually acquired after birth.
- Immune deficiency is commonly acquired and is commonly due to diseases such as HIV, malignancies particularly blood dyscrasias, and TB.
- Iatrogenic causes such as cancer chemotherapy also lead to suppressed immune status.

Suppressed immunity in these patients predisposes them to OIs. Not only these individuals acquire unusual infections, often the presentation of these infections is atypical. Atypical presentation of unusual infections makes establishing a timely diagnosis and management a difficult task. This chapter discusses these patient populations individually.

TRANSPLANT RECIPIENTS

Infection is a leading cause of death among patients receiving solid organ transplants. Among infections, lower respiratory tract infection is the most common site closely followed by skin, blood leading to bacteremia, urinary tract infection, etc. Type of infections, causative organisms, and frequency of infections after transplant follow a predictable time course. Infections are, therefore, classified on the basis of time after transplant. Infections occurring within 30 days, 30 days–6 months, and after 65 months after transplant.[1]

Infections within 30 Days of Transplant

These infections occur due to technical or surgical issues related to transplant such as surgical site skin infections (SSIs), pneumonia, upper respiratory tract infections, uncomplicated or complicated cystitis, graft pyelonephritis, vascular catheter-related infections, and herpes simplex viral infections and are usually healthcare associated or nosocomial. Pneumonia is the most common infection in postrenal transplant recipient. Reactivation of fungal or viral infections can also occur in the absence of adequate prophylaxis.

Infections within 30 Days–6 Months of Transplant

After 30 days, nosocomial infections subside and give rise to an increase in number of OIs. These include infections by uncommon protozoa, viruses, and fungi.

Infections after 6 Months of Transplant

After 6 months, transplant recipient experiences an increase in community-acquired infections or there can be reactivation of indolent fungi and viruses. **Flowchart 1** summarizes timeline of various infections in immunocompromised host.

Flowchart 1: Timeline of infections in immunocompromised transplant recipient.

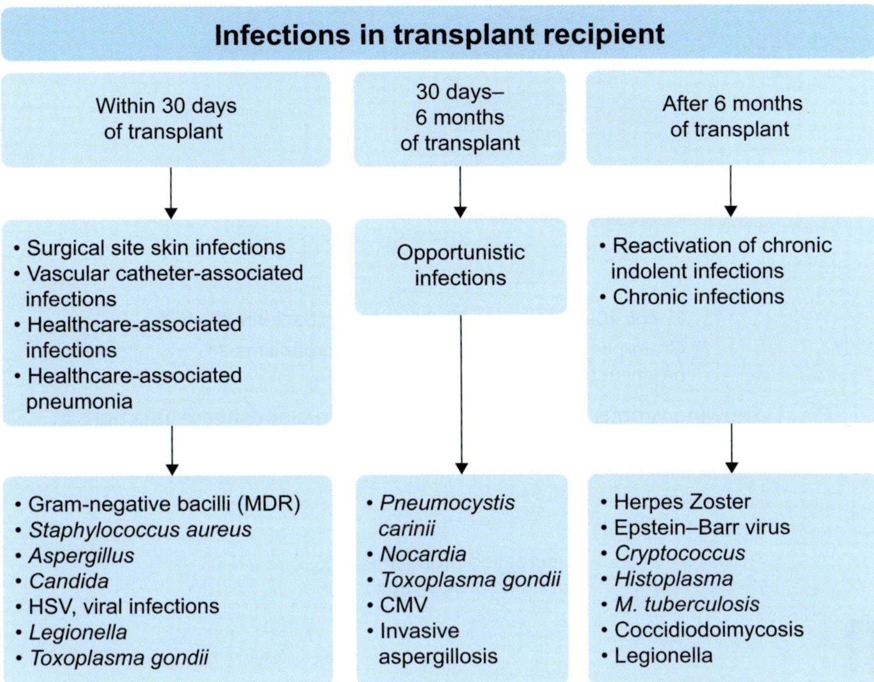

(CMV: cytomegalovirus, HSV: herpes simplex virus, MDR: multidrug resistant)

PATIENTS RECEIVING CANCER CHEMOTHERAPY

Patients receiving cancer chemotherapy develop infections due to coexisting neutropenia. Patients with neutrophil counts below 1,000/mm^3 lasting for >1 week often develop increased likelihood of infections. Neutropenia also hampers the characteristic manifestations of these infections.[2] For example, neutropenic patients acquire pneumonia without fever, sputum production, and characteristic radiographic features (atypical presentation) on chest X-ray. Patients with defects in T cell-mediated immunity often acquire organisms such as *Salmonella species, Histoplasma capsulatum, Pneumocystis carinii, Leishmania species*, and cytomegalovirus (CMV). On the other hand, patients with B-cell defects lead to increase predisposition to *Streptococcus pneumoniae, Haemophilus influenzae,* and *Neisseria meningitidis*. B-cell defects are commonly seen in patients with multiple myeloma, bone marrow transplant, chronic lymphocytic leukemia, etc., presence of catheters such as intravascular, intraperitoneal, intracranial, and intravesical also increases the likelihood of blood stream infections. **Figure 1** demonstrates various bacteria implicated in cancer chemotherapy recipients. The most common causative organism is *Escherichia coli*, accounting for 40–60% isolates, closely followed by other

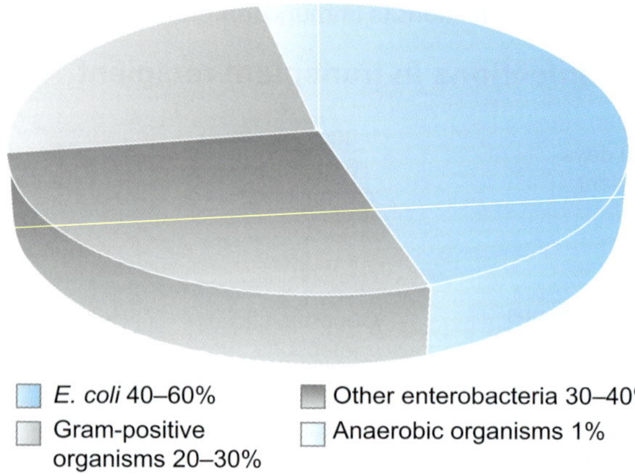

Fig. 1: Showing various microorganisms isolated in bloodstream infections in neutropenic cancer patients.

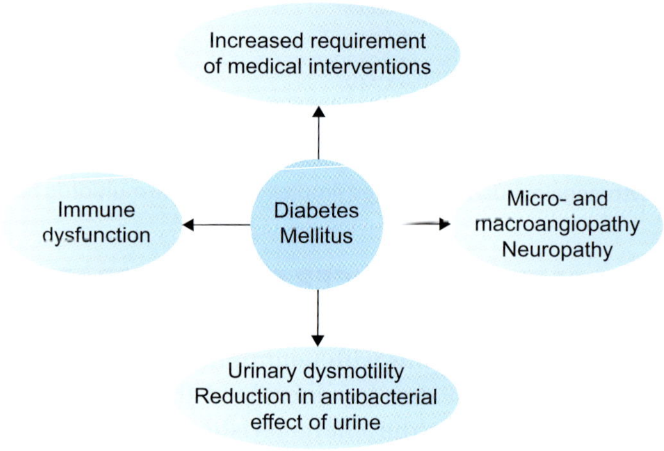

Fig. 2: Factors leading to increased risk of infections in diabetic patients.

gram-negative organisms from *Enterobacteriaceae*, e.g., *Acinetobacter baumannii, Klebsiella pneumoniae,* and *Pseudomonas aeruginosa* gram-positive organisms, e.g., *Staphylococcus aureus, Enterococci, Streptococcus,* and anaerobes constitute the remaining 30% isolates.[6]

Diabetes Mellitus

Patients with diabetes mellitus are more likely to have frequent infections in greater severity as compared to nondiabetic counterparts. This is perhaps due to the fact that hyperglycemia favors growth of microbes, host immune defense mechanisms are weakened, and concurrent microangiopathy increases oxidative stress. **Figure 2** enumerates several factors leading to increased predisposition of infections in diabetics. Lower respiratory tract infection (pneumonia) is by far the most common infections in patients with diabetes. The most common causative organism of pneumonia in these patients is *S. pneumoniae*. Diabetics are six times more likely to have greater severity of pneumonia and are more likely to require hospitalization.[3] Urinary tract infections (asymptomatic bacteriuria, pyelonephritis, etc.) are four to five times more likely in diabetics as compared to general population. **Box 1** enlists commonly occurring infections in diabetic patients.

Tuberculosis

Tuberculosis is one of the most common OIs in transplant recipients and neutropenic patients. Risk of acquiring TB is particularly higher in the first year after transplant and more so in patients undergoing lung transplants. TB is also the major cause of death in patients infected with HIV/AIDS (acquired immunodeficiency syndrome). The presentation of TB in immunocompromised patients is often asymptomatic (diagnosed on surveillance cultures) or is atypical presentation (absence of apical cavities in pulmonary TB). The clinical presentation of TB is governed by the degree

BOX 1: List of Infections in diabetic patients.

- *Respiratory infections:*
  - *Streptococcus pneumoniae*
  - Influenza, H1N1
  - Tuberculosis
- *Urinary tract infections:*
  - Asymptomatic bacteriuria
  - Pyelonephritis
  - Emphysematous pyelonephritis
  - Cystitis
  - Emphysematous cystitis
  - Perinephric abscesses
- *Gastrointestinal and liver infections:*
  - Oral and esophageal candidiasis
  - Emphysematous cholecystitis
- *Skin and soft tissue infections:*
  - Foot infection
  - Necrotizing fasciitis
  - Fournier's gangrene
- *Head and neck infections:*
  - Mucormycosis
  - Otitis media and externa
  - Malignant otitis externa
- *Other:*
  - HIV/AIDS

(HIV: human immunodeficiency virus; AIDS: acquired immunodeficiency virus) of immunosuppression. If the immunosuppression is profound (CD4 counts <50 cells/mm^3), patients present with extrapulmonary or disseminated TB. Patients with better immunological reserve tend to present with pulmonary or localized TB infection. Pulmonary cavitations are less common with increasing severity of immunosuppression.

PATIENTS WITH HUMAN IMMUNODEFICIENCY VIRUS/ ACQUIRED IMMUNODEFICIENCY VIRUS

Respiratory failure is the most common cause of intensive care unit (ICU) admission in patients with HIV/AIDS. Pneumonia secondary to *Pneumocystis jirovecii* (PCP) is the most common OI in patients with HIV/AIDS, closely followed by cerebral toxoplasmosis and TB.[4] Other common OIs in HIV/AIDS are *Cryptococcus neoformans* meningitis, histoplasmosis, disseminated *Mycobacterium avium intracellulare* complex disease, CMV infection, and progressive multifocal leukoencephalopathy (PML). PCP manifests as hypoxemia with bilateral pulmonary infiltrates on chest radiograph. **Flowchart 2** summarizes the spectrum of infections in patients with HIV/AIDS.

INFECTION PREVENTION STRATEGIES

A systematic approach to care of the immunocompromised individuals, tailored to the individual patient's needs, is crucial to reduce the risk of infection. Key components of infection prevention strategies include here.

Flowchart 2: The spectrum of patients treated with HIV.

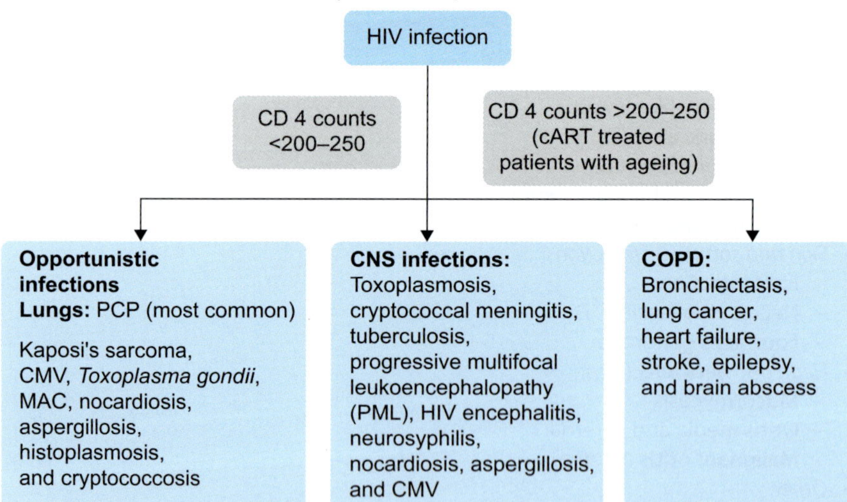

(CMV: Cytomegalovirus; COPD: chronic obstructive pulmonary disease; MAC: *Mycobacterium avium* intracellulare complex; PCP: *Pneumocystis jirovecii* pneumonia)

Recognition and Risk Assessment of the Compromised Host

Identifying the various causes of defects in patients body's defense mechanism as described above and assessing the level of immunosuppression, best evaluates a patient's risk of infection and helps in determining appropriate preventive measures.

Immunization

Vaccination is one of the most efficient ways to prevent infections in immunocompromised patients. Although, vaccinations is less effective compared to immune competent patients due to decreased cellular as well as humoral immunogenicity. This suboptimal response is still beneficial and provides protection from preventable infectious diseases.

Killed, inactivated, component and recombinant vaccines are found to be safe, well tolerated and highly recommended as they cannot cause infection. In contrast, live vaccines are mostly contraindicated in immunocompromised patients as they themselves can lead to infection. Live vaccines include oral polio, measles, mumps, and rubella (MMR), *Varicella*, oral typhoid, and BCG vaccine. Live vaccines should be delayed for 3–6 months postchemotherapy. In patients with planned immunosuppression such as patients planed for chemotherapy/solid organ transplantation, immunization should be completed at least 2 weeks prior for killed vaccine and 4 weeks prior for live vaccine.[5] **Table 1** gives the latest recommendation from Infectious Diseases Society of America (IDSA) for vaccination of immunocompromised host.

TABLE 1: The latest recommendation from IDSA for vaccination of immunocompromised host.

Vaccine	*Indications*	*Schedule*
Inactive influenza vaccine (IIV)	All immunocompromised patients except those receiving intensive chemotherapy and anti B-cell antibodies	Annual
Pneumococcal • Pneumococcal conjugate vaccine (PCV 13) • Pneumococcal polysaccharide vaccine (PPSV 23)	 • All immunocompromised patients • All immunocompromised patients	• Single dose • ≥8 weeks after PCV13, and a second dose of PPSV23 should be given 5 years later

Contd...

Contd...

Vaccine	*Indications*	*Schedule*
Hemophilus influenza B (HIB)	• Human immunodeficiency virus (HIV)-infected children >59 months who have not received HIB, not for HIV infected adults • Asplenia/sickle cell disease • 6–12 months after hematopoietic stem cell transplantation (HSCT)	• Single dose • Single dose • Three doses
Meningococcal	• HIV-infected children 11–18 years • Asplenia/sickle cell disease • 6–12 months after HSCT to 11–18 years • Patients with primary complement deficiencies	Two doses with 2 months interval with booster every 5 years
Hep B vaccine	• All HIV patients, consider high dose conc (40 µg) for adults. Repeat if post vaccination titers for anti HBs <10 mIU/mL • 6–12 months after HSCT • Adult patients with chronic inflammatory disease on immunosuppressive therapy • All antihepatitis B surface antibodies (HBs) negative solid organ transplant candidates • Chronic hepatitis B-infected recipients 2–6 months after liver transplant	Hep B vaccine series (three doses)
Varicella vaccine	• Avoid in all highly immunocompromised patients except in HIV without severe immunosuppression or chronic granulomatous disease	Two doses separated by 3 months interval
Measles, mumps, and rubella (MMR) vaccine	Avoid in all except in clinically stable HIV-infected children aged 1–13 years without severe immunosuppression and HIV-infected patients aged ≥14 years without measles immunity and with a CD4 T-cell lymphocyte count ≥200/mm and in measles-seronegative patients 24 months after HSCT patients if they have no chronic graft versus host disease and are not on immunosuppression	Two dose series

Antibiotic Prophylaxis Against Endogenous Infections

Using antimicrobial agents to prevent the reactivation of latent infections depends on the most common pathogens causing OIs. Trimethoprim-sulfamethoxazole (TMP-SMX) is a broad-spectrum antibiotic used as first-line agent in the prophylaxis of OIs, particularly *P. carinii* pneumonia (PCP), in immunosuppressed patients.[7]

Antifungal prophylaxis is advised for high-risk patients, particularly those anticipated to undergo significant and prolonged neutropenia. This condition is characterized by a neutrophil count of <100 neutrophils/µL for a duration exceeding 7 days. Herpes simplex virus-seropositive patients undergoing allogeneic hematopoietic stem cell transplantation (HSCT) or leukemia induction therapy should receive antiviral prophylaxis, such as acyclovir. For patients at high risk of hepatitis B virus reactivation, treatment with a nucleoside reverse transcription inhibitor (e.g., entecavir or tenofovir) is recommended.

Reduction of Exposure to Exogenous Pathogens and Targeted Hygiene Practices

Handwashing with soap and water and rigorous hand hygiene practices by patient visitors and healthcare workers is an important modality for prevention of infection. Five moments of hand hygiene as designed by World Health Organization (WHO) should be strictly followed. Close monitoring of patients with invasive devices to prevent ventilator-associated pneumonia (VAP), catheter-associated urinary tract infection (CAUTI), and central line-associated bloodstream infection (CLABSI).

Provide Protected Controlled Environment

The immunocompromised patient should be isolated in a single dedicated room with positive air pressure and high-efficiency particulate air (HEPA) filter. Personnel entering the room must be wearing sterile gown and gloves. Only sterile products, food, and water should be allowed. Regular surface cleaning and disinfection is necessary.[8]

MONITORING AND EARLY DETECTION OF INFECTIONS

Critical care physician plays an important role in establishing a structured approach in monitoring and surveillance of immunocompromised patients. This approach helps in timely diagnosis and management of complications.

- *Clinical assessment:* Patients should be regularly screened for signs of infection such as fever, cough, sputum production, tachypnea, skin lesions, and neurological changes.
- *Investigations:* Blood culture, sputum, and urine samples can be analyzed to diagnose OIs.
- *Imaging studies:* Detailed evaluation of organs can be done by chest X-ray and CT scan of concerned organ such as chest, abdomen, and pelvis, and MRI scan of brain in case of neurological changes.

- *Screening tests:* Organisms such as *Mycobacterium tuberculosis*, hepatitis B virus, hepatitis C virus, and HIV should be screened with the help of screening tests, e.g., tuberculin test [purified piperidine derivative (PPD)] is routinely used for *M. tuberculosis*. Window period of 3 months is present between infection and detection using PPD test.
- *Measurement of load of microorganism:* Monitoring of infection load of CMV, EBV (Epstein–Barr virus), etc., by nucleic acid amplification tests (NAAT) minimizes the clinical impact of infection. Viral load helps in distinguishing between active and latent infection.
- *Specific monitoring techniques for different types of infections*:
    - *Bacterial infections:* Blood culture, Gram staining for specific pathogens such as Ziehl–Neilson staining for acid fast bacilli.
    - *Fungal infections:* Cultures in fungal medium, detection of cell wall components with the help of beta-D-glucan assay, galactomannan, etc.
    - *Parasitic infections:* Blood and stool specimens can be utilized for detection of parasitic infections.

CONCLUSION

Immunocompromised patients are highly vulnerable to a wide range of infections that often present atypically and progress rapidly. Early recognition of risk factors, meticulous monitoring, timely diagnostic evaluation, and appropriate prophylactic strategies are essential to improving outcomes. Tailored vaccination, antimicrobial prophylaxis, strict hygiene measures, and controlled environments play a crucial role in prevention. A structured, patient-specific approach enables clinicians to detect infections early, reduce complications, and provide comprehensive care to this complex and high-risk population.

REFERENCES

1. Risi GF, Tomascak V. Prevention of infection in the immunocompromised host. Am J Infect Control. 1998;26(6):594-606.
2. Islas-Muñoz B, Volkow-Fernández P, Ibanes-Gutiérrez C, Villamar-Ramírez A, Vilar-Compte D, Cornejo-Juárez P. Bloodstream infections in cancer patients. Risk factors associated with mortality. Int J Infect Dis. 2018;71:59-64.
3. Casqueiro J, Casqueiro J, Alves C. Infections in patients with diabetes mellitus: A review of pathogenesis. Indian J Endocrinol Metab. 2012; 16 Suppl 1(Suppl1):S27-36.
4. Rosen MJ, Narasimhan M. Critical care of immunocompromised patients: Human immunodeficiency virus. Crit Care Med. 2006;34(Suppl):S245-50.
5. Rubin LG, Levin MJ, Ljungman P, Davies EG, Avery R, Tomblyn M, et al., 2013 IDSA Clinical Practice Guideline for Vaccination of the Immunocompromised Host. *Clin Infect Dis*. 2014;58(3):309-18.

6. Taplitz RA, Kennedy EB, Bow EJ, Crews J, Gleason C, Hawley DK, et al. Antimicrobial Prophylaxis for Adult Patients With Cancer-Related Immunosuppression: ASCO and IDSA Clinical Practice Guideline Update. J Clin Oncol. 2018;36(30):3043-54.
7. Lee WI, Lam L, Bacchi S, Jiang M, Inglis JM, Smith W, et al. Antibiotic prophylaxis in immunosuppressed patients - Missed opportunities from trimethoprim-sulfamethoxazole allergy label. World Allergy Organ J. 2024;17(1):100856.
8. Risi GF, Tomascak V. Prevention of infection in the immunocompromised host. Am J Infect Control. 1998;26(6):594–606.

17

CHAPTER

Improving Healthcare Practices: Strategies for Integrating Adult Vaccination in Intensive Care Unit Settings

Prashant Narayan Walse, Samvveda Shirish Samel

LEARNING OBJECTIVES

- High mortality and morbidity (influenza, pneumonia, typhoid, and cervical cancer).
- Epidemiological shift in the prevalence of vaccine preventable diseases (VPDs) among adults in India.
- Immunosenescence.
- Increased vulnerability of elderly for VPDs due to comorbidities immunosuppression in adults.
- Increased hospitalization cost.
- Increase in the antimicrobial resistance.

INTRODUCTION

Vaccination is among the most cost-effective public health interventions whose significance has been stressed by global eradication of small pox and the near elimination of polio. The World Health Organization (WHO) had launched the global Expanded Program of Immunization (EPI) in 1974 following which most of the countries followed up with their National Immunization Programs (NIPs). India launched EPI in 1978 and relabeled as Universal Immunization Program (UIP) in 1985. The UIP has aimed to achieve universal coverage of the pediatric population and pregnant women with vaccines. Tetanus toxoid vaccination was the only adult vaccine initially with latter inclusion of Japanese encephalitis (JE) vaccination in the endemic areas. Adolescent vaccination program is anticipated to become an integral part of UIP with the inclusion of Rubella and human papillomavirus (HPV) vaccine with catch-up campaigns for second dose of measles and rubella vaccines.[1]

The adult immunization depends upon the vaccination history in the childhood. The guidelines for adult vaccination have regional variations unlike the pediatric immunization guidelines, given by the Indian Academy of Pediatrics and the NIP.

The important guidelines followed for adult vaccination are:

- The Centers for Disease Control and Prevention Advisory Committee on Immunization Practices (ACIP) guidelines[2]
- World Health Organization (WHO) guidelines[2]
- Expert panel guidelines—Association of Physicians of India[2]

Along with the Indian Consensus guidelines on adult immunization in association with:

- Cardiological Society of India (CSI)[3]
- Clinical Infectious Diseases Society (CIDS)[3]
- Federation of Obstetric and Gynaecological Societies of India (FOGSI)[3]
- Geriatric Society of India (GSI)[3]
- Heart Failure Association of India (HFAI)[3]
- Indian Association of Preventive and Social Medicine (IAPSM)[3]
- Indian Chest Society (ICS)[3]
- Indian Medical Association (IMA)[3]
- Indian Rheumatology Association (IRA)[3]
- Indian Society of Critical Care Medicine (ISCCM)[3]
- Indian Society of Nephrology (ISN)[3]
- Indian Society of Oncology (ISO)[3]
- Research Society for Study of Diabetes in India (RSSDI)[3]

BURDEN OF VACCINE PREVENTABLE DISEASES IN INDIA

The current WHO and CDC recommendations on adult vaccination are provided in **Table 1**.[4]

During the last 15 years, India has seen a substantial outbreaks of VPDs in adults with 95% of associated fatalities. A 2005–2006 Kerala outbreak of meningococcal disease reported a mortality rate of 14.6%. Narayan et al. mentioned 51.1 deaths per 100,000 populations due to influenza-associated respiratory illness in the population above 65 years of age during 2010–2013 with 2,913 deaths out of 66,146 seasonal Influenza A cases from 2017 to 2023. A South Indian study shows that pneumonia contributes to 39% of hospitalizations in adults above 18 years with a mortality of 19%, escalating to 30% in the age group of 50–60 years. Gurav et al. reported 50% of JE virus infection among all acute encephalitis cases wherein 75% infected were adults. Cervical cancer has a mortality of 60% making it the second among the cancer-related fatalities in India.[5]

Clarke et al. highlighted that India had the highest global burden of diphtheria with more cases reported in the population aged >15 years. Similarly, measles which was considered as a pediatric disease but an outbreak in Karnataka reported higher number of cases in the population between 21 and 25 years of age. However, these studies were isolated investigations with no validated information.[6]

IMPORTANCE OF ADULT VACCINATION

The VPDs have a significant burden on the healthcare system, especially in the absence of guidelines. The treatment costs are substantially higher per episode in immunocompromised (IC) patients. A US based retrospective

TABLE 1: VPD burden in Southeast Asia region and WHO/CDC standing on adult vaccination.

VPDs	*Burden of VPDs in population of South and Southeast Asia*		*Base year*	*WHO standing adult vaccination*	*CDC recommendation adult vaccination*
	Incidence	*Mortality*			
Typhoid	148–160/100,000 in ≥15 years	CFR-1%	2010	High-risk population	Travelers to South Asia
Hepatitis B	138,000 cases/annum	30,000 deaths/ annum		High-risk population if not previously immunized	All adults aged 19–59 years. For 60 years and older with risk factor
Hepatitis A	400,000 cases/annum	800 deaths/ annum		Basis—incidence of acute hepatitis A, change in the endemicity from high-to-intermediate, and consideration of cost-effectiveness	If not vaccinated previously and want to be protected
Diphtheria	0.52/100,000 (All ages)		2019	To be completed in childhood given in combination with tetanus toxoid	After primary immunization, booster every 10 years in combination with tetanus (Td)
Varicella	40–60% of adults remain susceptible			Vaccinate adults without evidence of varicella immunity	Vaccinate who never had chickenpox and were never vaccinated
Cervical cancer	17.8/100,000	10/100,000	2018	Age >15 years, recommended only if feasible, affordable, cost-effective, and does not divert resources from vaccination of the primary target population or from effective cervical cancer screening programs	Recommended through age 26 years, from 27 to 45 years on discussion with their clinician

Contd...

Contd…

VPDs	*Burden of VPDs in population of South and Southeast Asia*		*Base year*	*WHO standing adult vaccination*	*CDC recommendation adult vaccination*
	Incidence	*Mortality*			
Measles	1.49/100,000	39,100 deaths		Measles vaccination should be routinely administered to potentially susceptible, asymptomatic HIV adults	For adults who do not have presumptive evidence of immunity
Rubella	10,361 Rubella cases with 361 congenital rubella syndrome		2016	Women of child-bearing age if not previously vaccinated	
Lower respiratory tract infection	*Episodes:* 45.9–48.8/1,000 population (All age group)	30.8–34.7/100,000 (All age group)		*Pneumococcal vaccine:* In resource-limited settings not recommended for adults for routine immunization *Influenza vaccine:* Pregnant women should have the highest priority, elderly persons ≥65 years of age, individuals with specific chronic medical conditions, and healthcare workers	Age 19–64 years with certain chronic medical conditions or other risk factors. Age 65 years or older recommended for all
Meningococcal disease	40–60 case/100,000	Case fatality Rate—10%		Recommended with conjugate vaccines preferred over polysaccharide vaccines	High-risk adults

(CDC: Centers for Disease Control and Prevention; CFR: case fatality ratio; HIV: human immunodeficiency virus; VPD: vaccine-preventable diseases; WHO: World Health Organization) study mentions that invasive pneumococcal disease (IPD) poses a 23.4-fold higher costs amounting to $58.5 million per 100,000 patient years in IC patients, driven by a higher morbidity and mortality patterns, frequent and longer hospitalization, and need for additional specialized care. Another USA data states that the risk of all-cause pneumonia and IPD was 3.6 and 4.6-fold higher in IC populations compared with the general population.[6]

In addition to progressive functional decline attributable to immunosenescence, the immune response in the geriatric population is compromised by comorbidities such as diabetes mellitus, hypertension, obesity, frailty, stress, and malignancy contributing to increased susceptibility to infectious diseases, some of which can be VPDs. The presence of one or two comorbidities is associated with a 40- to 150-fold increase in the epidemiology of influenza or pneumonia.[6,7]

Vaccination is considered as a prevention and control measure, but often overlooked as an antimicrobial stewardship (AMS) strategy as vaccines can reduce AMR by reducing the incidence of bacterial infections and inappropriate use of antimicrobials.[8]

A US study reported that 50% of the antibiotic prescriptions were inappropriately given for respiratory illnesses associated with viral pathogens such as influenza with data from outpatient/ambulatory hospital patient visits.[9]

On the other hand, evidence from a systematic review shows that influenza vaccination can reduce antibiotic use among healthy adults by nearly one-third.[10]

Among diabetic patients, influenza increases the risk of hospitalization and intensive care unit (ICU) admission by 3–6-fold and 4-fold, respectively[11,12] with an increased risk of myocardial infarction six times higher within the 1st week of laboratory confirmed influenza owing to the virus induced thrombophilia state and thrombosis of preexisting atherosclerotic plaque leading to acute coronary occlusion.[13]

Overall incidence rate per 100,000 population of adult pneumococcal disease of pneumococcal pneumonia is 8.8 in healthy adults, 51.4 in adults with diabetes, 62.9 in adults with chronic lung disease, and 93.7 in adults with chronic heart disease.[14]

Adults who die of VPDs each year is 350-fold higher versus the corresponding figure for children due to the inability of childhood vaccination to offer long-term benefits, as well as the changing disease epidemiology with the emergence and reemergence of certain diseases (tuberculosis, malaria).[15,16]

The immune status in cancer patients have been compromised due to chronic inflammation, impaired and/or decreased function of the hematopoietic cells, and immunosuppressant medications. Still advanced treatments in cancer patients have led to improved survival. However, cancer therapies make individuals prone to certain infections. They may have lower seroconversion rates after vaccination. According to American

Society of Clinical Oncology (ASCO) guidelines it is important that these patients should receive seasonal and risk-based vaccines (preferably 2–4 weeks) prior to the initiation of treatment applying to the under- or unvaccinated adults. In cancer patients not immunized prior to therapy, vaccination should occur at least 3 months after discontinuation of immunosuppressive therapy. Live attenuated vaccines (LAVs) are not recommended; however, in some patients who are not severely IC, LAVs may be considered with a lack of comprehensive and nationally adopted vaccination in Indian guidelines.[6]

IMMUNIZATION FOR HEALTHCARE WORKERS

The prevention of the vaccine-preventable diseases (VPDs) and healthcare-associated infections among healthcare workers (HCWs) is important for the safety of HCWs, patients, and the broader community. With accordance to WHO, HCWs should be vaccinated as per the countries individual policy with special consideration to outbreak-prone VPDs: tuberculosis (TB), hepatitis B virus (HBV), poliomyelitis, diphtheria, measles, rubella, meningococcal disease, influenza, varicella, pertussis, and corona virus disease of 2019 (COVID-19) being added in 2022. Despite this, there are suboptimal rates observed due to access barriers to vaccines, lack of specific policy, low uptake of vaccines, and vaccine hesitancy which are needed to be emphasized.[17,18]

The vaccination of the HCWs especially for hepatitis B vaccine have been localized at the level of large institutions during the last decade.[1]

UNMET NEED FOR IMMUNIZATION IN ADULT POPULATION

There would be increased pressure on the healthcare system due to significant burden from noncommunicable diseases and VPDs. Achievement of optimal vaccination coverage has been a challenge in the developing countries where majority of the population is subjected to the crowded living situations, poor diet, limited access to healthcare, and substandard sanitation systems, increasing the risk for spread of infectious disease and limited surveillance of VPDs.[6]

DISEASE BURDEN OF COMORBID AND IMMUNOCOMPROMISED POPULATION IN INDIA

The projection of India being the most populous country in the world is coming up very shortly with the population of adults aged ≥60 years growing at a rate three times faster than that of the total population and accounting for 19% of the global population by 2050. The most common subpopulations contributing to the IC population in India include cancer, autoimmune diseases, transplant patients (renal followed by liver, heart, lung, and

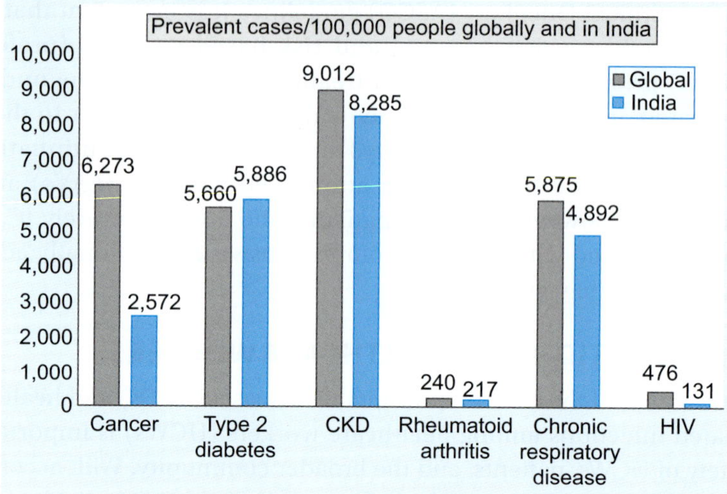

Fig. 1: Prevalent cases/100,000 people globally and in India—2019.[2]
(CKD: Chronic kidney disease; HIV: Human immunodeficiency virus)

hematopoietic stem cell), diabetes mellitus (DM), chronic kidney disease (CKD), and human immunodeficiency virus (HIV) **(Fig. 1)**.[6]

RECOMMENDED ADULT IMMUNIZATION SCHEDULE (FIGS. 2A AND B)[19]

Adult immunization: A framework for prevention **Figures 2A and B** presents the standardized U.S immunization schedule providing a critical evidence based framework for adult vaccination. While specific to the U.S context, these guidelines serve as an essential reference for developing risk based and age stratified vaccination strategies in India, particularly for high risk groups and the growing elderly population.

Vaccines in Adult Immunization

Influenza Vaccine

There are seasonal epidemics and pandemics due to the influenza virus undergoing frequent mutations, thus WHO recommending the development of seasonal vaccines twice a year (for Northern and Southern hemisphere) as per the circulating virus strains. As per the review published in Indian Journal of Medical Research 2024, about 33% of the total 1,219 patients with severe acute respiratory illness (SARI) were positive for influenza viruses in Kashmir. About 6.8% of the influenza positive patients were vaccinated, whereas 8.6% among the influenza negative counterpart. Vaccine effectiveness (VE) for any influenza strain was found to be 13% due to genetic mismatch between the circulating strain and the vaccine strain.[20]

Vaccine ▼ Age group ▶	19–21 years	22–26 years	27–49 years	50–59 years	60–64 years	≥65 years
Influenza [2,*]	1 dose annually					
Tetanus, diphtheria, pertussis(Td/Tdap) [3,*]	Substitute 1–time dose of Tdap for Td booster; then boost with Td every 10 years					
Varicella [4,*]	2 doses					
Human papillomavirus (HPV) female [5,*]	3 doses					
Human papillomavirus (HPV) male [5,*]	3 doses					
Zoster[6]					1 dose	
Measles, mumps, rubella (MMR) [7,*]	1 or 2 doses					
Pneumococcal 13–valent conjugate (PCV13) [8,*]	1–time dose					
Pneumococcal polysaccharide (PPSV23) [8,*]	1 or 2 doses					1 dose
Meningococcal [9,*]	1 or more doses					
Hepatitis A [10,*]	2 doses					
Hepatitis B [11,*]	3 doses					
Haemophilus influenzae type b (Hib)[12,*]	1 or 3 doses					

*Covered by the vaccine injury compensation program

For all persons in this category who meet the age requirements and who lack documentation of vaccination or have no evidence of previous infection;zoster vaccine recommended regardless of prior episode of zoster

Recommended if some other risk factor is present (e.g., on the basis of medical, occupational, lifestyle, or other indication)

No recommendation

U.S. Department of Health and Human Services
Centers for disease Control and prevention

Report all clinically significant postvaccination reactions to the Vaccine Adverse Event Reporting System (VAERS). Reporting forms and instructions on filing a VAERS report are available at www.vaers.hhs.gov or by telephone, 800-822-7967. Information on how to file a Vaccine Injury Compensation Program claim is available at www.hrsa.gov/vaccinecompensation or by telephone, 800-338-2382. To file a claim for vaccine injury, contact the U.S. Court of Federal Claims, 717 Madison Place, NW, Washington, DC 20005; telephone, 202-357-6400.
Additional information about the vaccines in this schedule, extent of available data, and contraindications for vaccination is also available at www.cdc.gov/vaccines or from the CDC-INFO Contact Center at 800-CDC-INFO (800-232-4636) in English and Spanish, 8:00 am. - 8:00 pm. Eastern Time, Monday-Friday, excluding holidays.
Use of trade names and commercial sources is for identification only and does not imply endorsement by the U.S. Department of Health and Human Services.

The recommendations in this schedule were approved by the Centers for Disease Control and Prevention's (CDC) Advisory Committee on Immunization Practices (ACIP), American Academy of Family Physicians (AAFP), American College of Physicians (ACP), American College of Obstetricians and Gynecologists (ACOG), and American College of Nurse-Midwives (ACNM).

Fig. 2A

Vaccine ▼ / Indication ▶	Pregnancy	Immuno-compromising conditions (excluding human immunodeficiency virus[HIV])[4,6,7,8,13]	HIV infection CD4+ T lymphocyte count[4,6,7,8,13] <200 cells/μL	HIV infection CD4+ T lymphocyte count ≥200 cells/μL	Men who have sex with men (MSM)	Kidney failure end-stage renal disease, receipt of hemodialysis	Heart disease, chronic lung disease, chronic alcoholism	Asplenia (including elective splenectomy and persistent complement component deficiencies)[8,12]	Chronic liver disease	Diabetes	Health care personnel
Influenza[2,*]	1 dose IIV annually				1 dose IIV or LAIV annually	1 dose IIV annually					1 dose IIV or LAIV annually
Tetanus, diphtheria, pertussis(Td/Tdap)[3,*]	1 dose Tdap each pregnancy	Substitute 1–time dose of Tdap for Td booster; then boost with Td every 10 years									
Varicella[4,*]	Contraindicated			2 doses							
Human papillomavirus(HPV)Female[5,*]		3 doses through age 26 years				3 doses through age 26 years					
Human papillomavirus(HPV)Male[5,*]		3 doses through age 26 years				3 doses through age 21 years					
Zoster[6]	Contraindicated				1 doses						
Measles, mumps, rubella(MMR)[7,*]	Contraindicated			1 or 2 doses							
Pneumococcal 13–valent conjugate (PCV13)[8,*]		1 dose									
Pneumococcal (PPSV23)8	1 or 2 doses										
Meningococcal[9,*]	1 or more doses										
Hepatitis A[10,*]	2 doses										
Hepatitis B[11,*]	3 doses										
Haemophilus influenzae type B (Hib)[12,*]		Post– HSCT recipients only	1 or 3 doses								

* Covered by the vaccine injury compensation program

- (blue) For all persons in this category who meet the age requirements and who lack documentation of vaccination or have no evidence of previous infection; zoster vaccine recommended regardless of prior episode of zoster
- (grey) Recommmended if some other risk factor is present (e.g.,on the basis of medical, occupational, lifestyle, or other indication)
- (white) No recommendation

U.S. Department of Health and Human Services
Centers for disease Control and prevention

These schedules indicate the recommended age groups and medical indications for which administration of currently licensed vaccines is commonly indicated for adults ages 19 years and older, as of February 1, 2015. For all vaccines being recommended on the Adult Immunization Schedule: a vaccine series does not need to be restarted, regardless of the time that has elapsed between doses. Licensed combination vaccines may be used whenever any components of the combination are indicated and when the vaccine's other components are not contraindicated. For detailed recommendations on all vaccines, including those used primarily for travelers or that are issued during the year, consult the manufacturers' package inserts and the complete statements from the Advisory Committee on Immunization Practices (www.cdc.gov/vaccines/hcp/acip-recs/index.html). Use of trade names and commercial sources is for identification only and does not imply endorsement by the U.S. Department of Health and Human Services.

The recommendations in this schedule were approved by the Centers for Disease Control and Prevention's (CDC) Advisory Committee on Immunization Practices (ACIP), American Academy of Family Physicians (AAFP), American College of Physicians (ACP), American College of Obstetricians and Gynecologists (ACOG), and American College of Nurse-Midwives (ACNM).

Fig. 2B

Figs. 2A and B: Adult Immunisation Guidelines (US 2015): (A) (by age) : Age based routine schedule for adults >19 years; (B) (by risk): recommendations for adults by comorbidities, immunocomprising conditions or specific risk factors. While based on US (ACIP) guidelines, this framework provides a critical reference for developing standardized adult vaccination schedules in India, particularly for high risk and elderly populations.
Source: Adapted from the Advisory Committee on Immunization Practices.

Phylogenetic analysis of hemagglutinin (HA) gene from India are matching with the WHO recommended Vaccine component of Southern hemisphere (SH) 2024 thus making it prudent to use SH 2024 quadrivalent vaccine in the coming season.

Japanese Encephalitis, Measles, Rubella Vaccines

The overall VE for JE was 77% in a case control study in Assam while a study from Pune highlighted the waning of immunity following childhood measles immunization and the need of adult vaccination. A study from a pediatric ophthalmology hospital in Madurai showed a significant risk among the HCWs to rubella as one-tenth of the HCWs were found to be seronegative and thus vulnerable and vaccinating them with RA 27/3 rubella vaccine would mount a protective response.[20]

Pneumococcal Vaccination

The vaccine is indicated for all individuals aged ≥65 years while can be administered for adults between 19- and 64-years including diabetes mellitus, chronic liver disease, chronic lung disease, increased risk of meningitis (cerebrospinal fluid leak, cochlear implant), IC conditions (HIV infection, hematologic malignancies) and impaired immunocompetence (functional or anatomic asplenia, nephrotic syndrome, and chronic renal illness).[5]

Venkitakrishnan et al. showed that there was a significant decrease in the multilobar consolidation in the vaccinated group ($p = 0.0001$) while fever, leukocytosis, elevated C-reactive protein and ICU care, inotropic support, and assisted ventilation was significantly higher in the unvaccinated group patients with exacerbation of chronic obstructive pulmonary disease (COPD), thus concluding that prior immunization with pneumococcal conjugate vaccine ameliorates the severity of exacerbation in COPD patients needing hospitalization.[21]

IMMUNIZATION POLICIES IN INDIA

There is no clear mandate on adult vaccination in India by National Technical Advisory Group on Immunization (NTAGI).

There needs an approach to assess risk factors and comorbidities among adults and have a phase wise coverage with the provision of subsidized vaccines and support for people living in hard-to-reach areas and tribal groups through the Ayushman Bharat scheme.[22]

There is an exhaustive consensus in 2024 by the Association of Physicians of India (API), in collaboration with the "Societies of Subject Experts" **(Table 2 and Box 1)**.[23]

TABLE 2: Indian consensus on recommendation of adult vaccines based on age.[23]

Age group (year)	*Recommended vaccines*
18–49	Chicken pox, cholera (at risk), COVID-19 (pandemic or epidemic), HBV, HPV, influenza, MMR, meningococcal, rabies (postexposure), TdaP (every 10 years), yellow fever (travelling to an endemic country), when there is additional risk factors—typhoid, Japanese encephalitis (JE), HIB, HAV, rabies (preexposure)
50–64	HBV, influenza, meningococcal, pneumococcal, TdaP (every 10 years), shingles, rabies (postexposure), COVID-19 (pandemic or epidemic), yellow fever (travelling to an endemic country), when there is additional risk factors typhoid, JE, HIB, HAV, HIB, cholera, rabies (preexposure)
≥65	HBV, influenza, pneumococcal, TdaP (every 10 years), shingles, RSV (above 60 years of age) rabies (postexposure), COVID-19 (pandemic or epidemic), yellow fever (travelling to an endemic country), when there is additional risk factors-typhoid, JE, HIB, HAV, rabies (preexposure)

(COVID-19: Corona virus disease of 2019; MMR: Measles, mumps, rubella; HIB: Hemophilus influenza B; HAV: hepatitis A virus; HPV: Human papillomavirus; RSV: Respiratory syncytial virus; Tdap: Tetanus, diphtheria, and pertussis)

BOX 1: Adult vaccination for special population as per API and CDC guidelines.[5]

- *Adults with compromised immune systems:* HIV/AIDS, neoplastic disorders post-transplantation states chronic medical conditions (hepatic, cardiovascular, respiratory, or metabolic diseases, pregnancy, aging or consuming alcohol, healthcare professionals, and travelers traveling to regions with endemic diseases
- *Influenza vaccine:* In all high-risk groups single dose of inactivated influenza vaccine or quadrivalent recombinant influenza vaccine (RIV4) annually. LAIV can be given among travelers and HCPs in the age group 18–49 years (API) and 19–49 years (CDC)
- *Pneumococcal vaccine:* 18–49 years one dose of PCV 13 and one dose of PPSV23 after a gap of 8 weeks to be administered in immunocompromised adults, individuals with asplenia, and kidney failure. In all the other high-risk groups one dose of PCV13 is followed by one dose of PPSV23 after 1 year (API). In the age group 19–64 years, who have not received a PCV13, PCV15, or PCV20 or unknown previous vaccination history one dose of PCV15 followed by one dose of PPSV23 at least after 1 year (at least 8 weeks apart for adults with immunocompromising condition, cochlear implant, or cerebrospinal fluid leak) (CDC)
- *Diphtheria pertussis and tetanus vaccine:* In each pregnancy, one dose of Tdap is recommended. In other high-risk groups Tdap one dose and then Td/Tdap at 1 month and between 6 and 12 months. Followed by Td/Tdap every 10 years
- *Hepatitis A vaccine:* Recommended for individuals with HIV infection and alcoholism, travelers, HCPs, immunocompromised individuals, and pregnant females if there is an additional risk. Two-dose series HepA (6–18 months apart) or three-dose series with HepA-HepB (0, 1, 3–6 months) (API)

Contd...

Contd...

- Two-dose series HepA or three-dose series HepA–HepB (0, 1, and 6 months). *In travelers:* Three doses (at 0, 7, and 21–30 days) followed by a booster dose at 12 months (CDC)
- *Hepatitis B vaccine:* Recommended in all high-risk group individuals—three doses (0, 1, and 6 months) (API), CDC—two-dose schedule (at least 4 weeks apart); Three-dose schedule at 0, 1, and 6 months; Three-dose schedule HepA-HepB at 0, 1, and 6 months; Four-dose series accelerated schedule of three doses (at 0, 7, and 21–30 days), a booster dose at 12 months
- *Cholera vaccine:* Travelers (18–64 years) at high risk and given based on benefit-risk evaluation in HCPs. Two doses (at least after 2 weeks) (API) and CDC: Recommended in travelers (18–64 years) CVD 103-HgR 1 dose if traveling to areas of active cholera transmission
- *Yellow fever vaccine: Travelers as a single dose.*
- *Rabies vaccine (not used in routine cases):* Used in people at risk of exposure, all animal bite victims of category II and III. API: Preexposure prophylaxis—three doses (0, 7, and 21–28 days); For postexposure—four doses (0, 3, 7, and between 14 and 28 days); For elderly postexposure—five doses (0, 3, 7, 14, and 28 days) CDC: Preexposure prophylaxis—two doses (0 and 7 days); Postexposure prophylaxis—4 (0, 3, 7, and 14 days) doses. Vaccinated—need only two doses of rabies vaccine after an exposure
- *Polio vaccine:* Recommended in travelers and HCPs (in contact with an infected person)
- API: Vaccinated—One dose IPV; Unvaccinated: Three doses (0, 1, 6–12 months) CDC: Unvaccinated—three doses (0, 1, 6–12 months). Accelerated schedule if protection needed for ≥ 8 weeks (three doses of IPV at least 4 weeks apart) in vaccinated—one dose IPV
- *Meningococcal (conjugate vaccine):* Recommended in HIV infection, asplenia, complement deficiency—two doses (at least after 8 weeks). Travelers (Haj pilgrimage) need single dose. Revaccination after every 5 years if risk persists

(AIDS: Acquired immunodeficiency syndrome; API: The Association of Physicians of India; CDC: Centre for disease control; HCP: Healthcare professional; HepA: Hepatitis A; HepA-HepB: HepA-hepatitis B; HIV: Human immunodeficiency virus; IPV: Inactivated polio vaccine; LAIV: Live attenuated influenza vaccine; PCV: Pneumococcal conjugate vaccine; PPSV: Pneumococcal polysaccharide vaccine; Td: Diphtheria (reduced dose) and tetanus vaccine; Tdap: Diphtheria, tetanus and acellular pertussis vaccine)

FUTURE BREAKTHROUGH

The immunization target is expected to reach 95% or beyond for the target age group with improved coverage of the childhood immunization program. Few steps can be introduced, helping to achieve this target:

- Recommendations for adult vaccination by NTAGI.
- Improved recording and reporting system for VPDs with age group wise data.
- Public and healthcare provider education and awareness on increased utilization of vaccines.

- Systematic mechanisms for vaccination of high-risk adult population.
- More operational research on understanding acceptance and practice toward adult vaccination.
- Education of healthcare providers and members of professional association.
- Inclusion of vaccination for all age groups into package of services offered through government primary healthcare facilities and that of health and wellness centers (HWCs) under Ayushman Bharat program of India.[1]

CONCLUSION

There has been a significant improvement in the vaccination programs both globally and in India since >4 decades after EPI and UIP with higher coverage and more sustained coverage resulting in epidemiological shift with the disease prevalence in higher age group. The traditional childhood vaccination programs all over the world are transitioning toward "child and adolescent vaccination programs" with adult vaccination being a next step to maximize the full benefits.[1]

Vaccination programs in India would need a focus on:
- Increasing awareness around vaccine-preventable diseases among adults and HCWs.
- Actively engaging healthcare systems and community-based organizations.
- Developing and producing affordable, safe, and country-appropriate vaccines with effective communication strategies and tools.[20]

SUMMARY

Previously, the main focus of the vaccination has been for the pregnancy and pediatric subpopulation. But now the time has come where it needs to be shifted to the vulnerable geriatric and IC group due to decline in intrinsic resilience.

Adult immunization should now be considered as a novel healthcare priority incorporating the WHO framework of promoting healthy aging.[24]

REFERENCES

1. Lahariya C, Bhardwaj P. Adult vaccination in India: Status and the way forward. U.S. National Library of Medicine. 2020;16(7):1508-10.
2. Guidelines for vaccination in normal adults in India. Indian J Nephrol. 2016; 26(1):S7-14.
3. Apiindia.org. Indian consensus guideline on adult immunization. [Online] Available from https://apiindia.org/reader/Indian%20Consensus%20 Guideline%20on%20Adult%20Immunization [Last accessed August, 2025].

4. Faujdar DS, Kaushik SK, Sharma P, Yadav AK. Need to study the health impact and economics of adult vaccination with India in Focus. Indian J Community Med. 2022;47(4):471-5.
5. Gupta M, Bansal A, Mehta A, Sharma N. Need and rationale of the adult immunisation in India: A review. Preventive Medicine: Research & Reviews. 2024;2(2):76-86.
6. Vaid A, Rastogi N, Doherty TM, San Martin P, Chugh Y. Review of the unmet medical need for vaccination in adults with immunocompromising conditions: An Indian perspective. Hum Vaccin Immunother. 2023;19(2).
7. Bianchi FP, Tafuri S. Vaccination of elderly people affected by chronic diseases: A challenge for public health. Vaccines (Basel). 2022;10(5):641.
8. Xu W, Wong G, Hwang YY, Larbi A. The untwining of immunosenescence and aging. Semin Immunopathol. 2020;42(5):559-72.
9. Jansen KU, Knirsch C, Anderson AS. The role of vaccines in preventing bacterial antimicrobial resistance. Nat Med. 2018;24(1):10-9.
10. Fleming-Dutra KE, Hersh AL, Shapiro DJ, Bartoces M, Enns EA, File TM Jr, et al. Prevalence of inappropriate antibiotic prescriptions among US ambulatory care visits, 2010-2011. JAMA. 2016;315(17):1864.
11. Bonanni P, Sacco C, Donato R, Capei R. Lifelong vaccination as a key disease prevention strategy. Clin Microbiol Infect. 2014;20(5):32-6.
12. Peleg AY, Weerarathna T, McCarthy JS, Davis TME. Common infections in diabetes: pathogenesis, management and relationship to glycemic control. Diabetes Metab Res Rev. 2007;23(1):3-13.
13. llard R, Leclerc P, Tremblay C, Tannenbaum T-N. Diabetes and the severity of pandemic influenza A (H1N1) infection. Diabetes Care. 2010;33(7):1491-3.
14. Kwong JC, Schwartz KL, Campitelli MA, Chung H, Crowcroft NS, Karnauchow T. Acute myocardial infarction after laboratory confirmed influenza infection. N Engl J Med. 2018;378(4):345-53.
15. Buckley BS, Henschke N, Bergman H, Skidmore B, Klemm EJ, Villanueva G, et al. Impact of vaccination on antibiotic usage: a systematic review and meta-analysis. Clin Microbiol Infect. 2019;25(10):1213-25.
16. Bonanni P, Bonaccorsi G, Lorini C, Santomauro F, Tiscione E, Boccalini S, et al. Focusing on the implementation of 21st century vaccines for adults. Vaccine. 2018;36(36):5358-65.
17. Kyaw MH, Rose CE Jr, Fry AM, Singleton JA, Moore Z, Zell ER, et al. The influence of chronic illnesses on the incidence of invasive pneumococcal disease in adults. J Infect Dis. 2005;192(3):377-86.
18. Hasan T, Lynch M, King C, Wehbe C, Plymoth M, Islam MS, et al. Vaccine-preventable disease outbreaks among healthcare workers: A scoping review. Clin Infect Dis. 2024;79(2):555-61.
19. Kim DK, Bridges CB, Harriman KH, on behalf of the Advisory Committee on Immunization Practices. Advisory committee on immunization practices recommended immunization schedule for adults aged 19 years or older: United States, 2015. Ann Intern Med. 2015;162(3):214-23.
20. Bhattacharyya A, Shahabuddin SM. Adult vaccination in India: A rapid review of current status & implementation challenges. Indian J Med Res. 2024;160 (3 & 4):279-92.

21. Venkitakrishnan R, Vijay A, Ramachandran D, Cleetus M, Nirmal AS, John S. Severity of exacerbation in pneumococcal vaccinated versus unvaccinated patients with exacerbation of chronic obstructive pulmonary disease: A post hoc analysis of presentation status of the subjects of HOPE chronic obstructive pulmonary disease study. J Advanced Lung Health. 2024;4(2):77-85.
22. Singh D, Sinha A, Kanungo S, Pati S. Disparities in coverage of adult immunization among older adults in India. Vaccines (Basel).2022;10(12):2124.
23. Dash R, Agrawal A, Nagvekar V, Lele J, Di Pasquale A, Kolhapure S, et al. Towards adult vaccination in India: a narrative literature review. Hum Vaccin Immunother. 2020;16(4):991-1001.
24. Vora A, Pasquale AD, Kolhapure S, Agrawal A. Vaccination in older adults: An underutilized opportunity to promote healthy aging in India. Drugs & Aging, Springer International Publishing. 2021;38:469-79.

18

CHAPTER

Infection Control during Pandemics and Outbreaks

Shaik Arif Pasha, Naseema Shaik, Siva Prabodh Vuddandi

LEARNING OBJECTIVES

- ICU Infection epidemiology.
- Core prevention practices.
- Environmental and engineering controls.
- Prevention of device-associated infections.
- Outbreak management.

INTRODUCTION

Pandemics will continue to force critical care units to act outside their normal processes. The practices are drawn from the existing Centers for Disease Control and Prevention (CDC) recommendations and represent fundamental standards of care that are not expected to change based on emerging evidence or technology or practice changes and are applicable across the continuum of healthcare settings. Intensive care units (ICUs) face significant challenges in infection control, requiring a multidisciplinary approach, heightened awareness, and constant vigilance among healthcare workers (HCW).[1]

EPIDEMIOLOGY OF INTENSIVE CARE UNIT'S INFECTIONS DURING PANDEMICS AND OUTBREAKS

During pandemics and outbreaks, ICUs are crucial for managing critically ill patients but are also high-risk areas for healthcare-associated infections (HAIs), which can worsen outcomes. Understanding ICU infection epidemiology is essential to enhance care and prevent pathogen spread.[2]

Common Pathogens in Intensive Care Unit Settings during Pandemics

During pandemics and outbreaks, ICUs often encounter a surge in infections caused by the following pathogens **(Table 1)**:

Source of Infection

Based on carrier status, types of infections in ICU have been divided into the following categories:

- *Primary endogenous infections:* Occur early (within 1st week of ICU admission), often brought into the ICU by the patient (e.g., *Streptococcus pneumoniae* infection).

TABLE 1: Types of pathogens.

Bacteria	*Viruses*	*Fungi*
Multidrug-resistant organisms (MDROs): • *Klebsiella pneumoniae* • *Pseudomonas aeruginosa* • *Acinetobacter baumannii* • *Methicillin-resistant Staphylococcus aureus (MRSA),* • *Vancomycin resistant enterococci (VRE)* • *Carbapenem resistant Enterobacteriaceae (CRE)* • *Clostridium difficile*	• Pandemic-causing viruses such as SARS-CoV-2 (COVID-19), Influenza A (H1N1), and Middle East Respiratory Syndrome Coronavirus (MERS-CoV) • Cytomegalovirus (CMV)	• *Candida* species • *Aspergillus* species • *Candida auris* (multi-antifungal resistant)

- *Secondary endogenous infections:* Occur after 1 week of ICU stay, caused by aerobic multidrug-resistant (MDR) organisms colonizing on the skin surface.
- *Exogenous infections:* ICU-acquired infections caused by MDR nosocomial pathogens, transmitted through HCWs' hands or contaminated surfaces, and are more feasible to control through high-level hygiene compliance.

Modes of Transmission

The ICU infections are transmitted through various routes, including:

- *Direct contact:* Contaminated hands of HCW, inadequately sterilized medical equipment.[3]
- *Airborne transmission:* Aerosolized particles from infected patients, particularly for pathogens such as severe acute respiratory syndrome coronavirus 2 (SARS-CoV-2) and Influenza.[4]
- *Droplet transmission:* Larger respiratory droplets during procedures like intubation or suctioning.[5]
- *Fecal-oral transmission:* Contaminated surfaces.
- *Environmental contamination:* Pathogens persisting on surfaces such as bedrails, ventilators, and monitors.[6]

RISK FACTORS IN INTENSIVE CARE UNIT SETTINGS

The ICU patients are more likely to get infections than ward patients for a number of reasons:

- *Severity of illness:* ICU patients' severe diseases deplete energy supplies, lower immune function, and increase susceptibility to colonization by exogenous organisms.

- *Immunosuppression:* Pain, anxiety, and isolation (physiological stressors) can weaken the immune system and make patients more vulnerable to infections.
- *Increased device use:* Central lines, catheters, and ventilators increase infection risk.
- *Prolonged hospital stays:* Longer ICU stays heighten exposure risks.
- *Age and comorbidity:* Elderly patients and those with conditions like diabetes are more susceptible.
- *Indiscriminate antibiotic use:* Overprescribing broad-spectrum antibiotics promotes resistance.
- *Stress ulcer prophylaxis:* Routine antacid and proton pump inhibitor use may increase infection risk.
- *Sleep deprivation:* Inadequate sleep exacerbates stress and potentially alters immune function.
- *Malnutrition:* Hypoalbuminemia and inadequate calorie intake increase susceptibility to infections.
- *Understaffing:* Inadequate nurse-to-patient ratios compromise infection control practices.

LESSONS LEARNED FROM PAST PANDEMICS

- *Enhanced infection prevention measures:*
  - Universal masking, enhanced hand hygiene, and use of personal protective equipment (PPE) were critical during the COVID-19 pandemic.[7]
  - Rigorous disinfection protocols for equipment and environmental surfaces.[8]
- *Surveillance and early detection:* Implementation of rapid diagnostic tools for early pathogen detection.[9] Real-time surveillance systems to monitor infection trends.[4]
- *Antimicrobial stewardship:*
  - Judicious use of antibiotics and antifungals to prevent resistance.[10]
  - Education of HCW on appropriate antimicrobial use.[11]
- *Healthcare system resilience:*
  - Investment in ICU infrastructure and staffing.[12]
  - Establishment of surge capacity plans to handle increased patient loads.[13]
- ***Research and collaboration:***
  - International collaboration in sharing data and resources.[14]
  - Accelerated development of vaccines and therapeutics.[15]

KEY INFECTION PREVENTION STRATEGIES

Standard Precautions

Healthcare workers should adhere to standard precautions when providing patient care. These safety measures are given in the following text.

Hand Hygiene

Importance and Techniques

Hand hygiene is the most fundamental practice of infection prevention. The World Health Organization (WHO) recommends:

- *Hand rub:* Alcohol-based 70–80% ethyl alcohol or 0.5–4% chlorhexidine hand-rub should be available at every bedside and as a pocket hand-rub. Hand-rub should be used whenever there is WHO's indication of "My Five Moments for Hand Hygiene" **(Fig. 1)**.
- *Handwash* with 4% chlorhexidine is preferred for *Clostridium difficile* infection. Washbasins should be elbow/foot-operated and placed near the ICU entrance and at key points within the ICU to provide ease of access to caregivers **(Table 2)**.

Strategies to Improve Adherence

- *Behavioral interventions:* Use of reminders and visual aids **(Fig. 2)**.

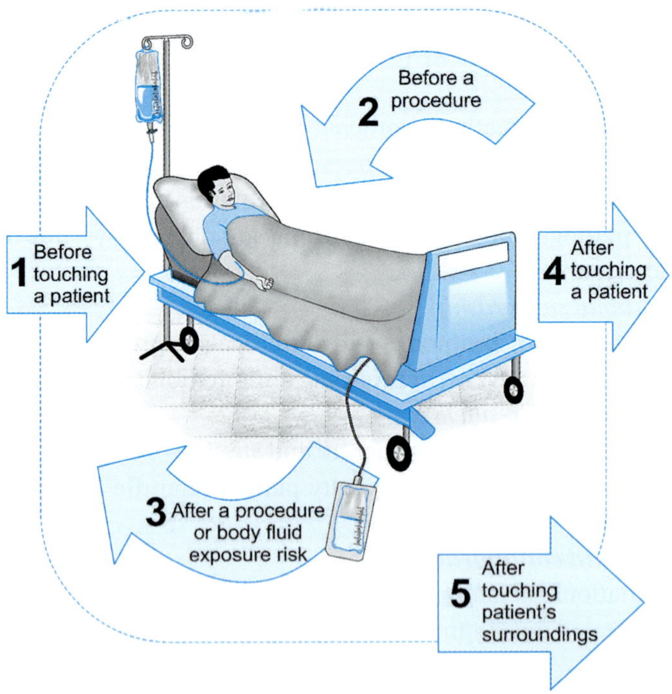

Fig. 1: My five moments for hand hygiene.
Source: World Health Organization (WHO).

TABLE 2: Indications for using hand rub, hand wash, and hand scrub.

Indications for using hand rub (20–30 seconds)	*Indications for using hand wash (40–60 seconds)*	*Indications for using hand scrub (3–5 minutes)*
• During five moments of hand hygiene • During routine rounds • In emergencies • When hands are not visibly soiled	• Visible dirt, blood, or body fluids • Potential exposure to spore forming organisms (e.g., *Clostridium difficile*); nonenveloped viruses (e.g. Norovirus, rotavirus, enteroviruses) • Handling patients having diarrhea • After using restroom • Before handling medication or food • After removal of gloves	Prior to any surgical procedure

- *Automated monitoring:* Real-time feedback systems for hand hygiene compliance include technologies such as wearable sensors that track hand movements, badges with proximity detection to remind users of hygiene practices, and software solutions integrated with hospital monitoring systems. These tools provide immediate data and alerts, ensuring adherence in ICU settings.[1]

Personal Protective Equipment

Appropriate PPE, including eye and face protection, gloves, and gowns, must be worn during procedures that may generate splashes or sprays of blood, body fluids, secretions, or excretions, or cause soiling of clothing **(Fig. 3)**.

- *Donning (wearing):* Gown first → Mask or respirator → Goggles or face shield → Gloves
- *Doffing (removing):* Gloves first → Face shield or goggles → Gown → Mask or respirator.

Challenges and Solutions in Maintaining Personal Protective Equipment Supplies

- *Challenges:* Supply shortages during peak outbreaks.
- *Solutions:* Stockpiling, local manufacturing, and implementing reusable PPE options where feasible.[3]

Training and Compliance Monitoring

- *Training:* Regular simulations and competency assessments.
- *Monitoring:* Use of infection control teams to oversee adherence.

Transmission-based Precautions

In addition to standard precautions, transmission-based precautions should be followed for patients with diseases having specific transmission modes **(Fig. 4)**.

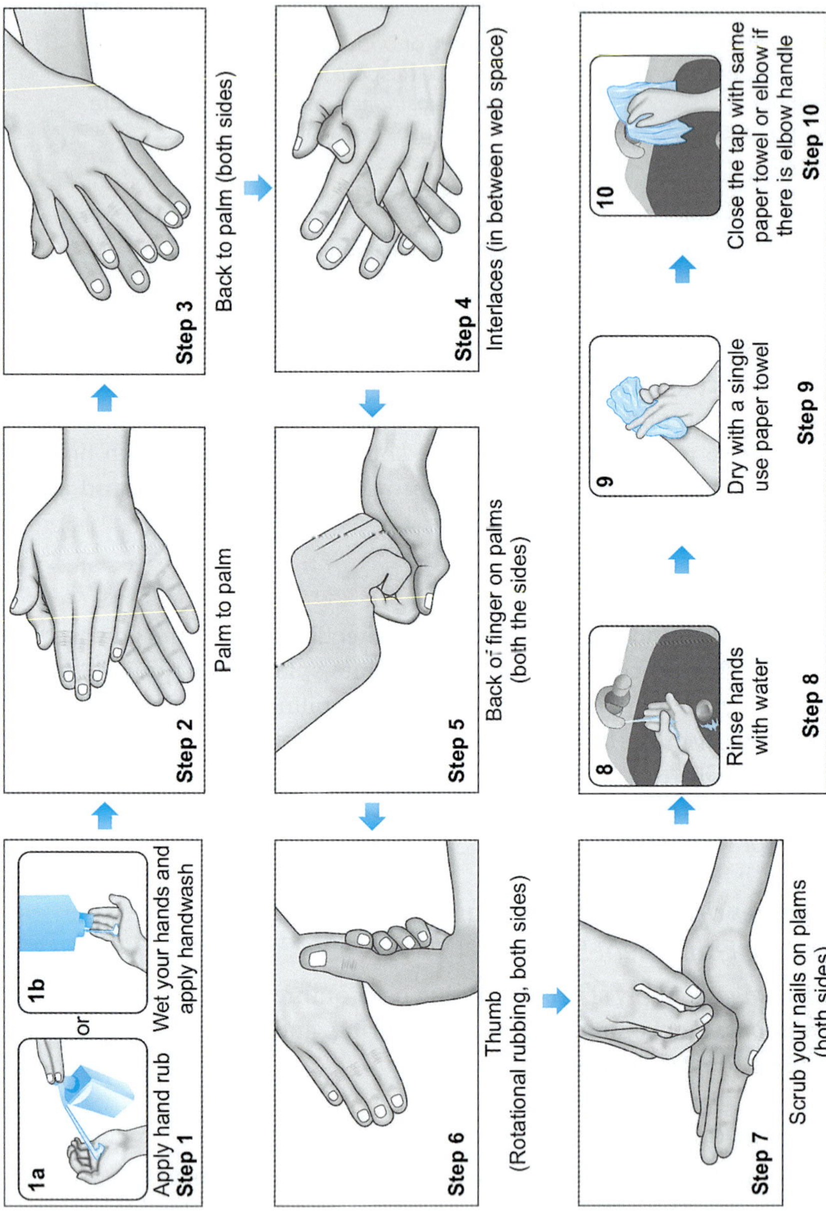

Fig. 2: Steps of hand hygiene.

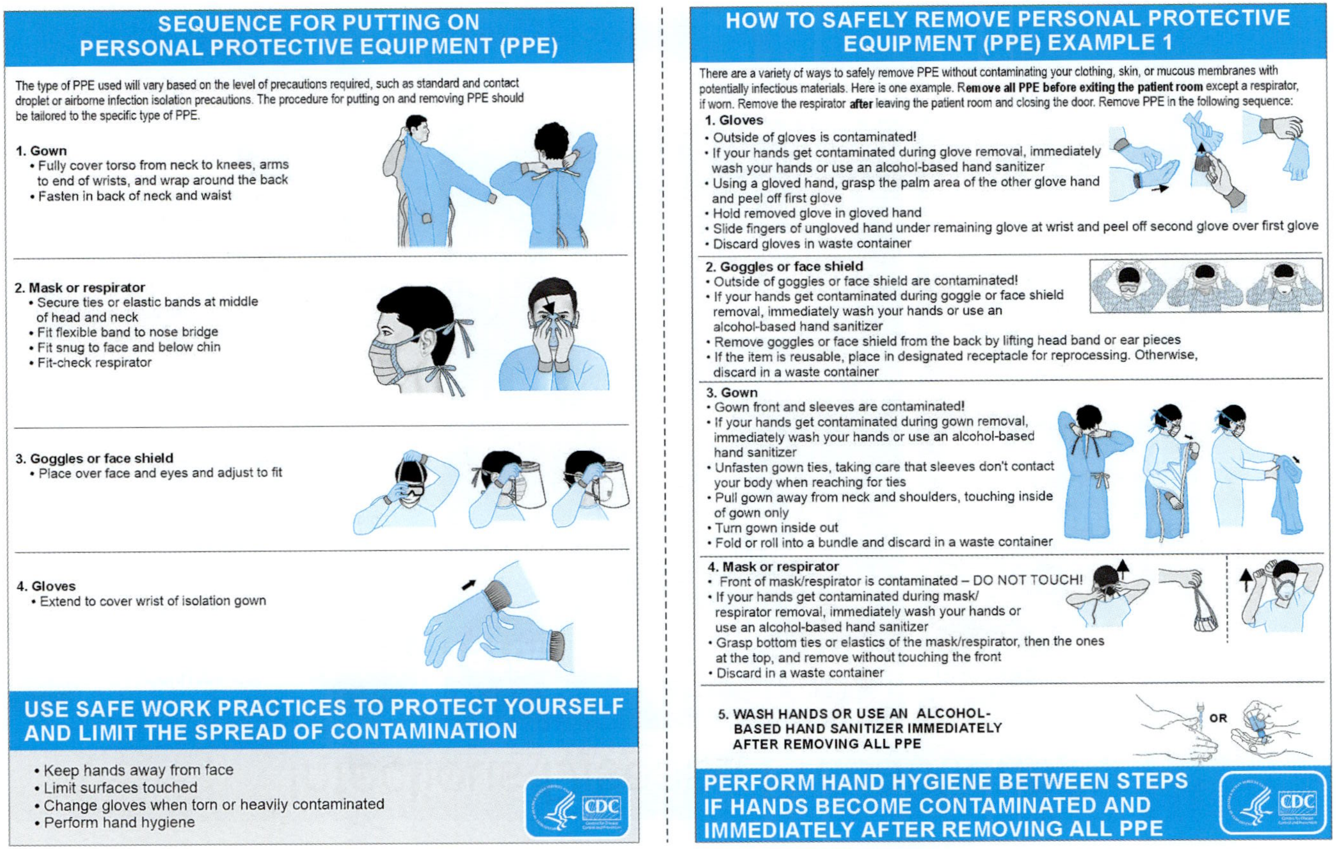

Fig. 3: Donning and doffing of personal protective equipment (PPE).

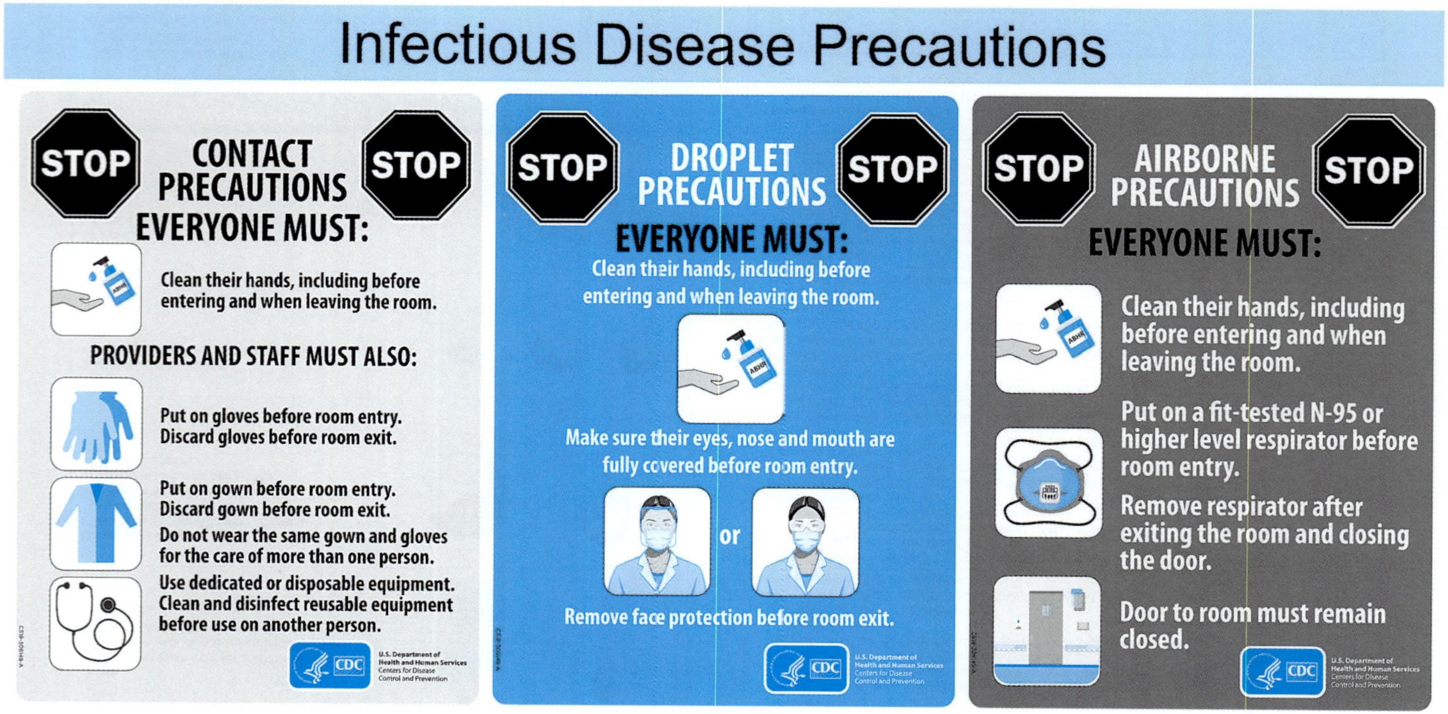

Fig. 4: Transmission-based precautions.

Contact Precautions

Implemented for patients with infectious agents spread via direct or indirect contact during care **(Fig. 5)**.

- *Direct transmission:* Person-to-person transfer without an intermediate object (e.g., contaminated hands or body fluids).
- *Indirect transmission:* Transfer via contaminated objects (e.g., clothes, devices, and surfaces).
- *Pathogens:* Methicillin-resistant *Staphylococcus aureus (MRSA), carbapenem resistant Enterobacteriaceae (CRE), vancomycin resistant enterococci (VRE), MDR Gram-negative bacilli, conjunctivitis agents, Group A Streptococcus, scabies, C. difficile, rotavirus, and hepatitis A and E.*
- *Infection control measures*
  - *Hand hygiene:* Strict adherence to prevent contact transmission.
  - *PPE:* Gloves, gowns; optional masks/eyewear for splashes.
  - *Equipment:* Use single-patient devices or clean/disinfect shared ones.
  - *Patient placement:* Prefer isolation rooms with bathroom; cohort if necessary, with spatial separation (>3 feet).
  - *Patient transfer:* Limit to essential purposes; if necessary HCW must wear PPE.
  - *ICU cleaning:* Frequent cleaning with detergent and disinfected with sodium hypochlorite (0.5%), especially of high-touch surfaces.

Droplet Precautions

Prevent the spread of agents via respiratory droplets (>5 μm) that require close contact (<3 feet). Droplets settle on surfaces, enabling contact transmission.

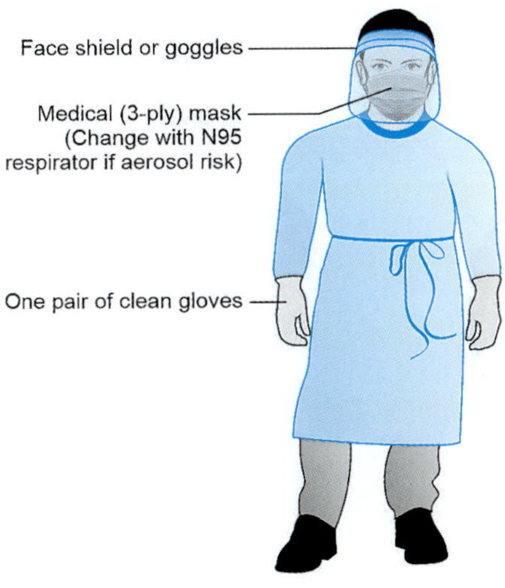

Fig. 5: Personal protective equipment recommended for healthcare workers while giving care in pandemic situations.

- *Pathogens:* Influenza, SARS-CoV2, mumps, rubella, etc.
- *Infection control measures:*
  - *Hand hygiene:* Essential to minimize contact transmission.
  - *PPE:* Surgical masks (for source control) and N95 respirator during aerosol generating procedures (AGPs); gloves, gowns, and eyewear for splashes.
  - *Patient placement:* Isolation rooms preferred; cohort or spatial separation of >3 feet with curtains in between beds if needed.
  - *Patient transfer:* Minimal, with patients wearing masks.
  - *Disinfection:* Disinfect daily all surfaces, equipment, and patient care items before use by another patient.
  - *Cough etiquette:* Cover nose/mouth, use tissues, and maintain distance (>1 meter). Hand hygiene should be done **(Fig. 6)**.

Airborne Precautions

Airborne transmission occurs when infectious agents are carried in fine aerosol particles (<5 μm). These aerosols are produced during certain aerosol-generating procedures—such as intubation, suctioning, bronchoscopy, tracheostomy care, and sputum induction. Because of their very small size,

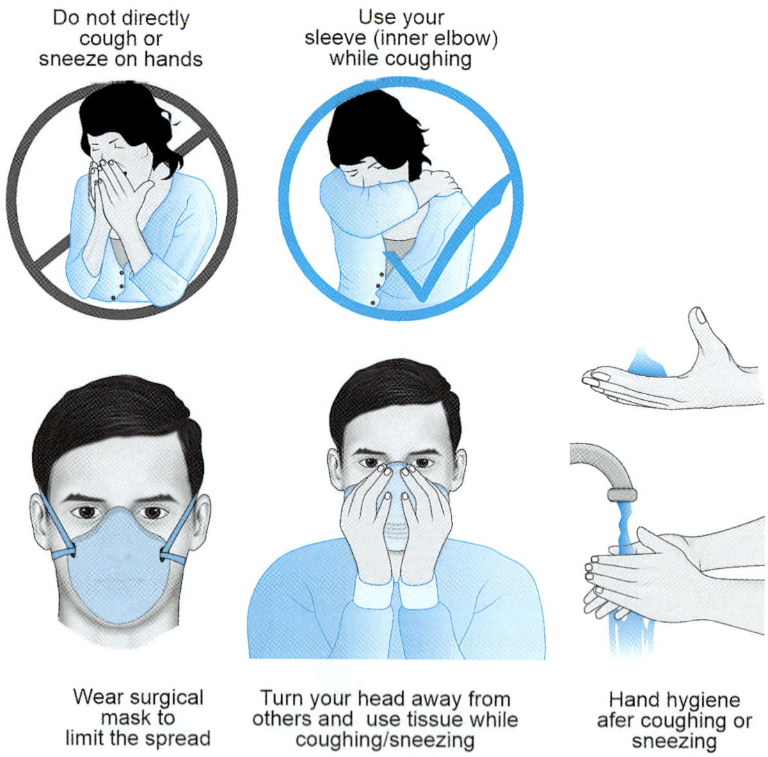

Fig. 6: Respiratory hygiene/cough etiquette.

these particles can remain suspended in the air for extended periods and may travel farther distances with air currents, increasing the risk of transmission.

- *Pathogens:* TB, measles, smallpox, and aspergillus.
- *Aerosol-generating procedures (AGPs):* Intubation, suctioning, cardiopulmonary resuscitation (CPR), and bronchoscopy.
- *Infection control measures:*
  - *PPE:* N95 respirators or higher with fit checking every time; gloves, gowns, and eyewear as needed.
  - *Patient placement:* Use airborne infection isolation rooms (AIIRs) with negative pressure ultraviolet germicidal irradiation (UVGI) and filtration.
  - *Patient transfer:* Minimize; patients wear masks, lesions covered.
  - *Visitor and staff restrictions:* Limit entry; ensure proper PPE use.
  - *Medication preparation* areas should be separate from patient care areas and maintained as clean areas.
  - *Soiled linen and waste storage:* The collected bedside trash should be kept apart from the places used for direct care and clean medication. All linens used for ICU patients should be cleaned with laundry detergent at 60–90°C, then soaked for about half an hour in 0.1% sodium hypochlorite before being dried.
  - *Sharps discarding* containers within easy access to each bed.
  - *Traffic low and accessibility:* Locate the ICU near the operating theater (OT) and emergency department for accessibility, while separating it from main ward areas. Implement policies to control traffic flow and minimize contamination sources from visitors, staff, and equipment.
  - Keep *windows* closed to control airborne risks. Avoid having plants and flowers in the ICU vicinity.

ENVIRONMENTAL LEANING AND INFECTION IN INTENSIVE CARE UNIT SETTINGS

In ICUs, stringent cleaning and disinfection protocols are critical to prevent healthcare-associated infections (HAIs). Effective environmental cleaning and disinfection protocols, incorporating advanced technologies such as ultraviolet (UV) light and hydrogen peroxide vapor, play a pivotal role in minimizing microbial contamination.[16]

Standard Cleaning and Disinfection Protocols

- *Routine cleaning:* Cleaning should be performed daily using detergents and disinfectants approved by the healthcare facility. High-touch surfaces, including bed rails, monitors, intravenous (IV) poles, and doorknobs, must be prioritized.
- *Terminal cleaning:* Terminal cleaning involves thorough cleaning and disinfection of all surfaces after patient discharge. Guidelines from the

CDC emphasize the use of Environmental Protection Agency (EPA)-registered hospital-grade disinfectants.

- *Chemical disinfectants:* Common agents include sodium hypochlorite, quaternary ammonium compounds, and hydrogen peroxide. Proper dilution and contact times must be adhered to for efficacy.

Ultraviolet Germicidal Irradiation

For disinfection where ventilation is inadequate along with negative pressure ventilation **(Fig. 7)**.

Mechanism of action: Ultraviolet germicidal irradiation (UVGI) utilizes ultraviolet-C (UV-C) light with wavelengths between 200–280 nm to inactivate microorganisms. UV-C damages the deoxyribonucleic acid (DNA) or ribonucleic acid (RNA) of pathogens, leading to the disruption of their replication and rendering them nonviable. This makes UVGI effective against bacteria, viruses, and fungi, including drug-resistant strains.

Intensity and exposure: The intensity of UV-C light is measured in microwatts per square centimeter ($\mu W/cm^2$). Recommended exposure times and intensity levels depend on the pathogen's resistance, typically guided by manufacturer instructions and validated studies. For example, UV-C light with an intensity of 100 $\mu W/cm^2$ may require an exposure time of 10–15 minutes to inactivate common pathogens such as MRSA or *C. difficile*. Far-UVC (222 nm) at 50 $\mu W/cm^2$ has been shown to reduce microbial load significantly within 5–10 minutes in experimental setups. Specific exposure parameters vary and must align with environmental conditions and device calibration.[17,18]

Placement: UVGI can be wall mounted installed at least > 2.5 meters (> 8 feet) from floor. UVGI devices can be installed as fixed overhead units or deployed as mobile units within ICUs. Placement must ensure optimal line-of-sight exposure to surfaces and air.

Ensure unobstructed airflow between the UV bulb and the air to be disinfected. Use transparent plastic covers to protect bulbs while

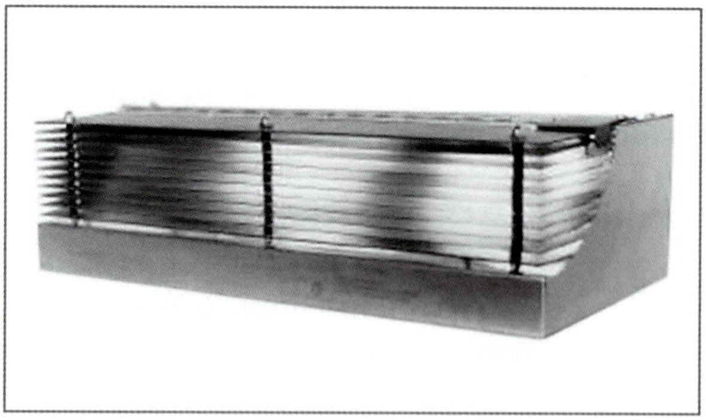

Fig. 7: Wall-mounted ultraviolet germicidal irradiation.

maintaining effectiveness. Secure on/off switches out of patients' reach. Apply nonreflective coatings (e.g., titanium dioxide) to walls and ceilings. Display clear warning signs near UVGI fixtures and on surrounding walls.

These guidelines ensure the safe and effective use of UVGI technology in reducing microorganisms and promoting a healthier environment.

Installation guidelines: Install units in areas with minimal shadowing to maximize efficacy. Conduct room mapping to identify high-touch zones and critical surfaces. Fixed UV-C systems may require integration with HVAC systems for air disinfection. Mobile units should be used systematically, ensuring comprehensive coverage through programmed pathways.

Maintenance-lamp replacement: UV-C lamps degrade over time and typically require replacement after 9,000–12,000 hours of use.

Surface cleaning: Lamps and reflective surfaces must be cleaned regularly with spirit to prevent dust accumulation, which can impede UV-C output (violet blue glow).

Monitoring: Install sensors to measure UV-C intensity and ensure consistent performance.

Calibration: Periodic calibration of devices ensures alignment with manufacturer specifications.

Limitations: Direct exposure can harm skin and eyes; safety measures such as shields and motion detectors are necessary. UV-C is ineffective on soiled surfaces; precleaning is essential.

Ventilation and Role of Negative Pressure Rooms

Ventilation in ICU settings: Effective ventilation systems in ICU settings are essential to control airborne transmission of pathogens. Ventilation ensures adequate air exchange, minimizes contaminant buildup, and maintains optimal indoor air quality.

Air changes per hour (ACH): Guidelines recommend at least 12 ACH for new ICU constructions and six ACH for existing facilities.

Filtration: High-efficiency particulate air (HEPA) filters are used to remove particles as small as 0.3 microns, including airborne bacteria and viruses.

Monitoring: Continuous monitoring of air quality parameters, such as carbon dioxide levels and particle counts, is critical to ensure system effectiveness.

Negative pressure rooms: Negative pressure rooms are designed to prevent the spread of airborne infections by creating a pressure differential between the room and adjacent areas.

Mechanism: Air flows into the room from hallways or adjoining spaces, preventing contaminated air from escaping. The air is then filtered through HEPA systems and exhausted outside the building.

Applications: Negative pressure rooms are particularly essential for patients with airborne diseases, such as TB or COVID-19.

Standards: The CDC and American Society of Heating, Refrigerating, and Air-Conditioning Engineers (ASHRAE) recommend maintaining a minimum pressure differential of 2.5 Pascals (Pa) between the isolation room and adjacent spaces.[7,19]

Installation and Maintenance

Design considerations: Proper room sealing, anterooms, and monitoring systems are critical to maintain pressure differentials.

Regular inspections: Systems should be inspected and tested regularly to ensure compliance with standards.

Backup systems: Emergency backup systems are recommended to maintain negative pressure during power outages.

Recent advances-smart ventilation systems: Integration with Internet of Things (IoT) technologies for real-time monitoring and adjustments.

UV-C integrated systems: Combining HEPA filtration with UV-C light for enhanced air disinfection.

Energy efficiency: Modern systems focus on energy efficiency without compromising airflow or filtration standards.[20,21]

FILTRATION

High-efficiency Particulate Air Filters and Portable Air Cleaning Devices in Intensive Care Unit

Importance of Air Purification in ICUs: ICUs require rigorous infection control measures to protect vulnerable patients from airborne pathogens. High-Efficiency Particulate Air (HEPA) filters and portable air cleaning devices can play a crucial role in reducing airborne pathogens and improving patient outcomes.

High-efficiency Particulate Air Filters

Capture 99.97% of particles: HEPA filters remove airborne pollutants, allergens, and bacteria as small as 0.3 microns. By removing airborne pathogens, HEPA filters help reduce the risk of HAIs in ICU patients.

Portable Air Cleaning Devices

- *Flexibility and convenience:* Portable devices are easy-to-move and place in different areas of the ICU.
- *Improved air quality:* Portable air cleaners help remove airborne pollutants, allergens, and bacteria, promoting a healthier environment.
- *Reduced risk of HAIs:* Portable devices can help reduce the risk of HAIs by removing airborne pathogens.
- *Device placement:* Place portable air cleaners in areas where they can most effectively capture airborne pathogens.
- *Filter selection:* Choose devices with HEPA filters or those with antimicrobial properties.
- *Maintenance and upkeep:* Regularly maintain and replace filters to ensure the device remains effective.
- ***Integration with existing infection control measures:*** Use HEPA filters and portable air cleaners as part of a comprehensive infection control strategy.[22]

BUNDLE CARE APPROACH FOR PREVENTION OF DEVICE-ASSOCIATED INFECTIONS IN INTENSIVE CARE UNIT

Device-associated infections (DAIs) are a significant concern in ICU settings, where patients are more vulnerable to infections due to their critical condition. The majority of DAIs are:

- Central line-associated bloodstream infections (CLABSI) **(Table 3)**
- Catheter-associated urinary tract infections (CAUTI) **(Table 4)**
- Ventilator-associated pneumonia (VAP) **(Box 1)**

By adhering to the bundle care approach and following strict aseptic techniques, ICU staff can significantly reduce the risk of DAIs and improve patient outcomes.[2]

TABLE 3: Bundle care central line.

Insertion bundle	*Maintenance bundle*
• Hand hygiene both prior to and following central line insertion • Wear the most sterile PPE possible, including a mask, gown, drapes, gloves, and a cap • *Insertion site:* Subclavian preferable; femoral • Preparing the skin using antiseptics like chlorhexidine • After using antiseptics, skin needs to be totally dry • Apply dressing that is semi-permeable • Document information and insertion time	• Aseptic central line care every day while handling • It is necessary to practice hand hygiene • Decontamination of the hub with alcohol • Monitoring local infection symptoms on a daily basis • Using 2% chlorhexidine to change the dressing • A daily evaluation of the central line's preparedness for removal needs to be recorded

TABLE 4: Bundle care for urinary catheter.

Insertion bundle	*Maintenance bundle*
• Only in cases with appropriate indication (such as acute urine retention) can a catheter be inserted • For catheter insertion, only sterile supplies are utilized • The catheter is implanted using a stringent asepsis and nontouch procedure • Use a closed drainage system • A suitable-sized catheter must be used • The catheter must be correctly fastened using the plaster-tube-plaster procedure following installation	• Regular daily catheter care (also known as vaginal or meatal care) requires stringent aseptic precautions, including hand washing and single-use gloves • The catheter is always correctly secured • The drainage bag needs to be below the bladder level and always above the floor • The closed drainage system is constantly in use • The following procedures must be followed while collecting urine from a bag: Hand washing, changing gloves between patients, using a different jug for every bag, and disinfecting the outlet with alcohol swabs • A daily evaluation of the catheter's preparedness for removal needs to be recorded

BOX 1: Maintenance bundle for mechanical ventilators.

- Hand hygiene adherence
- Raising the bed's head by 30–45° will stop oropharyngeal aspiration into the respiratory system
- Using a 2% chlorhexidine solution for daily dental care
- Every day, the necessity for prophylactic treatment for peptic ulcer disease (PUD) should be evaluated; if necessary, only sucralfate should be administered
- If necessary, prophylactic treatment for deep vein thrombosis (DVT) should be given
- A daily evaluation of the preparedness to remove the mechanical ventilator needs to be recorded

OUTBREAK MANAGEMENT IN INTENSIVE CARE UNITS[2,23]

Guidelines for outbreak control must be reviewed periodically and updated every 2 years. Epidemiological steps are described briefly below.

Preparation

- *Establish an outbreak control team:* Identify key personnel, including infection control specialists, ICU staff, and hospital administrators.
- *Develop an outbreak management plan:* Create a comprehensive plan outlining procedures for identifying, containing, and managing outbreaks.
- *Conduct regular surveillance:* Monitor ICU patients and staff for signs of infection or illness.

Identification

- *Recognize unusual patterns or clusters:* Identify unexpected increases in infections, illnesses, or deaths among ICU patients or staff.
- *Alert the outbreak control team:* Notify team members of potential outbreaks and initiate an investigation.

Investigation

- *Gather data:* Collect information on affected patients and staff, including demographic data, medical history, and treatment details.
- *Identify potential sources:* Investigate possible sources of the outbreak, such as contaminated equipment, environmental surfaces, or staff.
- *Perform laboratory testing:* Conduct laboratory tests to confirm the diagnosis and identify the causative agent.

Control and Containment

- *Implement infection control measures:* Enforce strict infection control protocols, including hand hygiene, PPE, and isolation precautions.
- *Isolate affected patients:* Separate affected patients from others to prevent further transmission.
- *Restrict staff movement:* Limit staff movement between affected and nonaffected areas.
- *Clean and disinfect:* Thoroughly clean and disinfect affected areas, equipment, and surfaces.

Communication and Collaboration

- *Notify stakeholders:* Inform hospital administrators, public health authorities, and other relevant stakeholders of the outbreak.
- *Collaborate with experts:* Seek guidance from infection control experts, epidemiologists, and other specialists as needed.
- *Keep patients and families informed:* Provide regular updates to patients and their families on the outbreak and control measures.

Evaluation and Review

- *Monitor the outbreak:* Continuously monitor the outbreak to assess the effectiveness of control measures.
- *Review and revise protocols:* Evaluate the outbreak response and revise protocols as needed to prevent future outbreaks.
- *Conduct an outbreak report:* Document the outbreak, including causes, control measures, and outcomes, to inform future outbreak management.[11]

CONCLUSION

Pandemics and outbreaks expose the ICU to heightened infection risks and demand exceptional vigilance from healthcare teams. Effective control depends on consistent application of standard precautions, appropriate use of PPE, and strict hand-hygiene practices. Strengthening environmental and engineering measures such as thorough disinfection, UV-based decontamination, optimized ventilation, and HEPA filtration—further limits transmission in critical-care areas. Device-related infections can be markedly reduced through adherence to evidence-based bundle care. A structured outbreak-management approach that emphasizes rapid detection, coordinated response, and continuous review is essential to contain spread and protect both patients and staff. By integrating these strategies, ICUs can maintain safe care delivery even during public-health emergencies.

REFERENCES

1. Centers for Disease Control and Prevention (CDC). CDC's Core Infection Prevention and Control Practices for Safe Healthcare Delivery in All Settings. [Online] Available from https://www.cdc.gov/infection-control/hcp/core-practices/index.html [Last accessed August, 2025].
2. Shastry AS, R Dheepashree. Essential of hospital infection control, 1st edition. New Delhi: Jaypee Brothers Medical Publishers; 2019.
3. Allegranzi B, Nejad SB, Combescure C, Combescure C, Graafmans W, Attar H, et al. Burden of endemic healthcare-associated infection in developing countries: systematic review and meta-analysis. Lancet. 2011;377(9761):228-41.
4. Klompas M, Baker MA, Rhee C. Airborne transmission of SARS-CoV-2: theoretical considerations and available evidence. JAMA. 2020;324(5):441-2.
5. Tran K, Cimon K, Severn M, Pessoa-Silva CL, Conly J. Aerosol generating procedures and risk of transmission of acute respiratory infections to healthcare workers: a systematic review. PloS One. 2012;7(4):e35797.
6. Tanner WD, Leecaster MK, Zhang Y, Stratford KM, Mayer J, Visnovsky LD, et al. Environmental contamination of contact precaution and non-contact precaution patient rooms in six acute care facilities. Clin Infect Dis. 2021;72(Suppl 1):S8-S16.
7. Centers for Disease Control and Prevention (CDC). (2020). COVID-19: How to Protect Yourself & Others. [Online] Available from https://www.cdc.gov/covid/prevention/index.html [Last accessed August, 2025].
8. Donskey CJ. Beyond high-touch surfaces: portable equipment and floors as potential sources of transmission of health care-associated pathogens. Am J Infect Control. 2020;48(5S):A90-A95.
9. Banerjee A, Kulcsar K, Misra V, Frieman M, Mossman K. Bats and coronaviruses. Viruses. 2019;11(1):41.
10. Spellberg B, Bartlett JG, Gilbert DN. The future of antibiotics and resistance. N Engl J Med. 2020;382(4):299-303.
11. Baur D, Gladstone BP, Burkert F, Carrara E, Foschi F, Döbele S, et al. Effect of antibiotic stewardship on the incidence of infection and colonisation with

antibiotic-resistant bacteria and *Clostridium difficile* infection: a systematic review and meta-analysis. Lancet Infect Dis. 2017;17(9):990-1001.

12. Rubinson L, Vaughn F, Nelson S, Giordano S, Kallstrom T, Buckley T, et al. Mechanical ventilators in US acute care hospitals. Disaster Med Public Health Prep. 2010;4(3):199-206.
13. Christian MD, Devereaux AV, Dichter JR, Geiling JA, Rubinson L. Definitive care for the critically ill during a disaster: a framework for allocation of scarce resources in mass critical care: from a Task Force for Mass Critical Care summit meeting, January 26-27, 2007, Chicago, IL. Chest. 2008;133(5 Suppl):51S-66S.
14. Peeri NC, Shrestha N, Rahman MS, Zaki R, Tan Z, Bibi S, et al. The SARS, MERS and novel coronavirus (COVID-19) epidemics, the newest and biggest global health threats: what lessons have we learned? Int J Epidemiol. 2020;49(3):717-26.
15. Sabin S, Gurwith M, Lock M, McVey D, MacLachlan I. Development of mRNA vaccines: scientific and regulatory issues. Vaccines (Basel). 2020;8(2):342.
16. Kampf G, Todt D, Pfaender S, Steinmann E. Persistence of coronaviruses on inanimate surfaces and their inactivation biocidal agents. J Hosp Infect. 2020;104(3):246-51.
17. Simmons S, Morgan M, Hopkins T, Helsabeck K, Stachowiak J, Stibich M. Impact of a multi-hospital intervention utilising a novel automated ultraviolet-C disinfection device on healthcare-associated infections. J Hosp Infect. 2021;107:133-40.
18. Buonanno M, Welch D, Shuryak I, Brenner DJ. Far-UVC light (222 nm): A new tool to reduce microbial contamination in ICU environments. Sci Rep. 2020;10(1):10285.
19. ASHRAE. ASHRAE Standard 170: Ventilation of Health Care Facilities. American Society of Heating, Refrigerating and Air-Conditioning Engineers; 2021. [Online] Available from https://www.mwhcec.org/wp-content/uploads/2023/11/D-11-14-2023-FINAL_-Std_170-2021-Wilson-Monroe.pdf [Last accessed August, 2025].
20. Escombe AR, Oeser CC, Gilman RH, Navincopa M, Ticona E, Pan W, et al. The role of ventilation in preventing airborne transmission in hospitals. Lancet Respir Med. 2020;8(10):931-4.
21. Beggs CB, Avital EJ. Upper-room ultraviolet air disinfection might help to reduce COVID-19 transmission in buildings: a feasibility study. PeerJ. 2020; 8:e10196
22. Centers for Disease Control and Prevention (CDC). Guidelines for Environmental Infection Control in Healthcare Facilities. CDC; 2020. [Online] Available from https://www.cdc.gov/infection-control/hcp/environmental-control/index.html [Last accessed August, 2025].
23. Centers for Disease Control and Prevention (CDC). Outbreak Investigations in Healthcare Settings. CDC Guidelines; 2020. [Online] Available from https://www.cdc.gov/healthcare-associated-infections/about/outbreak-investigations-in-healthcare.html [Last accessed August, 2025].

6

SECTION

Innovations and Future Directions

Section Editor: *Binila Chacko*

19

CHAPTER

Emerging Technologies and Innovations

Srinivas Samavedam, Afreen Kidwai Abdul Razak, Krishna K Chaitanya

LEARNING OBJECTIVES

- Understand the pathophysiological role of biomarkers.
- Learn the key aspects of using biomarkers for rapid diagnosis of infections.
- Know the novel tools that may be available for implementing infection control.
- Understand the role and limitations of machine learning in implementing infection control.

INTRODUCTION

Critical care, as a discipline, deals with patients afflicted with a wide variety of life-threatening conditions. Derangement of function is often seen in multiple organs at the same time. This derangement of function puts the life of the patient at immediate and persistent danger. Many support systems, devices, and gadgets are quite often needed to sustain the basic function of the compromised organs. In addition, multiple teams and medical professionals are closely involved in the care of such patients. Moreover, these patients often need to be transported out of the intensive care unit (ICU) for diagnostic and therapeutic procedures. These attributes put the patients at risk of acquiring infections inherent to a health care environment.

Traditionally, culture sensitivity reports have been used to tailor the antimicrobial prescriptions in ICUs. This approach still remains the yardstick of guided decision-making. However, the turnaround time of traditional culture methods ranges from 48 hours to five days. Clinical decision-making may sometimes have to be done in far less time. The search for the most definitive tool to help guide antimicrobial therapy continues. This is even more imperative in current times when the pipeline of newer classes of antimicrobials has run dry.

Several biomarkers have emerged and have been evaluated for their predictive and discriminative values. Although a biomarker that is exclusive to infection and sepsis remains elusive, some of them [C-reactive protein (CRP) and procalcitonin (PCT)] have found their way into well-validated and accepted algorithms related to antimicrobial stewardship (AMS). The availability of multiplex polymerase chain reaction (PCR) systems has added to the speed of organism detection and resistance pattern identification.

Big data analysis is the current norm for decision-making in most fields, including medicine in general and in ICUs in particular. Machine learning (ML) techniques promise to provide standard algorithms and decision-making trees for implementing AMS programs. This seems to be the way forward in personalized prescription of anti-microbials.

ROLE OF ARTIFICIAL INTELLIGENCE AND MACHINE LEARNING IN INFECTION DIAGNOSIS AND CONTROL

The application of artificial intelligence (AI) and ML in infection prevention in healthcare settings has evolved a lot. In the following sections, various models, data types, clustering algorithms, and clinical applications related to infection control will be discussed.

Early Warning Systems

Global Initiatives

- World Health Organization (WHO) Epidemic Intelligence from Open Sources (EIOS) system[1] represents a global collaboration between public health stakeholders with its "One Health" approach and focuses on early detection of public health threats from public sources.
- CDC's global robust surveillance systems supported electronic surveillance collaborations with over 45 countries,[2] with their focus on rapid response during health emergencies.[3]
- Early Warning Infectious Disease Surveillance Project (EWIDS) Program sponsored by the US-Mexico Border Health Commission, aims for cross-border early warning detection and operates within the Pandemic and All-Hazards Preparedness Act (PAHPA)[4] by involving local, state, and tribal health departments and providing epidemiology training.
- AI-powered Early Warning Systems supported by Trilateral's Health Cluster[5] have been supporting the development of AI-powered EWS, which can identify patterns and threats among vast amounts of data, enabling public authorities to anticipate and proactively manage public health crises and infectious diseases.

Implementation

- *Screening systems:* Temperature screening systems and data analysis systems are examples of this category. They help in screening large populations in the shortest possible time to identify potential carriers of infectious diseases.
- *Data sources:* Health records, social media data, and environmental data can be analyzed using ML algorithms to identify specific new patterns and presentations of disease, along with air quality indices, and help in predicting disease spread.

Detection of outbreaks: Clustering Algorithms are used for outbreak detection. Genuine outbreaks can be differentiated from random occurrences using likelihood ratio tests. These methods are often complemented by natural language processing, which extracts valuable inferences from unstructured data sources like clinical notes and research papers, enabling rapid information synthesis during critical early outbreak stages.

Disease-specific applications: El Morr et al. carried out a scoping review of all the models available for predicting outbreaks.[6] Several models for Dengue, Influenza, Malaria, and Cholera have shown a high level of efficiency in predicting outbreaks. Case surges during the COVID-19 pandemic were also predicted accurately by these models.

Clinical decision support systems: Elhaddad et al.[7-9] explored the useful impact of AI on Clinical Decision Support Systems (CDSS). AI models analyze real-time patient data, such as vital signs, laboratory results, and clinical notes, to detect early signs of sepsis. Predictive tools like ML algorithms can identify subtle changes in a patient's condition that may indicate the onset of sepsis hours before clinical symptoms become apparent. Reinforcement learning models can dynamically adjust treatment protocols for sepsis based on patient-specific responses, improving survival rates.

Personalized Intervention Recommendations

Data types for ML models: Machine learning models for infections have a variety of different data sources that feed into optimized user care. Clinical data, such as demographic details, medical history, laboratory results, and medication records, form the basis for personalized care. Microbiological data, like culture results or whole genome sequencing, further identify pathogen types and resistance profiles, leading to correct antibiotic selection. Epidemiological data, such as the prevalence of an infection and risk factors, help in prevention and treatment. Behavioral and socioeconomic data ensure that interventions remain practical and feasible. Lastly, genomic and proteomic data show genetic susceptibility to infections. Even environmental data on climate and sanitation increases the relevance of treatment recommendations.

Clinical applications of ML:

- Sepsis management in ICUs—prediction, early detection, and intervention
    - *Prediction:* Some models can analyze various risk factors such as patient demographics, medical history, and treatment protocols to identify patients at risk for developing HAIs.

Early detection and intervention: There are ML tools that can help improve diagnostic accuracy and reduce misdiagnosis and unnecessary treatment. ML models[10] can improve diagnostic accuracy by differentiating between acute inflammation and actual infections. This advancement can reduce the risk of misdiagnosis, unnecessary testing, and inappropriate treatments, thereby reducing healthcare costs.

Antimicrobial resistance and AI: Machine learning models can effectively predict resistance patterns, thus highlighting the potential for application of such models in diverse geographical settings to manage and control AMR.[11]

The application of unsupervised ML techniques,[12] such as K-means clustering and Principal Component Analysis (PCA), can be used to identify patterns in *AMR* gene data and new patterns in gene length and resistance classes that provide deeper insights into the mechanisms underlying AMR.

- *Personalized antibiotic therapy:* Machine learning models demonstrate high predictive performance in selecting appropriate antimicrobials and determining the optimal duration of therapy.[13]

  ProCCESs AWARE (Patient-centric Real-time Electronic Sepsis AwaREness), developed by Ambient Clinical Analytics in collaboration with Mayo Clinic, Rochester, is an advanced clinical decision support platform integrated with electronic medical records to support real-time decision-making in acute and critical care.[14]
  - Predicting infection risks in immunocompromised patients.
  - Various interventions for different types of infections.

  Machine learning algorithms vary in their approach based on the type of infection,[8,9] adapting to the unique characteristics and treatment requirements of bacterial, viral, or fungal infections.

  Based on the type of infections, ML can have various roles. In bacterial infections, the focus of ML could be to recommend antibiotics based on resistance patterns, minimizing unnecessary antibiotic use, and reducing resistance risks. In viral infections, ML may help in predicting viral shedding, disease progression, and response to antiviral treatments and can thereby help in personalizing antiviral therapy. In fungal infections, the focus of ML has been on predicting susceptibility to antifungal agents and customizing treatment strategies based on patient-specific data.
- *Role of AI and ML in resource allocation:* Critical challenges in healthcare operations, such as resource allocation, staffing, patient scheduling, and cost efficiency, can be overcome by a mixed-integer linear programming (MILP) model.[15] ML systems can optimize healthcare resource utilization through Staff Deployment Optimization by Real-time adjustment of staffing levels based on patient load and Optimization of infection control specialist coverage.

Digital Technology for Early Detection and Treatment

The concept of "digital biomarkers," where physiologic and behavioral parameters that may indicate the early onset of illness, such as high resting heart rate, low heart rate variability, decreased blood oxygen saturation, disturbed sleep, and decreased physical activity, can help in early detection and prevention of infections.

- *Bioelectronic wearables:* Researchers at the University of Chicago and the University of California, San Diego have developed a bioelectronic wearable patch that targets antibiotic-resistant bacteria.[16] This device operates by delivering a gentle electric zap that reduces the activity of harmful genes in infectious bacteria, thereby inhibiting their growth.
- *AI-based wearable sensors:* Wearable Health Technology has seen the integration of AI, specifically ML and deep learning techniques. These sensors can predict the onset of infections, by measuring physiological data such as heart rate and skin temperature. This predictive capability is critical for early intervention and prevention of infections.
- *Electrodeposition technology:* To address the risk of infections caused by microbial contamination and skin irritation, electrodeposition technology has been applied to wearable devices. This process enhances the functional properties of wearables while minimizing the risks of infection through improved material surfaces that are less prone to harboring bacteria.
- *RATE Project by the US Department of Defense (DoD):* The DoD expanded its Rapid Assessment of Threat Exposure (RATE) project,[17] which uses wearable technology to detect infectious diseases. This project gained traction during the COVID-19 pandemic and aims to monitor health metrics to manage readiness and prevent infections among users.
- *Wearable sweat biosensors:* Wearable sweat biosensors are being developed to detect biomarkers related to infections that can provide non-invasive monitoring of physiological changes, which may indicate the presence of an infection, allowing for timely and targeted responses.
- *Wearable technology for predicting viral infections:* Researchers at Stanford Medicine, in collaboration with Fitbit and Scripps Research,[18] are working on using data from smartwatches to predict the onset of viral infections. By monitoring indicators such as heart rate and skin temperature, these devices can detect early signs of infection and potentially prevent the spread of contagious diseases.

Use of Rapid Diagnostics and Biomarkers

Sepsis triggers the innate immune system when pattern recognition receptors (PRRs) on host cells recognize pathogen-associated molecular patterns (PAMPs) or damage-associated molecular patterns (DAMPs). This activation leads to the release of pro- and anti-inflammatory mediators and acute-phase proteins such as PCT, calprotectin, pro-adrenomedullin, pentraxin 3 (PTX3), and CRP.[19]

Several biomarkers are being actively researched for their potential diagnostic and prognostic value in sepsis. Some of the more commonly studied biomarkers are summarized below:

- *Monocyte chemoattractant protein-1 (MCP-1):* MCP-1 is a soluble chemokine released by monocytes, endothelial cells, and fibroblasts. It initiates the inflammatory cascade and recruits immune cells to sites of injury. Elevated MCP-1 levels have been associated with organ dysfunction and poor outcomes in sepsis.
- *Soluble triggering receptor expressed on myeloid cells-1 (sTREM-1):* Expressed on neutrophils and monocytes, sTREM-1 plays a crucial role in amplifying cytokine release and inflammatory signaling during sepsis. Elevated serum levels of sTREM-1 serve as a useful diagnostic marker.
- *Soluble urokinase plasminogen activator receptor (suPAR):* suPAR is expressed on various immune cells and participates in cellular migration, adhesion, and angiogenesis. Elevated serum suPAR levels have been correlated with increased mortality, with a meta-analysis reporting an area under the curve (AUC) of 0.838 for predicting sepsis.
- *CD64 on neutrophils:* CD64, a high-affinity Fc gamma receptor I, is minimally expressed on resting neutrophils but markedly upregulated during early immune activation. The CD64 index has been proposed as a reliable and rapid diagnostic marker for sepsis.

In addition to these biomarkers, *rapid diagnostic tools* are increasingly being employed to complement clinical assessment and biomarker data. Molecular methods such as *polymerase chain reaction* and *next-generation sequencing (NGS)* applied directly to clinical specimens or cultures can enable *rapid identification of causative pathogens,* significantly reducing the time to targeted antimicrobial therapy.

Emerging biomarkers, including microRNAs, long noncoding RNAs (lncRNAs), and the human microbiome, are gaining prominence for diagnosing and predicting sepsis outcomes.

DIAGNOSTIC BIOMARKERS

Presepsin (sCD14-subtype)

A glycopeptide derived from bacterial lipopolysaccharides, presepsin has a key role in bacterial phagocytosis and lysosomal cleavage. Presepsin has been suggested as a possible biomarker for sepsis diagnosis.[20] Studies have shown that presepsin levels were significantly higher in sepsis compared to noninfected patients, with an AUC of 0.937 for diagnosing sepsis, outperforming PCT (0.915), interleukin-6 (IL-6) (0.86), and CRP (0.85). It has been noted that presepsin levels can vary between gram-positive and gram-negative bacterial infections, providing additional diagnostic utility.

Pentraxin 3

Pentraxin 3 (PTX3) is a long pentraxin produced by monocytes, dendritic cells, and macrophages upon exposure to microbial components or inflammatory cytokines that influences cell extravasation, complement activity, and pathogen resistance.[21] PTX3 levels have been shown to correlate with organ dysfunction scores such as Sequential Organ Failure Assessment Score (SOFA) and APACHE II, with an AUC of 0.798 for predicting septic shock in a prospective study on 101 patients.[21]

Calprotectin

Calprotectin, composed of S100A8 and S100A9 subunits, is involved in inflammatory signaling via MAPK, NF-kB, and PI3K pathways. A prospective study has highlighted its superiority over PCT in distinguishing bacterial infections from viral ones, with an AUC of 0.907. Havelka et al. showed Calprotectin was particularly effective in identifying bacterial pneumonia from viral pneumonia.[22]

PROGNOSTIC BIOMARKERS

Adrenomedullin and Midregional Proadrenomedullin

- ADM, a vasodilatory peptide produced by endothelial and vascular smooth muscle cells, is unstable due to rapid degradation. MR-proADM, a more stable fragment, accurately reflects ADM activity.
- MR-proADM predicts sepsis-related organ dysfunction 24 hours before its onset and correlates with severity scores such as SOFA, Pitt, and CPIS in a prospective study.
- Biologically active ADM (bio-ADM) is measured by a double monoclonal sandwich immunoassay and was found to be higher in septic shock patients.
- The AdrenOSS-1 study demonstrated that Bio-ADM levels normalize rapidly (<70 pg/mL) in survivors, linking normalization to reduced 28-day mortality and improved cardiovascular outcomes.[23]

Noncoding Ribonucleic Acid

- MicroRNAs (miRNAs): made up of 20–24 nucleotides; miRNAs regulate immune response pathways. miR-150, for instance, correlates with immune-related genes like TNF-alpha, IL-10, and IL-18, serving as a prognostic marker in sepsis.
    - *Long noncoding RNAs (lncRNAs):* lncRNAs such as NEAT1 and MALAT1 regulate inflammatory responses and cytokine release. MALAT1 has an AUC of 0.910 for predicting sepsis, outperforming APACHE II (0.868) and lactate levels in a prospective cohort analysis of 120 septic patients.

- In a recent study involving 219 sample size of, it shows a good predictive value in diagnosing sepsis if the plasma samples of lncRNAs are taken within 24 hours of admission.[24]

Angiopoietin

- Angiopoietin-1 and Angiopoietin-2 regulate vascular permeability. Elevated angiopoietin-2 and an increased angiopoietin-2/1 ratio are linked to poor prognosis in sepsis.
- A retrospective cohort study in ICU patients showed an AUC of 0.736 for predicting 28-day mortality, comparable to the SOFA score (0.745).[25]

NOVEL INFECTION PREVENTION TOOLS

Detection and Monitoring Technologies[26]

- *Bacterial imaging:* The MolecuLight i:X, a medical imaging device used for identifying bacteria in wounds a bedside device utilizing violet light for bacterial detection in wounds (>104 CFU/g) that captures fluorescent images without patient contact, where red fluorescence indicates most bacteria and cyan fluorescence indicates Pseudomonas with a 95% accuracy. It showed 300–400% better sensitivity than standard methods and demonstrated improvement in healing outcomes with reduced antibiotic use.
- *Real-time visual feedback systems:* Highlight (Kinnos) Technology is a color-additive technology for disinfectant wipes, providing real-time visualization that produces transient color on wiped surfaces, where the Color fades after effective cleaning. It showed Improved room cleanliness by 69.2% with a reduced turnover time by 5.9%.
- *Bioluminescence detection:* Adenosine triphosphate (ATP) testing that utilizes the firefly luciferase reaction for contamination measurement helps in providing real-time results available in under one minute and has applications in food safety and healthcare settings. A recent advancement of Total adenylate (A3) testing helps in the simultaneous measurement of ATP, adenosine diphosphate (ADP), and adenosine monophosphate (AMP) with enhanced detection capabilities over traditional ATP-only methods.
    - *Limitations:*
        - Cannot identify specific contaminants.
        - Potential interference from cleaning chemicals.
- *Digital contact tracing technologies:* Digital contact tracing has demonstrated significant advantages over traditional methods, despite the very low quality of evidence on the following areas:
    - *Enhanced contact identification:*
        - Doubled contact identification during Ebola outbreaks using mobile applications.

    - Identified over three times more contacts (45 vs. 13) during pertussis outbreaks using radio-frequency identification compared to medical record searches.
  - *Key advantages include:*
    - Faster data entry
    - Reduced data loss risk
    - Improved handling of large datasets
  - *Challenges in resource-limited settings:*
    - Higher implementation costs
    - Internet connectivity issues
    - Potential privacy breach concerns
- *Real-time face mask detection systems:* Recent advancements in real-time face mask detection have produced remarkable results through multiple AI-powered systems. One significant development is a Static and Real-Time Video Detection Model that has achieved exceptional accuracy in mask detection. This system, trained on a comprehensive Kaggle dataset of approximately 4,000 images, effectively classifies subjects into "with mask" and "without mask" categories, achieving an impressive 98% performance accuracy rate.

Even more sophisticated is the MobileNetV2-Based Classification System, which represents a significant leap forward in detection technology. This advanced system integrates the FaceNet model as a feature extractor and employs a feedforward multilayer perceptron for enhanced accuracy. The system was trained on an extensive dataset of 13,359 images, carefully balanced with 52.9% showing faces with masks and 47.1% without masks. The performance metrics of this system are particularly noteworthy, achieving an exceptional 99.52% accuracy in recognizing individuals wearing masks and an even more impressive 99.96% accuracy in identifying those without masks. These cutting-edge systems demonstrate the remarkable potential of AI in enhancing public health monitoring capabilities.

Disinfection Technologies[27]

Ultraviolet-C Applications

Recent studies have demonstrated varying effectiveness across different settings:

- *Equipment decontamination:* Wall-mounted far UV-C technology showed:
  - 3 log10 CFU reduction of C. auris after 8-hour exposure.
  - 2 log10 CFU reduction in 4 hours on portable equipment.
  - 3 log10 reductions of MRSA on 6 of 8 device sites.
- *Environmental decontamination:* The Benefits of Enhanced Terminal Room (BETR) Disinfection Study demonstrated:

- 10–30% reduction in pathogen acquisition.
- Effective against rooms previously occupied by patients with MDROs or *Clostridium difficile*.
- Limited efficacy in immunocompromised populations.

- *Advanced air purification:* Advanced air purification technology (AAPT) utilizing UVGI (UV germicidal irradiation) technology demonstrated a significant reduction in airborne fungal and bacterial levels with a 39.5% decrease in patient length of stay, 23% cost savings, and a 39.6% reduction in facility-acquired infections.

Compliance Monitoring Systems

Hand Hygiene Monitoring

Innovative systems

- *Novel hand sanitizer alternatives:* CG-101 represents a groundbreaking advancement in skin protection technology, utilizing a carefully formulated composition of 5% w/w biocompatible ionic liquids derived from choline and geranic acid. This innovative protectant has demonstrated remarkable performance in both laboratory and clinical settings. Studies have shown its robust ability to inactivate a broad spectrum of pathogens, including bacteria and human coronavirus (hCoV229E), with a distinctive feature being its extended protection duration of up to 4 hours after a single application. This longevity significantly surpasses the effectiveness window of traditional 70% ethanol-based sanitizers. Rigorous clinical trials have validated multiple aspects of CG-101's efficacy and safety profile. The trials confirmed not only its compatibility with human skin but also provided substantial evidence of its sustained antimicrobial protection capabilities. Furthermore, the studies documented comprehensive validation of its effectiveness against various infectious diseases, establishing CG-101 as a promising alternative in settings requiring long-term antimicrobial protection.
- *AI-powered systems*:
  The Soapy Clean Machine[28] features:
  - Touchless operation
  - Integrated sensors (sonars, camera, and thermometer).
  - Real-time analysis of handwashing technique.
  - Personalized feedback based on WHO recommendations.
  - Data tracking through the "SoapyWisdom" platform

Automated monitoring: Studies of automated hand hygiene reminder systems (AHHRS) showed:

- Significantly higher observation capacity (265,505 versus 2,642 events, $p < 0.01$).
- Improved hand hygiene adherence over time ($p < 0.001$).
- Reduced cross-contamination events, particularly in ICU settings ($p < 0.05$).

Specialized infection prevention and control (IPAC) management platforms: HealthConnex IPAC Management platform features a specialized platform for skilled nursing and senior living facilities across North America. It helps in real-time infection trend visualization across units without any requirement for external tools. It has:

- *A centralized, interactive dashboard displaying comprehensive data on*:
  - Residents
  - Staff
  - Visitors
- *An automated reporting capability:*
  - Infection rates analysis
  - Treatment tracking
  - Compliance audit generation

Robotic Solutions for Infection Control

Autonomous Disinfection Systems

Smart cleaner:[29]

- Autonomous indoor disinfection robot
- Utilizes drymist hydrogen peroxide
- *Validated effectiveness in multiple settings*:
  - Hospitals
  - Hotels
  - Offices
  - Laboratories
- Third-party verified results

Specialized Function Robots

Door handle cleaning robot.[30]

Features:

- RGBD and wide-angle cameras
- Deep learning-based detection
- 88–92% real-time detection accuracy
- 18-minute cleaning cycle for four handles

Environmental Disinfection Robots

Surface-specific solutions:[31]

- *GeckoH13:*
  - Wall and ceiling cleaning capabilities
  - Pneumatic vacuum cup system
  - Steam cleaning functionality
- *Swingobot 2,000:*
  - 360° sensor system

    - 76% reduction in water/chemical usage
    - Automated performance reporting
- *XDBOT:*
    - 6-axis arm design
    - Lidar and HD camera navigation
    - Electrostatic nozzle system
- *Jasmin:*
    - Multidisinfectant compatibility
    - Autonomous navigation
    - Human detection capabilities
- *Breezy one:*
    - Large-scale facility focus.
    - EPA-registered disinfectant use.
    - 99.9999% pathogen elimination.
    - 2-hour treatment cycle.

Emerging Technologies

- *Antimicrobial materials:* Research on antimicrobial textiles has shown mixed results:
    - *Copper-impregnated linens*: No conclusive evidence of HAI reduction.
    - *Iodine-impregnated incision drapes*: Reduced contamination during knee arthroplasty
    - *Silver nanoparticle-treated cotton*: Demonstrated antibacterial activity against *Escherichia coli* and *Staphylococcus aureus*.
- Novel personal protective equipment:
  A new antiviral face mask using soap-coated polymer filaments showed:
    - Rapid virus inactivation within one minute
    - Effectiveness against SARS-CoV-2 and phage Φ6
    - No cytotoxicity in human keratinocytes
    - Potential adaptability for other protective clothing

Technology-enhanced Diagnostic and Treatment Tools

Mobile Applications for Clinical Use

Antibiotic susceptibility testing:[32]

- AI-powered smartphone application for disk diffusion measurement
- *Features:*
    - Camera-based analysis
    - High agreement with manual and automated systems
    - Offline functionality
    - User-friendly interface
- Particularly valuable for resource-limited settings

Automated Antibiotic Stewardship

AI-powered auditing system:

- Developed by DXC and Singapore Government Hospital
- *Capabilities:*
  - Real-time analysis of antibiotic use patterns
  - Antibiotic recommendation system
  - *Processing speed:* <1 second per case (vs. 20 minutes manually)
- Pending resolution of data challenges for full implementation

Advanced Predictive Technologies

Antimicrobial Resistance Tools

- *AI-powered development platforms:*
  - Multichannel deep neural network (DeepBLI)
  - ML algorithms
  - DeepBL Deep Learning-Assisted Photochromic Sensor
  - ML-random forest model
- Enhanced accuracy in identifying resistance genes through DeepARG methodology.

Biofilm Analysis

Biofilm-i Platform

- Web-based prediction tool for biofilm inhibition.
- *Features:*
  - Chemical similarity searching.
  - Analog generation.
  - First regression-based prediction tool.
- It has many advantages over classification-based methods.

Artificial Intelligence-enhanced Laboratory Diagnostics

Matrix-assisted Laser Desorption Ionization–Time of Flight Mass Artificial Intelligence Integration

- *Applications:*
  - Microbial identification
  - Strain typing
  - Antimicrobial resistance detection
- *Implementation features:*
  - Computational preprocessing
  - ML models (Random Forest and Deep Learning)
  - Local model training for regional pathogen profiles
- Challenges with grey-zone predictions (0.4–0.48 probability range)
- Specific issues with certain *S. aureus* strains

Personalized Antibiograms

In a study by Corbin et al., ML models were developed to create personalized antibiograms using data from Stanford and Boston. The following are the inferences from these validation studies:

- *Stanford dataset:* 8,342 infections.
  - *Boston dataset:* 15,806 urinary tract infections.
- *Performance metrics:*
  - *Stanford:* 85.9% coverage (comparable to clinicians at 84.3%).
  - *Boston:* 90.4% coverage (superior to clinicians at 88.1%).
- *Impact on antibiotic stewardship:*
  - 69% reduction in vancomycin + piperacillin/tazobactam use at Stanford.
  - 48% reduction in ciprofloxacin use in Boston.

Educational and Quality Improvement Tools

Project Firstline

The Centers for Disease Control and Prevention's Project Firstline represents an innovative educational framework implementing a microlearning approach to infection prevention and control education. This national training collaborative provides the healthcare and public health workforce with timely, accessible, and accurate infection control education through adaptable modules designed for various healthcare settings.

Novel Auditing Tools

Kamishibai cards (K-cards), a three-part auditing tool consisting of "Show me at bedside," "Show me on the computer," and "Ask" components, have demonstrated significant effectiveness in infection control. Implementation at a 953-bed level one trauma teaching hospital over 32 months (January 2017–August 2019) achieved:

- 50% reduction in infection rates.
- CLABSI rates decreased from 2.2 to 1.1 per 1,000 device days.
- CAUTI rates reduced from 2.2 to 1.3 per 1,000 device days.

Electronic Communication Systems

A mandatory electronic communication tool (MECT) based on clinical practice guidelines showed remarkable results in a historical cohort study at an academic tertiary medical center, with:

- CLABSI rate reduced to 0/1,000 catheter days.
- 84% decrease in premature PICC removals (from 16 to 2.5%; $p < 0.0001$).
- Total complication rate decreased from 45.5% to 24% ($p < 0.0001$).
- 25% reduction in radiology costs.

CONCLUSION

- Emerging technologies are reshaping infection prevention in critical care by enabling faster diagnosis, smarter surveillance, and more targeted interventions. Advances in AI, machine learning, digital wearables, rapid diagnostics, and novel biomarkers now allow earlier detection of sepsis, improved antimicrobial stewardship, and personalized therapeutic strategies. At the same time, innovations such as UV-C systems, autonomous disinfection robots, enhanced hand-hygiene platforms, and intelligent PPE strengthen environmental and procedural safety.
- Together, these tools represent a shift toward a more proactive, data-driven model of infection control. As integration and validation continue, these innovations hold the potential to significantly reduce healthcare-associated infections and improve ICU outcomes.

REFERENCES

1. Fanelli A, Schnitzler JC, De Nardi M, Donachie A, Capua I, Lanave G, et al. Epidemic intelligence data of Crimean-Congo haemorrhagic fever, European Region, 2012 to 2022: a new opportunity for risk mapping of neglected diseases. Euro Surveill. 2023;28(16):2200542.
2. Donelle L, Comer L, Hiebert B, Hall J, Shelley JJ, Smith MJ, et al. Use of digital technologies for public health surveillance during the COVID-19 pandemic: A scoping review. Digit Health. 2023;9:20552076231173220.
3. Bridget M, Gebru GN, Odongo GS, Hedberg C, Elduma AH, Kanu JS, et al. Digitalizing disease surveillance: experience from Sierra Leone. Health Policy and Planning. 2025;40(1):85-96.
4. Aceves B, Lopez-Galvez N, Rangel G, Gonzalez-Fagoaga E, Zapata-Garibay R, Rosales C. Virtual Seminar on Coronavirus 2019 for the US-Mexico Border Region: Building Opportunities for Communication and Collaboration. J Immigr Minor Health. 2021;23(4):879-82.
5. Piccinini F, Martinelli G, Carbonaro A. Reliability of Body Temperature Measurements Obtained with Contactless Infrared Point Thermometers Commonly Used during the COVID-19 Pandemic. Sensors (Basel). 2021;21(11):3794.
6. El Morr C, Ozdemir D, Asdaah Y, Saab A, El-Lahib Y, Sokhn ES. AI-based epidemic and pandemic early warning systems: A systematic scoping review. Health Informatics J. 2024;30(3):14604582241275844.
7. Elhaddad M, Hamam S. AI-Driven Clinical Decision Support Systems: An Ongoing Pursuit of Potential. Cureus. 2024;16(4):e57728.
8. Ghaddaripouri K, Ghaddaripouri M, Mousavi AS, Mousavi Baigi SF, Rezaei Sarsari M, Dahmardeh Kemmak F, et al. The effect of machine learning algorithms in the prediction, and diagnosis of meningitis: A systematic review. Health Sci Rep. 2024;7(2):e1893.
9. Peiffer-Smadja N, Dellière S, Rodriguez C, Birgand G, Lescure FX, Fourati S, et al. Machine learning in the clinical microbiology laboratory: has the time come for routine practice? Clin Microbiol Infect. 2020;26(10):1300-9.

10. De Corte T, Van Hoecke S, De Waele J. Artificial Intelligence in Infection Management in the ICU. Crit Care. 2022;26(1):79.
11. Nsubuga M, Galiwango R, Jjingo D, Mboowa G. Generalizability of machine learning in predicting antimicrobial resistance in E. coli: a multi-country case study in Africa. BMC Genomics. 2024;25(1):287.
12. Sakagianni A, Koufopoulou C, Koufopoulos P, Kalantzi S, Theodorakis N, Nikolaou M, et al. Data-Driven Approaches in Antimicrobial Resistance: Machine Learning Solutions. Antibiotics (Basel). 2024;13(11):1052.
13. Pinto-de-Sá R, Sousa-Pinto B, Costa-de-Oliveira S. Brave New World of Artificial Intelligence: Its Use in Antimicrobial Stewardship-A Systematic Review. Antibiotics (Basel). 2024;13(4):307.
14. Verhaeghe J, Corte TD, Waele JJ, Ongenae F, Hoecke SV. Designing a Pharmacokinetic Machine Learning Model for Optimizing Beta-Lactam Antimicrobial Dosing in Critically Ill Patients. International Conference on Medical and Health Informatics. 2024. DOI:10.1145/3673971.3673982.
15. Yinusa A, Faezipour, M. Optimizing Healthcare Delivery: A Model for Staffing, Patient Assignment, and Resource Allocation. Applied System Innovation. 2023;6(5):78.
16. Kim S, Eig E, Yue J, Yang A, Comerci C, Laune M, et al. Bioelectronic drug-free control of opportunistic pathogens through selective excitability. Device.2024;2(11):100596.
17. Conroy B, Silva I, Mehraci G, Damiano R, Gross B, Salvati E, et al. Real-time infection prediction with wearable physiological monitoring and AI to aid military workforce readiness during COVID-19. Sci Rep. 2022;12(1):3797.
18. Goergen CJ, Tweardy MJ, Steinhubl SR, Wegerich SW, Singh K, Mieloszyk RJ, et al. Detection and Monitoring of Viral Infections via Wearable Devices and Biometric Data. Annu Rev Biomed Eng. 2022;24:1-27.
19. Cho SY, Choi JH. Biomarkers of sepsis. Infect Chemother. 2014;46(1):1-12.
20. Ulla M, Pizzolato E, Lucchiari M, Loiacono M, Soardo F, Forno D, et al. Diagnostic and prognostic value of presepsin in the management of sepsis in the emergency department: a multicenter prospective study. Crit Care. 2013;17(4): R168.
21. Bottazzi B, Doni A, Garlanda C, Mantovani A. An integrated view of humoral innate immunity: pentraxins as a paradigm. Annu Rev Immunol. 2010;28:157-83.
22. Havelka A, Sejersen K, Venge P, Pauksens K, Larsson A. Calprotectin, a new biomarker for diagnosis of acute respiratory infections. Sci Rep. 2020;10(1):4208.
23. Mebazaa A, Geven C, Hollinger A, Wittebole X, Chousterman BG, Blet A, et al. Circulating adrenomedullin estimates survival and reversibility of organ failure in sepsis: the prospective observational multinational Adrenomedullin and Outcome in Sepsis and Septic Shock-1 (AdrenOSS-1) study. Crit Care. 2018;22(1):354.
24. Na L, Ding H, Xing E, Gao J, Liu B, Wang H, et al. Lnc-MEG3 acts as a potential biomarker for predicting increased disease risk, systemic inflammation, disease severity, and poor prognosis of sepsis via interacting with miR-21. J Clin Lab Anal. 2020;34:e23123.
25. Seol CH, Yong SH, Shin JH, Lee SH, Leem AY, Park SM, et al. The ratio of plasma angiopoietin-2 to angiopoietin-1 as a prognostic biomarker in patients with sepsis. Cytokine. 2020;129:155029.

26. Le L, Baer M, Briggs P, Bullock N, Cole W, DiMarco D, et al. Diagnostic Accuracy of Point-of-Care Fluorescence Imaging for the Detection of Bacterial Burden in Wounds: Results from the 350-Patient Fluorescence Imaging Assessment and Guidance Trial. Adv Wound Care (New Rochelle). 2021;10(3):123-36.
27. Memic S, Cadnum JL, Osborne A, Rutala WA, Donskey CJ. A novel approach for safe and automated implementation of far ultraviolet-C light decontamination in clinical areas. Antimicrobial Stewardship & Healthcare Epidemiology. 2024;4(1):e123.
28. Simioli F, Annunziata A, Coppola A, Iervolino A, Boccia M, Fiorentino G. Artificial intelligence for training and reporting infection prevention measures in critical wards. Front Public Health. 2024;12:1442188.
29. Ruan K, Wu Z, Xu Q. Smart Cleaner: A New Autonomous Indoor Disinfection Robot for Combating the COVID-19 Pandemic. Robotics. 2021;10(3):87.
30. Mochurad L, Hladun Y. Neural network-based algorithm for door handle recognition using RGBD cameras. Sci Rep. 2024;14(1):15759.
31. Holland J, Kingston L, McCarthy C, Armstrong E, O'Dwyer P, Merz F, et al. Service Robots in the Healthcare Sector. Robotics. 2021;10(1):47.
32. Pascucci M, Royer G, Adamek J, Asmar MA, Aristizabal D, Blanche L, et al. AI-based mobile application to fight antibiotic resistance. Nat Commun. 2021;12(1):1173.

20

CHAPTER

Future Directions and Research Opportunities

Bhuvna Ahuja, Kuldeep Singh, Swati Singh

LEARNING OBJECTIVES

- To evaluate the impact of global health disparities/healthcare inequities in low-resource settings.
- To evaluate the effect of integration of technology with clinical knowledge.
- To explore novel therapeutic interventions for prevention of infection in intensive care unit (ICU).
- To assess the role of advanced infection prevention strategies.
- To analyze the gaps in current infection prevention practices in ICUs.

INTRODUCTION

Infection prevention in healthcare settings, especially in intensive care units (ICUs), has advanced significantly over the past few decades. Healthcare-associated infections (HAIs) are a major cause of morbidity and mortality worldwide, with ICUs being particularly vulnerable due to the complexity of care, the high acuity of patients, and the use of invasive devices. Significant strides have been made in areas such as hand hygiene, antimicrobial stewardship, and infection control protocols. However, substantial gaps still exist in fully understanding the mechanisms behind infections as well as in optimizing interventions to reduce their impact, especially in resource-limited settings and in the face of emerging pathogens.

Research in this area can significantly improve patient recovery rates, reduce mortality, and shorten hospital stays. By focusing on more targeted, evidence-based interventions, researchers can help lower the overall burden of infections.

IMPACT OF GLOBAL HEALTH DISPARITIES ON INFECTION PREVENTION PRACTICES

Global health disparities pose a significant barrier to consistent and effective infection prevention. In high-income countries, infection prevention strategies may be better resourced and more robust, but in many low- and middle-income countries (LMICs), healthcare infrastructure, equipment, and infection control training may be inadequate. Furthermore, the global movement of patients, healthcare workers, and pathogens contributes to the spread of resistant infections, complicating prevention efforts. Understanding

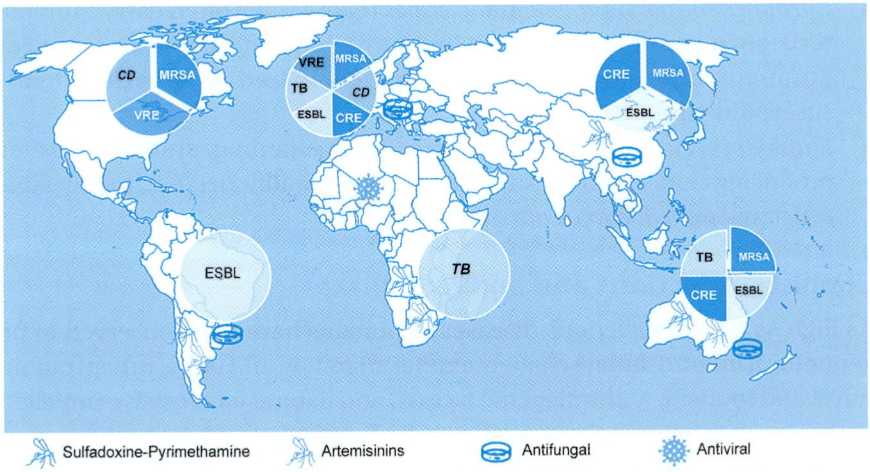

Fig. 1: Global distribution of the main multiresistant strains and antimicrobial resistance. (CD: *Clostridium difficile*; CRE: carbapenem-resistant Enterobacterales; ESBL: extended-spectrum beta-lactamase; MRSA: methicillin-resistant *Staphylococcus aureus*; VRE: vancomycin-resistant *Enterococcus*; Multidrug-resistant (MDR) TB is a form of tuberculosis caused by *Mycobacterium tuberculosis*

Source: Oliveira M, Antunes W, Mota S, Madureira-Carvalho Á, Dinis-Oliveira RJ, Dias da Silva D. An Overview of the Recent Advances in Antimicrobial Resistance. Microorganisms. 2024;12(9):1920.

how to tailor infection control practices to the specific needs and resources of different regions, while addressing inequalities in healthcare access, is global health improvement **(Fig. 1)**.

EMERGING PATHOGENS AND CHALLENGES

In the recent decades, the world has witnessed an alarming rise in novel pathogens and the reemergence of older ones. The movement of people, animals, and goods across borders has accelerated the transmission of infectious agents, turning localized outbreaks into global pandemics. Climate change has further expanded the habitat range of disease vectors. Meanwhile, many existing treatments have been rendered ineffective, compounding the challenges posed by these pathogens.

EMERGING THREATS

Multidrug-resistant Organisms

Multidrug-resistant organisms (MDROs) exhibit resistance to multiple antibiotics, making management of infections difficult and increasing the mortality rates, particularly in ICUs.

- *Candida auris:* A multidrug-resistant fungal pathogen that poses a risk for the already immunocompromised. It can survive on surfaces and resist disinfectants, making it challenging to control.

- *Carbapenem-resistant enterobacterales (CRE):* They often carry multiple resistance genes that limit treatment options and necessitate longer durations of costlier therapies when compared with carbapenem-susceptible strains.
- *Staphylococcus aureus, often referred to as* superbug, are notorious for producing clones with resistance to a range of antibiotics [e.g., methicillin-resistant *Staphylococcus aureus* (MRSA)].

Zoonotic Infections and Spillover Risks

As high as 60% of infectious diseases in humans have been observed to be zoonotic in origin. Climate change, animal migration and trade, urbanization, travel and tourism, anthropogenic factors, and natural factors have impelled the emergence, reemergence, and spread of zoonoses.

- The 2019 outbreak of COVID-19 [severe acute respiratory syndrome coronavirus 2 (SARS-CoV-2)] brought to the fore the devastating ramifications of zoonotic infections can have on economies and healthcare systems.
- A sizeable proportion of H5N1- and H7N9-infected patients as a consequence of high levels of plasma proinflammatory cytokines and chemokines, including develop bronchiolitis, pneumonia, and multiple organ dysfunctions.
- Resistant bacteria, genes, and antibiotics linger in various environmental reservoirs such as soil, water, and air. These areas become hot spots for genetic exchange among microbial communities, driving the evolution and spread of resistance traits. Human activities, including pharmaceutical manufacturing and improper disposal of medical waste, significantly contribute to environmental contamination with antimicrobial agents, further exacerbating the issue.
- Human-driven activities such as deforestation, expanding cities, and encroachment into previously untouched natural areas have heightened our interactions with wildlife and the diseases they may carry. Shifts in food production practices such as the growth of live animal markets and the clearing of forests for industrial agriculture also bring people into closer contact with animals. This increased proximity raises the risk of emerging infectious diseases.

RESPONSE STRATEGIES

Real-time Pathogen Detection and Rapid Diagnostics

Emerging culture-independent tests, such as polymerase chain reaction (PCR) and next-generation sequencing (NGS), aim at expediting the management of bloodstream infections (BSIs) by reducing turnaround times and/or improving diagnostic sensitivity.

- Molecular point-of-care testing (POCT) now allows for rapid, bedside detection of infections and precise antimicrobial use. For example, procalcitonin (PCT)-guided antibiotic stewardship using POCT can be adopted to decrease antimicrobial resistance (AMR).
- Genomic surveillance can help track mutations, predict resistance patterns, and guide vaccine development.

Vaccination and Global Surveillance Efforts

Vaccines are used prophylactically, decreasing the overall burden of infectious disease cases, and thus antibiotic use and AMR.

In the aftermath of COVID-19 pandemic, messenger ribonucleic acid (mRNA) technology, as a part of pandemic preparedness plans, has been recognized as a tool for accelerated vaccine development.

Global surveillance networks: Programs such as the Global Influenza Surveillance and Response System (GISRS) and World Health Organization's (WHO) Global Outbreak Alert and Response Network (GOARN) enable data sharing, pandemic preparedness and response, and quicker access to vaccines.

Enhancing the One Health Approach

The One Health approach recognizes the interconnectedness of human, animal, and environmental health. An integrated effort across disciplines is required for the better comprehension of emergence of pathogens.

The rise of emerging pathogens and the reemergence of the older ones pose significant threats to global health. MDROs, zoonotic infections, and viral outbreaks in ICUs highlight the vulnerabilities of modern healthcare systems.

To address these challenges, a multipronged approach involving early detection, vaccination programs, and the One Health framework is essential. Strengthening global surveillance systems and improving ICU preparedness will be crucial in combating future outbreaks.

- Real-time pathogen detection via PCR and NGS and molecular point-of-care tests help in early diagnosis of infections.
- Genomic surveillance use helps track mutations and predict resistance patterns.
- Vaccination reduces disease burden and AMR and enhances preparedness; mRNA technology aids faster vaccine development.

INFECTION CONTROL INNOVATIONS FOR INTENSIVE CARE UNITS

Infections acquired from health care are now receiving serious attention, especially in intensive care units where working with critically ill patients there are higher chances of antibiotic resistance and higher severity of infections. The current innovations in technology, diagnostic methods, and prevention have very significantly marked improvements in infection control practices in these units.

Innovative Technologies and Solutions

Artificial Intelligence and Machine Learning

Artificial intelligence (AI) predictive models for infections such as sepsis and ventilator-associated pneumonia (VAP) are now able to do patient data analysis for identifying early symptoms of these infections. Studies have proven efficiency in this area that machine learning algorithms reduce the delay to diagnosis and improve outcome-related results.[1]

Wearable Sensors

Wearable sensors provide continuous monitoring in most metabolic and physiological functions, using infection as the baseline marker for change in real-time data logging and survey for early interventions.[2]

Automated Disinfection Systems

Automated systems using ultraviolet C (UV-C) or hydrogen peroxide vaporizers have been effective in making the intensive care environment sterile and have also been shown to have their effect on the nature of contamination of surfaces. They also show a reduction in the transmission of MDROs.[3]

Advance Diagnostic Tools

Faster Pathogen Detection

Molecular methods such as PCR and next-generation sequencing (NGS) can hasten and increase accuracy in pathogen detection. These molecular methods ensure prompt initiation of treatment.[4]

Point-of-care Testing

Point-of-care testing offers quick and easy bedside analysis for infection markers such as PCT, thereby reducing the time-to-diagnose lengths.[5]

Metagenomic Sequencing

Metagenomics offers complete analysis and is also associated with the best diagnostics for organisms in their measurements inside the body.[6]

Novel Determinants of Prevention

Antimicrobial Coatings

The available surface coverings within ICUs have silver nanoparticles incorporated into antimicrobial coatings, which tend to reduce biofilm formation and colonization by pathogens.[7]

Probiotics

Probiotics can be given to ICU patients to prevent gastrointestinal colonization by pathogenic bacteria and thus to prevent subsequent infection.[8]

Selective Decontamination of the Digestive Tract (SDD)

The oropharyngeal application of some nonabsorbable antimicrobials to the intestinal tract effectively reduced the microbial load and thus the risk of infection.[9]

Best Practices of Hand Hygiene Enhancements

Automatic Monitoring Systems

Automatic monitoring systems are computerized automated hand hygiene monitoring systems that track compliance rates by healthcare workers, which in turn prevent cross infections.[10]

Touchless Dispensers

Touchless dispensers minimize the potential of cross contamination and encourage frequent use in effective hand hygiene practices **(Figs. 2A and B)**.[11]

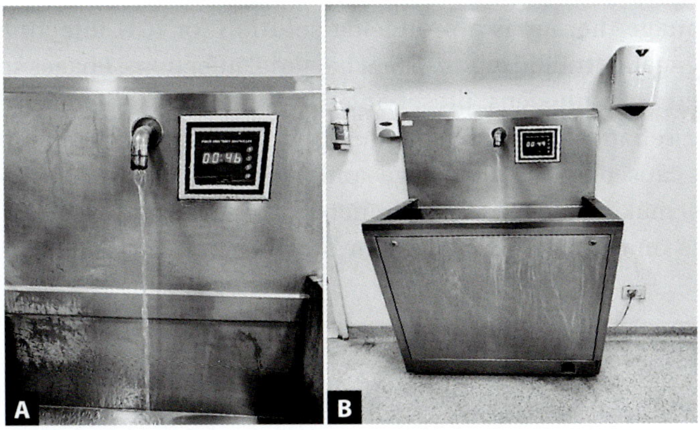

Figs. 2A and B: Modular handwashing sink in intensive care unit (ICU).

Antibiotic Stewardship

Artificial Intelligence Powered Decision Support

These AI tools help in prescribing drugs, i.e., antibiotics, rationally, thereby preventing misuse and resistance. Thus, these systems mine the patient's data and give appropriate regimens.[12]

Phage Therapy

Phage therapy is considered as a promising alternative to antibiotic therapy, targeting some specific drug-resistant bacteria.[13]

Data-based Surveillance Systems for Infections

Integrated Dashboards

Real-time dashboards integrate patient data from electronic health records (EHRs) into infection trends for early recognition.[14]

Predictive Analytics

Predictive models analyze patients' patterns and identify high risks for their possible prophylactic measures.[15]

Immunotherapy and Isolation Techniques

Monoclonal Antibodies

Targeted monoclonal antibodies neutralize bacterial toxins, significantly reducing the severity of the resulting infections.[16]

Bacteriophage Therapy

Bacteriophage therapy is a promising solution for ICU infection control, especially against multidrug-resistant bacterial infections. Phages specifically target bacterial pathogens, preserving the normal microbiota and reducing antibiotic reliance. Studies have demonstrated their efficacy in treating infections caused by MDROs. Phage–antibiotic synergy enhances therapeutic outcomes, making it a valuable adjunct in ICU settings. Continued research is focusing on engineering phages for broader and more effective bacterial coverage.[20]

Sepsivac

Sepsivac is an immunotherapy vaccine developed for sepsis caused by gram-negative bacterial infections. It is based on heat-killed Mycobacterium w (Mw), also known as Mycobacterium indicus pranii (MIP). They improve the immune response of the host and decrease the overstimulation of inflammation found in sepsis. Sepsivac administration also demonstrates the ability to decrease mortality and ICU-attending time due to immune dysregulation and infection.[18,19]

Isolation Pods and Negative Pressure Rooms

Portable isolation and negative pressure rooms can contain airborne pathogens and prevent cross contamination.[17]

Innovation in infection control in the ICU is changing the paradigms by which critical care is delivered. Such technologies integrated into an ICU would potentially yield great disease reduction, improvements in patient outcomes, and a host of other advantages such as new challenges posed by AMR. Future investigations will proceed toward personalized medicine for treatment and microbial-based therapy for further improving prevention and control.[18,19]

- Global surveillance systems (GISRS, GOARN) facilitate timely outbreak responses.
- One Health approach integrates human, animal, and environmental health.
- AI-powered decision support systems optimize antibiotic prescription to prevent resistance.

GAPS IN CURRENT INFECTION PREVENTION KNOWLEDGE AND OPPORTUNITIES FOR RESEARCH IN HEALTHCARE, PARTICULARLY IN THE INTENSIVE CARE UNIT

- *Insufficient understanding of biofilm formation and AMR mechanisms in medical devices*: Medical devices such as catheters, ventilators, and prosthetics are essential in critical care but can serve as reservoirs for infections. Biofilm formation, where bacteria aggregate and form a protective layer on the surface of devices, is a significant contributor to device-related infections. However, there is still a limited understanding of how biofilms form in the ICU setting and how they contribute to AMR. Furthermore, biofilm-associated bacteria can be more resistant to antibiotics and disinfectants, complicating treatment and prevention strategies. Research into novel materials for devices and effective biofilm-targeting therapies is critical.
- *Antimicrobial resistance*: There is limited evidence on the effectiveness of antimicrobial stewardship in resource-limited settings. Antimicrobial stewardship programs have been widely adopted in high-resource settings to combat AMR by optimizing the use of antibiotics. However, there is a lack of robust evidence on how these programs perform in resource-limited environments, which often face challenges such as limited access to diagnostic testing, fewer trained personnel, and greater reliance on broad-spectrum antibiotics. More research is needed to develop context-specific stewardship models that can be effectively

implemented in LMICs while balancing the availability of essential treatments. Additionally, the increasing issue of antibiotic resistance in ICU settings underscores the importance of research aimed at optimizing antibiotic use, developing new therapies, and identifying alternative treatment strategies. This includes developing strategies for more accurate diagnosis, tailored antimicrobial therapies, and minimizing unnecessary antibiotic use.

- *Infection control practices*: Hand hygiene is one of the most effective and simple measures to prevent HAIs. Despite clear guidelines, compliance remains suboptimal in many ICUs due to various factors, including high workload, understaffing, and a lack of immediate feedback on hand hygiene practices. Behavioral change interventions aimed at improving hand hygiene adherence often fall short, and there is still a need for a deeper understanding of the psychological, cultural, and organizational barriers to consistent hand hygiene practices. Strategies that consider these factors, alongside technological innovations such as real-time monitoring systems, may help improve compliance rates. Future research can refine and innovate infection prevention measures, such as better protocols for hand hygiene, sterilization techniques, use of personal protective equipment, and environmental cleaning strategies. It can also explore the effectiveness of novel infection control technologies such as UV light or antimicrobial coatings on surfaces.
- *Personalized approaches to infection prevention*: A growing body of research suggests that infection prevention strategies may benefit from being personalized to individual patients, particularly in critical care settings. Factors such as a patient's genetic predisposition to infections, their immune system status, microbiome composition, and previous antibiotic use could influence their risk of developing HAIs. Personalized infection prevention could optimize the use of antibiotics, improve patient outcomes, and reduce the spread of resistant organisms. However, much more research is needed to identify genetic markers, biomarkers, and other individual characteristics that could inform tailored interventions. Long-term effectiveness of bundled interventions for infection control bundled interventions, such as the "central line bundle" or "ventilator bundle," have been successful in reducing certain types of infections in ICUs. However, there is limited long-term data on the sustained effectiveness of these bundled approaches across diverse healthcare settings, especially in environments with fluctuating resource availability. Additionally, while these bundles aim to standardize care and reduce infection rates, their success depends on consistent implementation, which may be challenging. More longitudinal studies are needed to assess the durability of these interventions and identify ways to improve their scalability and sustainability.

- Emerging pathogens, climate change, and global mobility accelerate disease spread.
- MDROs, such as *Candida auris* and MRSA, complicate infection management.
- Zoonotic infections contribute to 60% of human infectious diseases.

- *Advances in diagnostics*: Rapid, accurate diagnostic tools for detecting infections and determining pathogens, including resistance profiles, are crucial for timely interventions. Research into improving molecular diagnostic methods, point-of-care tests, and AI-based diagnostic algorithms can lead to quicker identification and better targeted treatments.
- *Microbiome research*: There is a growing interest in the ICU microbiome as alterations in gut, skin, and respiratory microbiota may play a role in infection susceptibility. Future studies could explore microbiome-targeted interventions, such as probiotics or microbiota modulation, to reduce infections or improve recovery.
- *Integration of technology and clinical knowledge*: AI and machine learning can play a role in predicting infection risk, monitoring early signs of infection, and improving decision-making for clinicians. Future research could examine how these technologies can integrate with existing clinical workflows for proactive infection prevention.

CONCLUSION

Infection prevention is a critical area in healthcare, particularly in ICUs where patients are most vulnerable. While substantial progress has been made in understanding and addressing HAIs, significant gaps remain in our knowledge. Areas such as biofilm resistance, antimicrobial stewardship in resource-limited settings, optimizing hand hygiene compliance, and addressing global health disparities need further exploration. Future studies should focus on personalized infection prevention strategies and the long-term effectiveness of bundled interventions. By closing these gaps, we can continue to improve patient safety, reduce the burden of infections, and enhance the quality of care globally. Future research in ICU infection prevention holds the promise of developing more efficient, personalized, and scientifically grounded strategies to reduce infections, improve patient care, and combat the growing challenge of AMR.

REFERENCES

1. Ghassemi M, Naumann T, Schulam P, Beam AL, Chen IY, Ranganath R. Opportunities in machine learning for healthcare. Nat Med. 2018;25(1): 30-6.
2. Wang L, Zhou M, Li Y, Liu F, Cai X, Zhao J. Wearable sensors for infection detection: Current advances and challenges. Biosens Bioelectron. 2023;210:114443.

3. Nerandzic MM, Cadnum JL, Eckart KE, Donskey CJ. Evaluation of an automated ultraviolet radiation device for decontamination of *Clostridium difficile* and other healthcare-associated pathogens. BMC Infect Dis. 2020;10:197.
4. Gu W, Miller S, Chiu CY. Clinical metagenomic next-generation sequencing for pathogen detection. Annu Rev Pathol. 2019;14:319-38.
5. Plebani M. Point-of-care testing: Future perspectives. Clin Chem Lab Med. 2018;56(3):308-17.
6. Simner PJ, Miller S, Carroll KC. Understanding the promises and hurdles of metagenomic next-generation sequencing as a diagnostic tool for infectious diseases. Clin Infect Dis. 2018;66(5):778-88.
7. Salwiczek M, Qu Y, Gardiner J, Strugnell R, Lithgow T, McLean KM, et al. Emerging rules for effective antimicrobial coatings. Trends Biotechnol. 2014;32(2): 82-90.
8. van den Nieuwboer M, Claassen E. Probiotics and gastrointestinal diseases in older adults. Curr Opin Clin Nutr Metab Care. 2019;22(1):29-36.
9. de Smet AMGA, Kluytmans JAJW, Cooper BS, Mascini EM, Benus RF, van der Werf TS, et al. Decontamination of the digestive tract and oropharynx in ICU patients. Lancet Infect Dis. 2011;11(5):372-80.
10. Srigley JA, Furness CD, Baker GR, Gardam M. Quantification of the Hawthorne effect in hand hygiene compliance monitoring using an electronic monitoring system: A retrospective cohort study. BMJ Qual Saf. 2014;23(12):974-80.
11. Boyce JM, Pittet D. Guideline for hand hygiene in health-care settings: Recommendations of the healthcare infection control practices advisory committee. MMWR Recomm Rep. 2002;51(RR-16):1-45.
12. Barlam TF, Cosgrove SE, Abbo LM, MacDougall C, Schuetz AN, Septimus EJ, et al. Implementing an antibiotic stewardship program. Clin Infect Dis. 2016; 62(10):e51-77.
13. Kortright KE, Chan BK, Koff JL, Turner PE. Phage therapy: A renewed approach to combat antibiotic-resistant bacteria. Cell Host Microbe. 2019;25(2):219-32.
14. Wenzel RP, Edmond MB. The impact of hospital-acquired infections on the ICU patient. Curr Opin Crit Care. 2001;7(4):305-9.
15. Vincent JL, Rello J, Marshall J, Silva E, Anzueto A, Martin CD, et al. International study of the prevalence and outcomes of infection in intensive care units. JAMA. 2009;302(21):2323-9.
16. Lyon GM, Karlen S, Edwards KM. Immunotherapy for bacterial infections: A promising path forward. J Infect Dis. 2020;222(1):13-8.
17. Hurst FP, Neff RT, Vogel WB, Turenne J. Negative pressure isolation rooms in ICUs: Design innovations and effectiveness. Am J Crit Care. 2018;27(6): 482-6.
18. Minz RW, Kumar A, Mehta Y, et al. Immune-modulation by Mycobacterium W in sepsis: A novel therapeutic approach. Crit Care Med. 2020;48(6):e453-61.
19. Chaudhry R, Maheshwari A, Talwar V. Mycobacterium W: A new therapeutic glory in tuberculosis and beyond. Indian J Med Res. 2020;151(5):441-6.
20. Abedon ST, García P, Mullany P. Phage therapy: Past, present and future. Front Microbiol. 2021;12:658679.

21

CHAPTER

Intensive Care Unit Layout and Design for Infection Prevention

Kamal P Bhutada

LEARNING OBJECTIVES

While designing and planning a hospital and its critical areas, engineers, architects, and planners play an important role. In an intensive care unit (ICU), where the patient's health is the primary concern, maintaining high indoor air quality is crucial for preventing secondary infections and controlling the spread of diseases. The indoor air quality is directly influenced by the ventilation system in place and the surrounding outdoor environmental conditions. The doctors who are directly responsible for infection prevention must know the basics of ICU planning and designing. This review aims to make doctors, especially critical care consultants, aware of:

- The planning of the ICU layout.
- The concept of isolation.
- The idea of differential pressures in ICUs.
- How the hospital and ICU ventilation system works.
- How to optimize the workflow in the ICU to help in the prevention of the spread of infections.

INTRODUCTION

The proportion of intensive care unit (ICU) beds in a hospital typically ranges from <10% to as high as 30% of the total number of hospital beds; however, infections acquired in the ICU account for a large proportion of nosocomial infections. The various nosocomial infections in the ICU are catheter-related bloodstream infections (CRBSIs), ventilator-associated events (VAEs), including ventilator-associated pneumonia (VAP), and catheter-associated urinary tract infections. These infections contribute to increased length of stay in the ICU, morbidity, and mortality. The rate of infections is higher in resource-limited countries like India than in developed countries.

A multicenter prospective cohort surveillance study conducted across 46 hospitals in Central and South America, India, Morocco, and Turkey revealed an overall infection rate of 14.7% (or 22.5 infections per 1,000 ICU days), significantly higher than infection rates in developed countries. A subsequent study by the same international group reported results from 98 ICUs from Latin America, Asia, Africa, and Europe. Even though device utilization was remarkably similar to that reported from ICUs in the United States, rates of device-associated nosocomial infection were markedly higher in the ICUs from resource-limited countries.

INTENSIVE CARE UNIT LAYOUT

The incidence of hospital-acquired infection has got direct relation with the space available per bed and the space between two successive beds. If the space per bed is less, the chances of hospital-acquired infections increase. Evidence suggests that ICU design can improve the quality of infection control.

Intensive care units can be dormitory-like or single accommodation cubicles or rooms.

Dormitory-like Intensive Care Unit

Recommended space per bed is 150–200 sq ft. A few guidelines recommend even higher space, up to 250 sq ft per bed.[1] There should be at least 100–150% additional area to accommodate the nursing station, storage area, staff movement area, teaching room, doctor and nurses' room, and toilets.

According to a review by O'Connell et al. (2,000), putting about 20 sq m between each bed space is one such design feature (i.e., one does not brush past patient beds and curtains as one makes their way around the ICU).

Single Accommodation/Cubicle Intensive Care Unit

The area should be 250 sq ft per room/cubicle.

If it is a single accommodation ICU, the following safety features are desirable as far as infection is concerned.

- Own bathroom (to prevent cross-contamination of shared facilities by patients with communicable diseases).
- Anteroom to facilitate isolation as needed.
- Individual wash basin with elbow-operated inside the room to promote handwashing by staff and visitors.
- Alcohol hand rub holders inside and outside the doors.
- Internal and external patient monitoring display equipment.
- Windows from the ICU work area into the patient room, with curtains to allow for privacy.

Certainly, a cubicle ICU is more desirable than a dormitory type for obvious reasons **(Fig. 1)**. However, it may not be possible because of many reasons, including economic reasons.

ISOLATION ROOMS

Isolation rooms are essential for patients with specific medical conditions or infections, typically affecting the skin, lungs, airways, or intestines. These rooms help prevent the transmission of infections to others. An isolation facility controls the airflow in a room. By doing this, it reduces the number of infectious particles in the air to such an extent that it reduces the risk of cross-infection in healthcare facilities. This is achieved by:

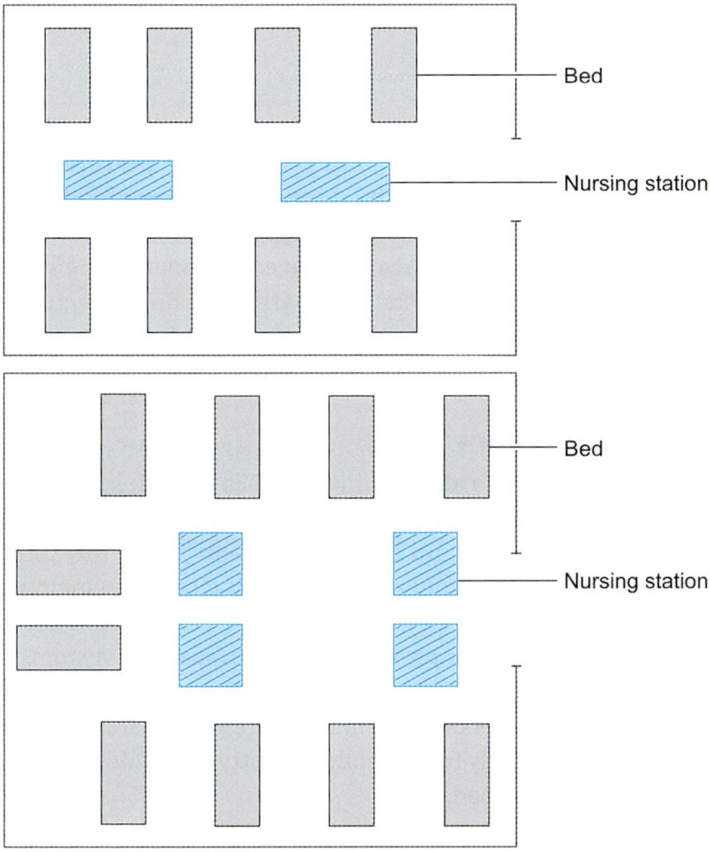

Fig. 1: Dormitory type ICU and cubicle ICU.

- Controlling the quantity and quality of air entering or exhausting a room
- Maintaining differential air pressure between adjacent areas
- Using air filters like high-efficiency particulate air (HEPA)
- By having different airflow patterns for different procedures.

Different Types of Isolation Facilities

- *Class S:* Standard air pressure is maintained using the air conditioner.
- *Class P:* It is a positive air pressure room. Immunocompromised patients, such as neutropenic patients, are kept here to protect them from airborne transmission of infections.
- *Class N:* It is a negative air pressure room. An infected patient is kept in such room where they may pose an infection risk for others.
- *Class Q:* It is a negative air pressure room where patients are kept for quarantine isolation.

  Usually, Classes P, N, and Q have additional anterooms.

  How are isolation rooms different than other patient care areas?

These rooms have a relatively high rate of air exchange compared to other patient care areas.

ANTEROOMS

It is an area attached to the isolation room where personal protective equipment (PPE) or clothing can be donned or removed before entering or exiting the isolation room. It is a controlled area where the transfer of equipment or people can take place without contaminating the surrounding health care areas. This area acts as a barrier against potential loss of pressurization when the isolation area door is opened. An anteroom cannot be shared between Class P and Class N isolation areas.

Design of an Anteroom (Fig. 2)

It should be large enough to allow storage of PPEs and other equipment, and it should also have a hand-washing facility. It should have two doors, one for entry into the anteroom and the other for entry from the anteroom to the isolation room. The entry door should be self-closing, swinging from the corridor to the anteroom. There should be a self-closing door between the anteroom and the isolation for providing access to staff and visitors. The door swings outwards in a negative-pressure room. It swings inwards in a positive-pressure room. This door is usually small. There is a separate door from the corridor to the room directly for the patient's entry. It should be large enough to allow movement of the bed.

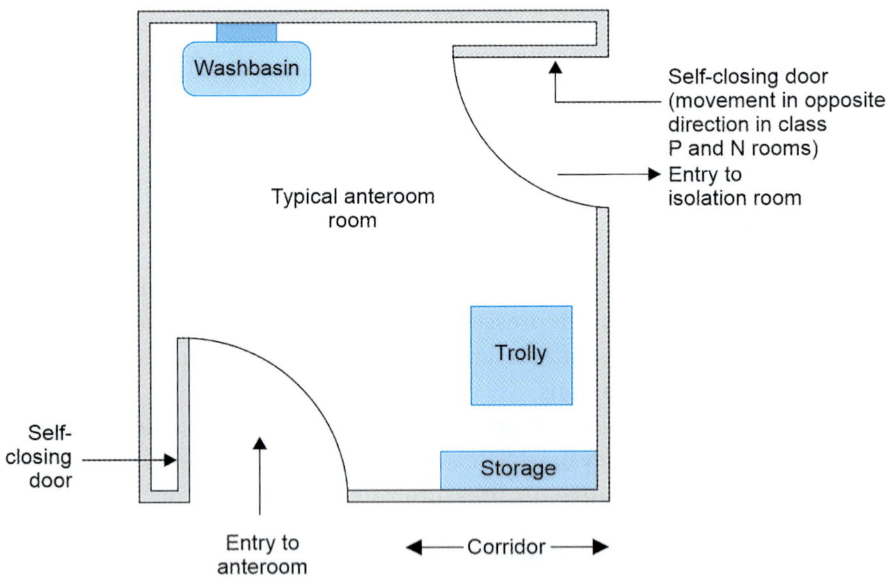

Fig. 2: Design of a typical anteroom.

Design of a Class N Isolation Room (Fig. 4)

The patient's room is strongly negatively pressured in relation to the adjacent corridor. Even the anteroom is negatively pressured in relation to the corridor. The patient's room is also negatively pressured in relation to the anteroom. Air flows from less negatively pressured areas to more negatively pressured areas **(Fig. 3)**. So, when the patient's entry door to the isolation room is opened, air flows from the corridor to the isolation room. So, there is no release or escape from organisms in the air from the room to the corridor.

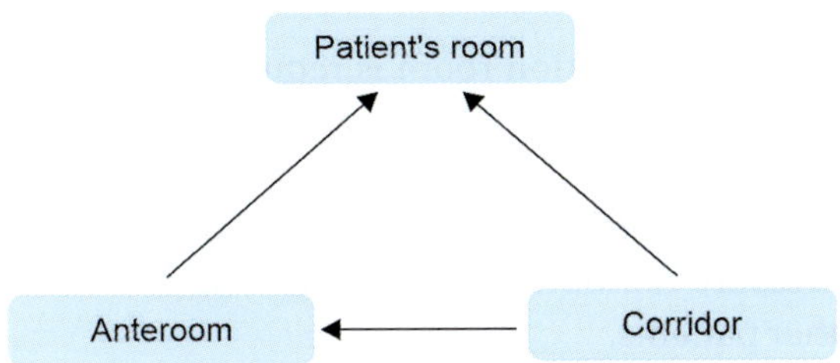

Fig. 3: Airflow directions for a class N room.

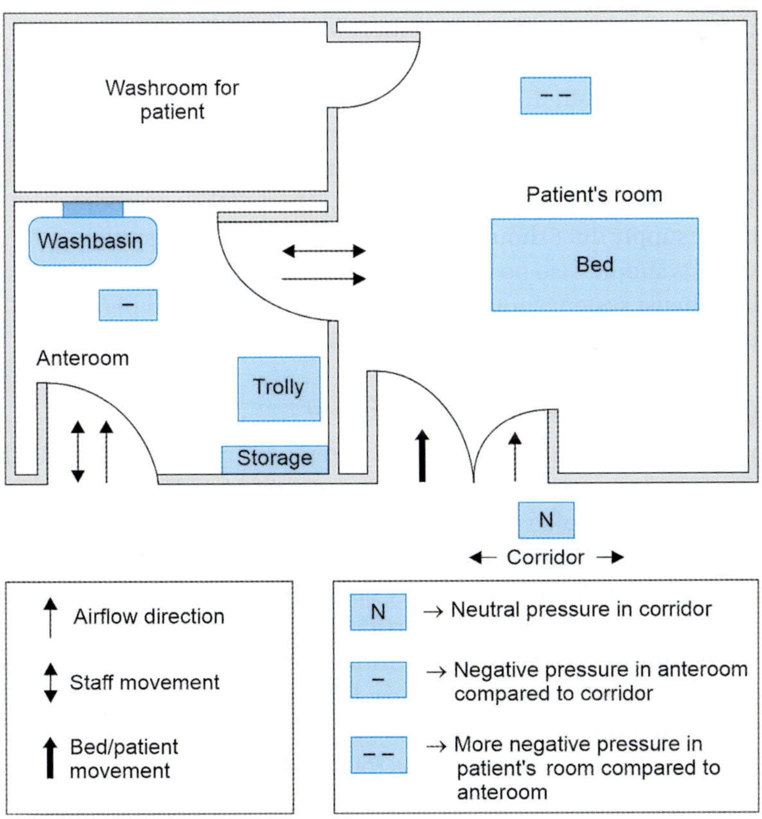

Fig. 4: Negative pressure room with anteroom (airflow and pressure gradient).

All class N rooms must be equipped with a permanently installed device or mechanism to continuously monitor the differential air pressure between the ICU and the corridor or adjacent areas.[2] A local visual indicator must be provided to show when negative differential pressure is being maintained. Such rooms should be provided with a dedicated exhaust system. Removing a quantity of air greater than that of the supply air maintains the negative pressure in an isolation room. The negative pressure ICU should have 12 air changes per hour, provided through a non-aspirating diffuser, with the temperature maintained between 22°C and 24°C and relative humidity between 40 and 60%.[3]

A negative-pressure isolation room is required for patients who require airborne droplet nuclei isolation. Examples include patients with chicken pox, measles, tuberculosis, hemagglutinin type 1 and neuraminidase type 1 (H1N1), and coronavirus disease 2019 (COVID-19). Placing patients in a negative-pressure room helps reduce the risk of transmitting airborne infections to other patients.

The location of the negative pressure isolation room should be such that the patient does not need to pass through other patient care areas.

A negative-pressure isolation room must have the following:
- Anteroom, which will also work as an airlock.
- Wash basin in both the anteroom and isolation room.
- Pressure gauges and alarms are used to monitor pressure loss.
- Bathroom and toilet facility for patients.
- Self-closing doors as described in the section of the anteroom.
- The air supply duct should be fitted with a HEPA filter system.
- Exhausts should also be provided with a HEPA filter.
- The exhaust system should be such that no air return is permitted.
- The exhaust should be around 200 mm above the floor level.

Design of Class P Isolation Room (Fig. 6)

The patient's room is strongly positively pressured in relation to the adjacent corridor. Even the anteroom is positively pressured in relation to the corridor. The patient's room is also positively pressured in relation to the anteroom. Air flows from a more positively pressured area to a less positively pressured area **(Fig. 5)**. So, when the patient's entry door to the isolation room is opened, air flows from the isolation room corridor. So, there is no entry of organisms in the air from the corridor to the room. A properly balanced, positively pressured room will prevent air entry from the corridor into the patient's room and anteroom.

Like class N rooms, class P rooms must have a pressure gauge and alarm system, preferably connected to the hospital alarm system.

Positive pressure isolation rooms are used to isolate immunocompromised patients, for example, neutropenic and some transplant patients. It reduces

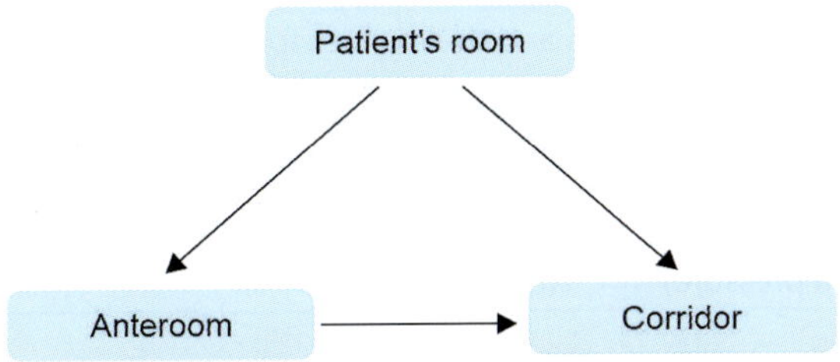

Fig. 5: Airflow direction for class P room.

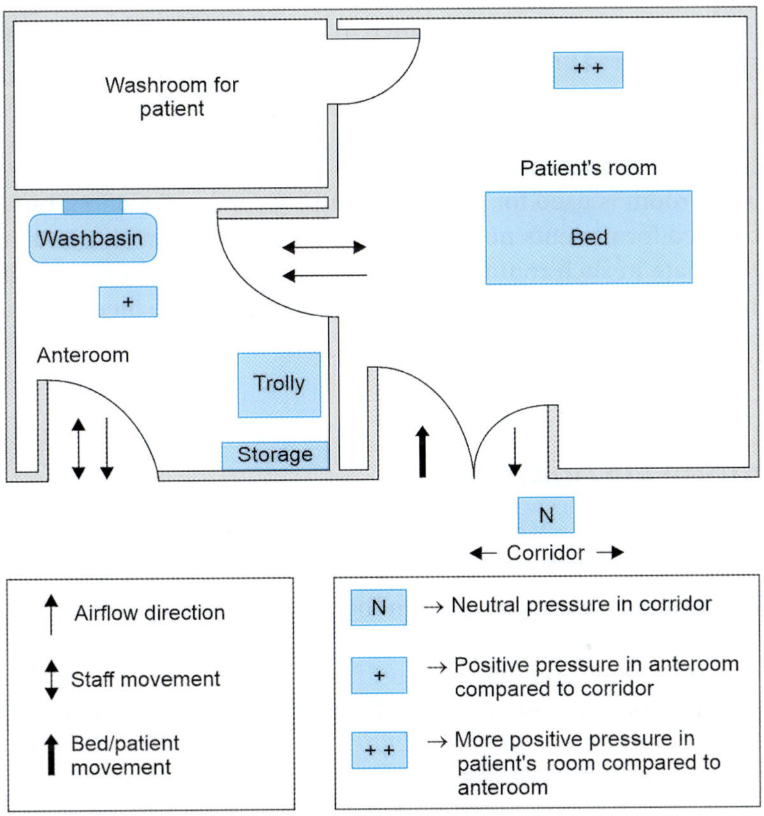

Fig. 6: Positive pressure room with anteroom (airflow and pressure gradient).

the risk of airborne transmission of infection to a susceptible patient. These rooms are also known as "protective isolation units" or "protective environment" rooms (PE rooms).

A positive pressure isolation room must have the following:

- Anteroom, which will also work as an airlock.
- Wash basin in both the anteroom and isolation room.
- Pressure gauge and alarm to monitor pressure loss.
- Bathroom and toilet facility for patients.

TABLE 1: Types of pressurization and their values for the anteroom and isolation.

Type of pressurization	*Anteroom*	*Isolation*
Class N (negative pressure)	−5 Pa	−10 Pa
Class P (positive pressure)	+5 Pa	+10 Pa
Class S (standard pressure)	Not required	

- Self-closing doors as described in the section of the anteroom.
- The air supply duct should be fitted with a HEPA filter system.
- The exhaust should be at around 200 mm above floor level.

A HEPA filter system is not required in the exhaust system as the exhaust air is not considered infectious.

Class S Isolation Room

It is also called a standard pressure room.

Such a room is used for patients requiring contact isolation, but it can also be used for patients not requiring isolation. Normal air conditioning is appropriate in such rooms. A handwash basin in the room is desirable. A bathroom with toilet facilities for patients should also be there.

Recommended Pressure Gradient

Refer **Table 1**.

INDOOR AIR QUALITY

Factors Affecting Indoor Air Quality in the Intensive Care Unit

The following factors directly affect indoor air quality in the ICU:

- *Design factors:* They refer to all the components that characterize the inpatient room (room dimensions, furniture, etc.). The focus should be on dimensional aspects, room configuration, and door motion.
- *Management and cleaning activities:* They refer to management and maintenance activities, ventilation systems, cleaning, and disinfectant activities in the functional unit. The focus should be on ventilation systems, including heating, ventilation, and air conditioning (HVAC).
- *Human presence and activities:* They refer to the users, their health status, and the medical activities in the patient's room. The focus should be on human behavior, especially infection prevention practices.
- *Outdoor and microclimatic factors:* They refer mainly to outdoor air and other microclimatic factors. Although these factors can vary, these factors have a significant influence on indoor air quality.

ASHRAE 170 standards define the parameters mentioned above. The following values are essential in the ICU.

- The temperature in the ICU should be between 21°C and 24°C. At this temperature, patients usually feel more comfortable.
- Relative humidity in the ICUs and anterooms should range between 40 and 60%.
- For outdoor use, a minimum of two air changes per hour (ACH) is required, with a total of six ACH needed to ensure and maintain the desired air quality and circulation conditions.
- The outdoor airflow rates for ICUs are mostly 30% outdoor air intake unless specified for isolation rooms.
- Air velocity should vary between 0.05 and 0.25 m/s.
- The minimum pressure difference between the room and corridor and the room and toilet is usually about 2.5 Pa.

AIR FILTRATION SYSTEMS

What are HEPA Filters?

High-efficiency particulate air, short for "high-efficiency particulate air" filter, is a pleated mechanical air filter designed to capture at least 99.97% of airborne particles, such as dust, pollen, mold, and bacteria, that are 0.3 microns (μm) in size. The 0.3 μm specification represents the most penetrating particle size (MPPS), which is considered the worst-case scenario for filtration efficiency. Particles either larger or <0.3 μm are captured with even greater efficiency, ensuring that the filter performs at 99.97% or better for all particle sizes.

As air particles pass through the air filter, they are caught by three mechanisms: diffusion, interception, and impaction. Diffusion occurs in a HEPA filter when gas molecules <0.1 μm collide and are delayed in passing through the filter.

The air in ICUs must be free of harmful viruses and bacteria. To ensure this, HEPA filters are trusted to keep the air clean in many hospitals and intensive care facilities. Antimicrobial HEPA filters are commonly preferred because they are capable of killing harmful microbes upon contact.

Heating, Ventilation, and Air Conditioning System

A good HVAC system is required in ICUs to maintain good indoor air quality. It is an important nonpharmacological strategy in preventing hospital-acquired infections. The primary function of the HVAC system is to create a comfortable and safe environment for patients, ICU staff, and visitors. Key roles of the HVAC system include heating (to raise or maintain temperature), cooling (to lower or maintain temperature), humidifying (to add water vapor), dehumidifying (to remove water vapor and maintain air moisture), filtering (to eliminate dust particles, bacteria, viruses, and fungi), ventilating (to regulate air change rates between indoor and outdoor spaces), and air distribution (to control air velocity, flow patterns, movement direction, and distribution patterns). These functions result in air conditioning, which aids in preventing contamination and cross-contamination, as well as environmental protection and operator protection. Maintaining optimal indoor air quality (IAQ) is a crucial nonpharmacological approach in preventing hospital-acquired infections.

Clinical Importance of the Heating, Ventilation, and Air Conditioning System

Inefficient HVAC systems, including issues with temperature control, humidity control, air distribution, and filtration, are linked to the spread of airborne diseases. Lutz et al. documented an outbreak of Aspergillus infections among inpatients who had undergone surgery in the same operating room within 12 days.[4] Several studies have reported air samples testing positive for methicillin-resistant *Staphylococcus aureus* (MRSA), antibiotic-resistant *Acinetobacter anitratus*, and the airborne spread of carbapenem-resistant *Acinetobacter* species.[5-7]

The transmission of airborne diseases is influenced by several factors, including the characteristics of particles, such as size (droplets ≥5 μm; airborne pathogens ≤5 μm), type, lifespan, distance traveled, and the surrounding environment. Additionally, architectural design and host risk factors also play significant roles in the spread of these diseases.[8,9] Once bacteria, molds, or allergens enter a building, air handling systems (HVAC) play a critical role in controlling their spread and removing them from the system in both droplet-borne diseases (such as pertussis, influenza, coronavirus, and *Staphylococcus aureus*) and airborne diseases (including tuberculosis, *Aspergillus*, norovirus, and varicella-zoster virus). This is achieved through dilution ventilation, which reduces pathogen concentration, or exhaust ventilation, which removes the pathogens. However, if an HVAC system is not properly maintained, it can become a continuous source of contamination, as seen in the growth of molds and other fungi on damp and wet surfaces, such as cooling coils, humidifiers, condensate pans, and filters.

The aim of an air-handling system is to manage the spread of airborne and droplet-borne diseases and assist in their removal from the system. This is done in two ways: either by removing the pathogen from the system using exhaust ventilation or by diluting the pathogen using dilution ventilation.

Components of the Heating, Ventilation, and Air Conditioning System

The HVAC system has three components:

- Outdoor air intake and air exhaust ducts and controls.
- Air handling units (AHUs).
- Air distribution systems[10]

The air handling unit has an important role to play as far as infection prevention is concerned. AHU plays an important role in controlling the indoor air quality and temperature. Its function is to take in outside air, recondition it, and supply it as fresh air.[2] Various components of the AHU are:

- Compressor
- Fans
- Filters
- Drains and drain pans
- Ultraviolet (UV) light emitters or ultraviolet germicidal irradiation (UVGI)
- Noise attenuators

The benefits of the AHU room include:

- Improved ICU air quality
- Increased patient satisfaction
- Reduced energy consumption
- Extended equipment life
- Compliance with regulations

VENTILATION STRATEGIES FOR INTENSIVE CARE UNIT

The ventilation rates cover ventilation for comfort, as well as for asepsis and odor control in areas of intensive care that directly affect patient care. Specialized patient care areas, such as organ transplant units, burn units, and specialty procedure rooms, should have enhanced ventilation provisions to ensure effective air quality control as needed.

The design of the ventilation system should ensure that air flows from cleaner to less clean areas while maintaining the appropriate pressure balance between rooms and corridors and upholding the minimum air changes required in these areas. The number of air changes can be reduced when the ICU or ICU room is unoccupied, provided that measures are in place to restore the specified air changes whenever the space is in use. Adjustments should include provisions so that the direction of air movement remains the same when the number of air changes is reduced.

Air changes mentioned above are the minimum changes needed. To match the changing room conditions, including temperature and humidity, the number of air changes may have to be increased. Such provisions should always be there. Air from the ICU, where patients with pulmonary infections are treated, should not be recirculated. However, for airborne infection control, air may be recirculated within individual isolation rooms if HEPA filters are used. In this application, the return air shall be passed through the HEPA filters before it is introduced into any other spaces.

Rooms with reversible airflow systems designed to switch between protective environments and airborne infection isolation (AII) functions are not permitted.

Temperature Control in Intensive Care Unit

As highlighted in *Energy and Buildings*, the thermal environment has a significant impact on both physical and mental well-being. Defining a universal standard for comfort can be extremely difficult, as it is often dependent on personal preferences. A healthcare setting has dual issues. It needs to ensure the comfort of both of its patients, as it affects their health, as well as its staff, as it affects their productivity. Temperature, especially, plays a vital role in maintaining comfort for both patients and staff. Thermal comfort is a key aspect of indoor environmental quality that influences patients' healing processes and the well-being of medical staff. For patients, thermal comfort takes precedence due to their medical conditions and weakened immune systems.

Challenges in Identifying the Ideal Room Temperature for Intensive Care Unit

Hospitals are unique places, bringing together a wide variety of patients and staff. According to *Intelligent Buildings International*, general hospitals host 39 different functional groups, all contributing to inpatient care, treatment, diagnostics, and support services. With such a diverse mix of people and health conditions, each group has its own specific comfort needs. The diversity in the ICU increases in relation to the clinical condition of the patient. Addressing the thermal comfort of ICU occupants, which includes not only patients but also the staff working there, is a complex matter. The ASHRAE thermal comfort standard (ASHRAE 2017a) specifies a range of environmental and personal factors influenced by the occupants' activity levels and clothing insulation.

Why is Thermal Comfort Important for Patients?

ASHRAE thermal comfort standard (ASHRAE 2017a) requires a set of environmental and personal factors that depend on the occupants' activity levels and clothing insulation. Extreme temperatures, whether excessively high or low, can result in an uncomfortable thermal experience for the patients.

Temperature Ranges for Patient Comfort, Staff Efficiency

In ICUs, patient comfort is best achieved with a room temperature typically ranging from 21°C to 24°C (70–75°F). Some guidelines suggest slightly wider ranges, such as 18–25°C (64–77°F) in the UK and 16–25°C (61–77°F) in India. For burns units, a higher range of 21–32°C (70–90°F) has been suggested in Australia, according to a study.[10]

The Centers for Disease Control and Prevention (CDC) suggests the following temperature ranges for healthcare facilities based on the zone:

- Cool temperatures (68–73 °F or 20–23°C) are typically recommended for operating rooms, endoscopy suites, and clean workrooms.
- Warmer temperatures (75° F or 24°C) are advised in areas where patient comfort is a higher priority, such as patient rooms and delivery rooms.
- A standard temperature range of 70–75 °F (21–24 °C) is generally suitable for most other healthcare areas.

In some situations, flexibility may be necessary to ensure both thermal comfort and safety.

Water Quality in Intensive Care Unit

Water is essential for life. When taken for granted and assumed to be a safe commodity in ICUs, it can create many problems. Biofilm readily becomes established in complex water services, presenting a risk to vulnerable patients. Harbored within biofilms are opportunistic pathogens that can be transmitted via hand contact, splashing, aerosol, and indirect contact through medical equipment. Evidence linking the role of water services in the transmission of infection to patients in ICUs has increased in recent years.

Waterborne infections are common even in well-controlled healthcare systems, and equally concerning is the recognition that wastewater organisms are infecting patients.[11] Access to good quality potable water remains an unmet need in many low- to middle-income countries (LMICs). The infrastructure is often damaged or insufficient, resulting in irregular supply, contamination with fecal matter due to broken pipes, and significant water wastage. There are reports of water contaminated with fecal organisms in the most sophisticated healthcare systems.[12] If these issues are not addressed properly, the individual vulnerable patient is at risk of acquiring resistant organisms. It also threatens the wider population in the community due to the spread of highly antibiotic-resistant organisms.[13]

The Water, Sanitation, and Hygiene (WASH) program, World Health Organization (WHO), has published guidelines for the water quality, quantity, and access needed in healthcare facilities, along with methods for evaluating these facilities using the comprehensive WASHFIT tool.

What are the Risks of Water Services?

Opportunistic premise plumbing pathogens are waterborne microorganisms that naturally inhabit premise plumbing systems and can cause infections in individuals with risk factors and predisposing conditions, such as being over 70 years old, having cancer, or being immunocompromised. Recognized opportunistic pathogens that transmit via the water plumbing include *Legionella pneumophila*, *Mycobacterium avium* and other nontuberculous mycobacteria (NTM), and *Pseudomonas aeruginosa*. A recent study revealed an increase in the incidence of cases caused by *Legionella* spp.[14] These organisms invariably enter healthcare water systems in small numbers in the incoming mains water, and the water system should be designed and maintained to minimize microbial growth and biofilm formation.[15] Regulations require that water be safe for immunocompromised patients, and the microorganisms should be controlled in the water so that they do not multiply and cause disease. Therefore, we must train and educate staff, so they understand the risks of water and the consequences of their actions if transmission of infection through water is to be controlled.

In low- to middle-income countries, high levels of water contamination, often associated with low levels of chlorination, have been linked to outbreaks of bloodstream infections caused by Enterobacteriaceae, including *Klebsiella* and *Enterobacter* spp.

Patients can be exposed to waterborne organisms through activities such as showering, bathing, drinking, or when coming into contact with medical equipment (such as tube feed bags, endoscopes, and respiratory equipment) that have been rinsed with tap water.

What are the Routes of Transmission?

Water naturally aids in the dispersion of microorganisms. It does so by travelling a large distance and by forming biofilm. Splashing will disperse water droplets containing microorganisms at least 2 m from the outlet or surface of the sink/drain, and patients and medical equipment are frequently located within this splash zone.

Many times, organisms found their journey to the patients from the hand washing station and basin through the staff nurse and attendant's hands. Hand washing stations are used for many other purposes other than hand washing, including using the hand-wash basin as a shelf, washing equipment, and disposing of fluids. Controlling human behavior is a difficult task. Refillable spray cleaning bottles represent another example of risk, becoming an extension of the water system. In this case, filling the bottle with tap water led to the fluid being contaminated with *P. aeruginosa* (>108 organisms/L).[16]

SUGGESTED GUIDELINES

- Hospital potable water must have <1 coliform bacterium/100 mL. High bacteria levels in hospital water, dialysate water, sinks, faucets, or shower heads have been associated with outbreaks or hand colonization.[17]
- Hospital water should not be cultured routinely. Water culture should be done during clusters of infection, particularly in LMICs.
- Chlorine levels in hospital water should be tested periodically using national or local standards.
- To reduce the spread of multidrug-resistant gram-negative bacteria, handwashing sinks should be placed in the corridors or at the entrance to

the clinical areas. Alcohol-based hand rubs (ABHR) should be encouraged instead of soap and water.

- Water used for dialysis should be sampled monthly, ensuring that bacteria levels are below 200 bacteria/mL. Dialysate should also be cultured, with similar bacteria levels maintained.
- Nebulization devices and other semi-critical respiratory-care equipment should be designated for single-patient use only.
- Install drift eliminators and regularly clean the water storage tanks using an effective biocide, following the manufacturer's recommendations.
- If a confirmed nosocomial case of Legionnaires' disease is found, an epidemiological and environmental survey should be conducted. If repeated cases are found, decontamination procedures should be conducted.

WORKFLOW OPTIMIZATION IN THE INTENSIVE CARE UNIT FOR INFECTION PREVENTION

Healthcare professionals cannot afford to make even minor workflow mistakes when a patient is admitted to an ICU. A seamless ICU workflow allows doctors and the nursing staff to look after the patient with high precision. Even a simple mistake or breach in infection prevention protocols can lead to disastrous complications. A single episode of nosocomial infection can result in increased length of stay, treatment cost, morbidity, and mortality.

Isolation rooms, the use of anterooms, and differential pressures must be carefully planned to ensure optimal air quality and ventilation. In the ICU, maintaining a proper temperature throughout the areas is crucial for both patient and staff comfort. This not only supports patient recovery but also enhances staff efficiency.

Intensive care unit workflow optimization is necessary for:

- Reducing errors
- Better patient outcome
- Cost-effective medical care
- Staff burnout prevention

WHAT ARE THE STRATEGIES FOR OPTIMIZING ICU WORKFLOW?

- *Fostering a culture of embracing change:* The only change that is permanent. So, staff must be ready to adopt changing guidelines and protocols, which will help improve patient outcomes.
- *Have a clear triage protocol:* This will avoid unnecessary ICU admissions.
- *Standardizing clinical pathways:* This avoids variability in patient care. This will prevent minor mistakes and breaches in protocols.

- *Continuing education and training of staff:* It should be a continuous process. As medical science is evolving rapidly, simulation-based training should be implemented in the ICU at each level. It will improve the critical care given to patients and safety.

INNOVATIONS IN INTENSIVE CARE UNIT INFECTION CONTROL RESEARCH

The first dictum of medical practice is "first do no harm." With advancing technology, infection control practices are evolving. Electronic hand hygiene monitoring systems (EHHMSs) are one such tool that is helping hospitals monitor hand hygiene compliance among staff and doctors.[18] Though direct observation is the gold standard, it is labor-intensive, and there are limitations on sample size.

Another promising technology is antimicrobial textiles. In 2020, Fan et al. conducted a systematic review and meta-analysis of 6 studies and did not find conclusive evidence that copper-impregnated linens decreased HAIs.[19]

Post-COVID-19 pandemic, ultraviolet C devices are being increasingly used in many ICUs.

CONCLUSION

Designing a hospital and ICU is not a simple architecture. The requirements in the ICU are also different from those in non-critical areas of the hospital. The layout of the ICU is one area that has its own role in the control of the spread of infection in the ICU. Isolation rooms, anterooms, and differential pressures must be carefully planned to ensure optimal air quality and ventilation. An ICU presents the unique challenge of maintaining comfort for the health of patients as well as for the efficiency of the staff in a high-pressure environment. Water quality is a neglected area that must be addressed, especially in countries like India. Post-COVID-19 pandemic, new innovations are evolving in the field of infection prevention, which need to be adopted fast if studies prove their usefulness.

REFERENCES

1. Rungta N, Zirpe KG, Dixit SB, Mehta Y, Chaudhry D, Govil D, et al. Indian Society of Critical Care Medicine Experts Committee Consensus Statement on ICU Planning and Designing, 2020. Indian J Crit Care Med 2020;24(Suppl 1):S43-60.
2. McDowall R. Fundamentals of HVAC systems: SI edition, 1st edition. Atlanta, Ga Amsterdam Boston: American Society of Heating, Refrigerating and Air-Conditioning Engineers eLearning Elsevier; 2007.
3. Ashutosh Sharma, Ramesh Kumar K, Saroj K Patnaik. Air-conditioning guidelines for healthcare facilities during the covid pandemic. Int J Med Res Rev. 2021;9(2):107-11.

4. Lutz BD, Jin J, Rinaldi MG, Wickes BL, Huycke MM. Outbreak of invasive Aspergillus infection in surgical patients, associated with a contaminated air-handling system. Clin Infect Dis Off Publ Infect Dis Soc Am. 2003;37(6):786-93.
5. Rutala WA, Katz EB, Sherertz RJ, Sarubbi FA. Environmental study of a methicillin-resistant Staphylococcus aureus epidemic in a burn unit. J Clin Microbiol. 1983;18(3):683-8.
6. Allen KD, Green HT. Hospital outbreak of multi-resistant Acinetobacter anitratus: an airborne mode of spread? J Hosp Infect. 1987;9(2):110-9.
7. Das I, Lambert P, Hill D, Noy M, Bion J, Elliott T. Carbapenem-resistant Acinetobacter and role of curtains in an outbreak in intensive care units. J Hosp Infect. 2002;50(2):110-4.
8. Fernstrom A, Goldblatt M. Aerobiology and its role in the transmission of infectious diseases. J Pathog. 2013;2013:493960.
9. Morawska L. Droplet fate in indoor environments, or can we prevent the spread of infection? Indoor Air. 2006 Oct;16(5):335-47.
10. Saran S, Gurjar M, Baronia A, Sivapurapu V, Ghosh PS, Raju GM, et al. Heating, ventilation and air conditioning (HVAC) in intensive care unit. Crit Care. 2020;24(1):194.
11. Parra LM, Cantero M, Sierra J, Asensio Á, García FJ. A systematic review and meta-analysis of risk factors associated with acquisition of waterborne healthcare-associated infection or colonization in high-risk units. Infect Control Hosp Epidemiol. 2019;1-4.
12. Jung J, Choi HS, Lee JY, Ryu SH, Kim SK, Hong MJ, et al. Outbreak of carbapenemase-producing Enterobacteriaceae associated with a contaminated water dispenser and sink drains in the cardiology units of a Korean hospital. J Hosp Infect. 2020;104(4):476-83.
13. Ahmad M, Khan AU. Global economic impact of antibiotic resistance: A review. J Glob Antimicrob Resist. 2019;19:313-6.
14. Falkinham J, Pruden A, Edwards M. Opportunistic Premise Plumbing Pathogens: Increasingly Important Pathogens in Drinking Water. Pathogens. 2015;4(2):373-86.
15. England NHS. (2016). NHS England » Health Technical Memorandum 04-01: Safe water in healthcare premises. [Online] Available from https://www.england.nhs.uk/publication/safe-water-in-healthcare-premises-htm-04-01/ [Last accessed August, 2025].
16. Weinbren MJ. The handwash station: friend or fiend? J Hosp Infect. 2018;100(2):159-64.
17. World Health Organization. Guidelines for drinking-water quality, 4th edition, incorporating the 1st addendum. [Online] Available from https://www.who.int/publications/i/item/9789241549950 [Last accessed August, 2025].
18. Lin T, Lin C, Chen K, Hsu H. Information technology on hand hygiene compliance among health care professionals: A systematic review and meta-analysis. J Nurs Manag. 2021;29(6):1857-68.
19. Madden GR, Heon BE, Sifri CD. Effect of copper-impregnated linens on multidrug-resistant organism acquisition and *Clostridium difficile* infection at a long-term acute-care hospital. Infect Control Hosp Epidemiol. 2018;39(11):1384-6.

22

CHAPTER

Psychological (Cognitive) Aspects of Infection Prevention

Subhash Todi

LEARNING OBJECTIVES

- Describe different biases in implementing infection control practices.
- Describe Behavior modification strategies to overcome these biases.
- Describe corrections in the organizational factors that will help to overcome biases.
- Strategies to improve communication.
- Describe psychological interventions to improve infection control practices.

INTRODUCTION

Historically, prevention of infection with water borne cholera epidemic was first investigated by John Snow a British epidemiologist. In the year 1854, there was an outbreak of cholera which occurred in London. Many hundreds of patients died in the district of Soho in London. John Snow a British epidemiologist observed that most of the deaths due to cholera took place in households around a tubewell in Broad Street in Soho. Interestingly, there were no incidence of cholera in people working in a Brewery situated near the tubewell as they were surviving on beer. He surmised that the outbreak could be due to consumption of contaminated water from the tubewell. Stopping the use of the tubewell water, reduced the cholera incidence in Soho district and for the first time it was proven that cholera was a water borne disease. The brewery is still there named after John Snow and the tube well is also existing, albeit the handle is removed and kept in a museum as human behavior may cause people to pump the well and drink water from it.[1] This is one example of how human behavior can impact infection prevention. Another example is that of Dr Ignaz Semmelweis an Austrian physician, who observed in 1844, in his hospital, that a high rate of puerperal death was occurring after obstetrical delivery conducted by doctors, whereas the puerperal death was negligible in deliveries carried out by mid wives. He also noticed that the doctors used to perform autopsies before coming to perform deliveries. At that time germ theory of infection was not yet discovered and he surmised that doctors contaminated hands from autopsy procedure may be responsible for the puerperal sepsis and instituted a protocol of hand hygiene prior to delivery that drastically decreased the incidence of infection and maternal death. The tragic end to Prof Semmelweis was that the medical community did not believe him, his medical license was canceled and he was confined to an asylum where he suffered a premature death.[2] Another example of infection prevention affected by human behavior and also the behavioral aspects of disbelief even when evidence is presented. Psychosocial factors may play a pivotal role in implementing infection prevention in healthcare organization. Environmental and behavioral factors that can influence the spread of cholera in urban slums of Kolkata, India was described in 1986.[3] In recent times behavioral aspects of infection prevention sometimes overdone is highlighted by the corona virus disease (COVID) pandemic. In the article psychological aspects of infection prevention will be discussed.

COGNITIVE BIASES[4-6] (BOX 1)

Cognitive biases are systematic errors where the behavior can be influenced by the information received. There are many cognitive biases which can influence our behavior including infection prevention strategies. Antibiotic stewardship and infection control are two sides of the same coin and each influences the other. Some of the biases mentioned are applicable to antimicrobial stewardship which indirectly will effect infection control strategies.

- *Anchoring bias:* Premature decision making based on an information received earlier and a prefixed idea. For example, if a patient is afebrile, it may be perceived as if he is no more infectious and isolation precaution are not maintained. Debiasing strategies could be to not fixate on one aspect of the patient but to receive information from other parameters like white count, etc., before deciding on infectious potential of the patient.
- *Availability bias:* Overestimating events that are memorable. "Removing central lines every 7 days decreased infection rate in an individual patient." This should not be taken as a routine policy and proper audit and analysis of data will lead to proper infection control policy.
- *Commission bias:* The perception that doing something is better than doing nothing—multiple infection control practices like mouth washing an intubated patient with chlorhexidine leads to increasing incidence of pneumonia. Reviewing literature and guidelines will help to prevent adopting this policy. Some recommendations are more likely to be

BOX 1: Biases.

- Anchoring
- Availability
- Commission
- Confirmation
- Labeling
- IKEA effect
- Negative
- Impact
- Present
- Omission
- Familiarity

accepted if they increase the spectrum (Meropenem) and are less likely to be accepted if they recommend reducing the spectrum (Ceftriaxone). Sharing experiences about problems associated with antibiotic commission (*Clostridium difficile* infection, resistance) may alleviate this problem.

- *Confirmation bias:* Tendency to favor evidence that confirms the hypothesis and ignore evidence that refutes the hypothesis or confirms the alternative hypothesis. Symptoms of respiratory tract infection may be wrongly attributed to be of bacterial in etiology because of a positive sputum culture report. The possibility of viral etiology is not investigated, and bacterial colonization is not considered, thus limiting infection prevention possibilities. Use of other diagnostic modalities with more specificity may help to identify the problem.
- *Labeling bias:* Solidification of clinical suspicion as the diagnostic information passes from a patient to clinicians across departments. History of an allergy to an antibiotic (e.g., penicillin) reported by a patient is suboptimally investigated and sticks with the patient. History of an allergy to an antibiotic (e.g., penicillin) reported by a patient is suboptimally investigated and sticks with the patient. Standardized checklist and written handovers may prevent recurrence of this problem.
- *IKEA effect:* This effect is named after a Swedish furniture manufacturer company which identified that instead of selling furniture as a whole is less appealing to buyer than selling it in parts which they assemble themselves, which gives them a sense of ownership. Thus, rather than imposing an infection control policy on the staff, involving them to make a policy will be more appealing.
- *Negative bias:* Negative experiences make a greater impression than positive outcomes. Treatment failure with a narrow-spectrum agent is more likely to be remembered (e.g., nitrofurantoin for urinary tract infection) than positive clinical outcomes with the same agent. This may be overcome by providing evidence and statistical data (e.g., hospital antibiogram and outcome analysis data).
- *Impact bias:* Overestimating benefits and underestimating risks of a diagnostic test/treatment. Thinking that antibiotic resistance although a problem is driven by other prescribers may be the reason.
- *Present bias:* Favoring smaller immediate benefits over larger long-term benefits. Favoring immediate patient satisfaction due to perceived symptom relief, over long-term problems such as antimicrobial resistance (e.g., azithromycin for viral upper respiratory tract infection). This may be decreased by providing inputs about risks versus benefit.
- *Omission bias:* Preferring omission (inaction) over commission. A tendency of antibiotic stewards (clinical microbiologists and infectious disease physicians) toward antibiotic prescribing inaction rather than

action. This may be circumvented by clinical data feedback about patient outcomes along with motivating the team to draw out an achievable action plan and reinforcing small changes.[7]

- *Familiarity bias:* Over-reliance on a familiar tool. A tendency of antibiotic stewards to focus on antimicrobial stewardship rather than looking at the patient from a broader perspective. Involve feedback from stakeholders and encouragement to communicate on broader issues through multidisciplinary ward rounds, meetings, and newsletters.

BEHAVIOR MODIFICATION STRATEGIES[8] (FIG. 1)

Many behavioral modification strategies are described in the literature, but "one size does not fit all" and these need to be customized to the particular institution implementing the strategy based on the human resources available to them. Certain fundamental principles may be followed which are applicable to all strategies.

- *Top-down approach:* Change is unlikely to sustain without support of institution leadership. Strategies need discussion and agreement of hospital administration and clinical departmental leadership. However, it might be difficult to keep the leadership focused on a specific change objective, considering their involvement in a wide domain. Continuous and effective engagement with leadership is essential.
- *Bottom-up approach:* All stakeholders starting from the junior most staff need to be involved in order to bring a change in infection control strategy.
- *Clear guidelines:* It should be clear to everyone as regards why changes are needed and how they are going to be corrected, i.e., the drawbacks of the current strategy and the steps needed to correct them. This would entail

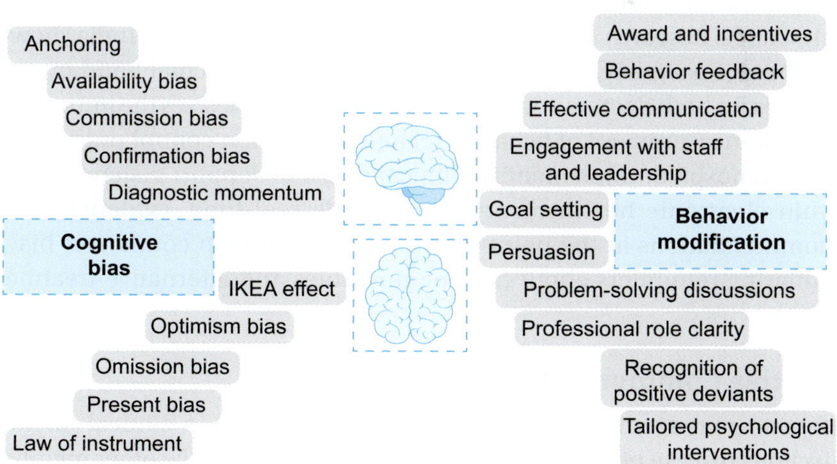

Fig. 1: Behavior modification strategy.

a series of meetings with the stakeholders which need to be carefully planned and executed.

- *Manage the sceptics:* In most organizations, there would be people who will resist changes, who need to be skillfully managed. This will include multi-modal strategies such as education, training, audit, feedback, use of media, opinion leaders, etc. Positive deviants need to be recognized, appreciated, and used as agents of change. An example of a positive deviant is a relatively junior nurse respectfully reminding a senior physician about his/her noncompliance to standard infection prevention and control practices (such as hand hygiene). As some setbacks are likely and perhaps inevitable, team leaders must focus and project small gains, which may be used to engage with and inspire others. Successes need to be shared in an open forum, and failures discussed in confidence. A positive change achieved in one department or area needs to be institutionalized through an effort to make a policy change in other departments within the institution. Comprehensive education program that emphasize importance of evidence-based practices can help mitigate cognitive biases. Regular training sessions that incorporate case studies and recent research findings can reinforce the need for adherence to guidelines and dangers of biases.

Organizational Factors and Professional Role Ambiguity

Despite having less than ideal knowledge about multidrug-resistant bacteria, nurses had an adequate understanding of correct Infection Prevention and Control (IPC) policies (cognition) or complying with the guideline (behavior). For example, lack of isolation rooms, a busy work environment, and the stress of the inability to implement guidelines into clinical practice (because of logistical or training inadequacy) are organizational factors that affect compliance. Research on hand hygiene from a cancer center in India showed that there is a significant gap between perceived and actual hand hygiene practices for both doctors and nurses.[8] This study emphasizes the importance of actual measurement of behavior related to infection control practices for staff in a hospital. Implementing clinical decision support systems (CDSS) within electronic health record can provide real-time, evidence-based recommendations at the point of care. These can help counteract biases by offering reminders about current guidelines and alternative treatment options.

Effective Communication[8]

Infection management discussions are mostly between clinical doctors, infectious disease physicians, clinical microbiologists. Sadly, other members (infection control nurses, bedside nurses, clinical pharmacists, and clinical pharmacologists) are often excluded from clinical discussions of infection management. Many clinicians may have low expectations about the contributions of IPC and antimicrobial stewardship program (AMSP) team members in the clinical management of the patient even when the primary problem is infection.

Psychological Intervention[9,10]

A cluster randomized controlled trial [PSYGIENE (PSYchological optimized hand hyGIENE promotion) trial] in Germany evaluated the effect of psychologically tailored hand hygiene interventions to improve hand hygiene compliance and thereby reduce multidrug-resistant infections. A number of behavior change techniques were used in the PSYCIENE trial and included: goal setting, behavior feedback, feedback of clinical outcome of healthcare worker behavior (e.g., healthcare-associated infection rates associated with hand hygiene compliance rates), instruction on how to perform the behavior (e.g., hand hygiene steps, and five moments of hand hygiene), information on psychological consequences of healthcare-associated infections (on patient, patient relatives, and primary physician), demonstration of behavior using ultraviolet light boxes, discussing effects of compliance and noncompliance, verbal persuasion, focus on past success, problem solving discussions, reflection and discussion on implementation intentions, active listening in feedback discussions, information about recognition by superiors, use of laminated information sheets as prompts/cues, rehearsal of specific behavior (hand hygiene), focusing on staff specific tasks (hand hygiene of a doctor before aseptic technique such as lumbar puncture), awards and incentives to staff, optimization of facilities and infrastructure (hand sanitizer and hand wash station availability), asking for team cooperation rather than individual cooperation, and situation specific reward (certification of a ward/department for the best compliance).

Discontinuation of needle recapping increased among nurses after specific behavior modification intervention packages following a stepped intervention model such as the announcement by nursing hierarchy (least improvement), use of posters and pamphlets (intermediate level of improvement), followed by use of in-service lectures (plus announcement plus posters). The last intervention had the maximum improvement. Understanding the attitude of healthcare workers through an anonymous questionnaire survey to assess the proportion of staff willing to change before intervention may help optimize intervention (hand wash versus hand rub) or intervention domain selection (different clinical departments). However, one needs to be careful while taking feedback, as the “discourse and narrative” about a problem may differ from the “actual practice” as found regarding simple hand hygiene practices. Participatory decision-making (PDM) and efforts to arrive at a consensus on infection control policy issues may ensure better compliance with standard practice recommendations. Implementation of even standard operating procedures may require the implementation of relatively unfamiliar ideas, policies, and products. The engagement of senior nursing staff as opinion leaders may facilitate implementation and sustainable adherence to practices. The use of education programs and engagement of opinion leaders have been shown to improve urinary care practices and reduce incorrect practices. The cognitive determinants of human behavior include many facets such as knowledge, motivation, intention, perception of threat, attitude, outcome expectancy, perceived self-efficacy and behavioral control, and social pressure.

CONCLUSION

Infection Prevention and Control in a healthcare organization are essential but resource-intensive activities. Even when well-established and universally accepted policies exist, behavior modifications at an organizational level require administrative and management support, dedicated funding, infrastructure, human resources, material resources, and consumables among other requirements to translate knowledge into practice. Conditioning human behavior and understanding cognitive biases are increasingly being recognized as key factors facilitating or hindering policy implementation. In this scenario, the role of psychiatrists, psychologists, and social and behavioral scientists are critically important, and AMSP/IPC professionals as well as healthcare administrators would be well advised to seek professional guidance in shaping organizational behavior and work culture. Implementing performance metrics that assess adherence to IPC and AMSP practices can create a sense of accountability. Regularly reviewing these metrics can help identify areas for improvement and encourage compliance.

REFERENCES

1. Tulchinsky TH. John Snow, Cholera, the Broad Street Pump; Waterborne Diseases Then and Now. Case Studies in Public Health. 2018:77-99.
2. Noakes TD, Borresen J, Hew-Butler T, Lambert MI, Jordaan E. Semmelweis and the aetiology of puerperal sepsis 160 years on: an historical review. Epidemiol Infect. 2008;136(1):1-9.
3. Deb BC, Sircar BK, Sengupta PG, De SP, Mondal SK, Gupta DN, et al. Studies on interventions to prevent El Tor cholera transmission in urban slums. Bull World Health Organ. 1986;64(1):127-31.
4. Tversky A, Kahneman D. Judgment under uncertainty: Heuristics and biases: Biases in judgments reveal some heuristics of thinking under uncertainty. Science. 1974;185(4157):1124-31.
5. Da Silva S, Gupta R, Monzani D. Editorial: Highlights in psychology: cognitive bias. Front Psychol. 2023;14:1242809.

6. Langford BJ, Daneman N, Leung V, Langford DJ. Cognitive bias: how understanding its impact on antibiotic prescribing decisions can help advance antimicrobial stewardship. JAC Antimicrob Resist. 2020;2:dlaa107.
7. Bearman G, Nori P. Implementing behaviour change in healthcare epidemiology and antimicrobial stewardship: The worst that can happen is you fail. Antimicrob Steward Healthc Epidemiol. 2023;3(1):e129.
8. Bonaconsa C, Mbamalu O, Surendran S, George A, Mendelson M, Charani E. Optimizing infection control and antimicrobial stewardship bedside discussion: a scoping review of existing evidence on effective healthcare communication in hospitals. Clin Microbiol Infect. 2024;30(3):336-52.
9. von Lengerke T, Ebadi E, Schock B, Krauth C, Lange K, Stahmeyer JT, et al. Impact of psychologically tailored hand hygiene interventions on nosocomial infections with multidrug-resistant organisms: results of the cluster-randomized controlled trial PSYGIENE. Antimicrob Resist Infect Control. 2019;8:56.
10. Pittet D. The Lowbury lecture: behaviour in infection control. J Hosp Infect. 2004;58(1):1-13.

7

SECTION

Practical Tools and Appendices

Section Editor: *Aruna Poojary*

23

CHAPTER

Interactive and Self-assessment Tools

Srikant Behera, Shailesh Kumar Sahu, Biswabikash Mohanty

LEARNING OBJECTIVES

- Infection control practice (IPC).
- Interactive and self-assessment tools in IPC.

INTRODUCTION

Hospital-acquired infections (HAIs) are a significant cause of morbidity and mortality in intensive care units (ICUs). The common nosocomial infections include hospital-acquired pneumonia, bloodstream infection, catheter-associated urinary tract infection, and surgical site infections. These infections affect patients and their caregivers, including the healthcare workers (HCWs), in a big way and increase the cost of treatment hugely. To handle these infections and treat them, the already overburdened healthcare system has to consume scarce resources, especially in resource-limited settings. Furthermore, the rise in resistance among microorganisms to commonly used antimicrobials poses more difficulties in treating them, and more so, the expense of treating these resistant infections is much higher. However, nosocomial infections can be prevented and controlled among hospital staff and patients through the proper implementation of infection control guidelines and policies. Developing nations spend a major portion of their healthcare budget in hospitals, including substantial expenditures for advanced diagnosis and treatment, equipment procurement, and for care of high-risk patients such as surgical patients or patients in intensive care units. Failure to prevent or control nosocomial infections limits the benefits of these expenditures and further compromises the hospital budget. Therefore, hospital infection control programs are required to reduce the risk of serious, yet preventable infections in *patients* and healthcare workers from both an economic and a clinical perspective.[1] But, implementation of infection prevention and control programs in low- and middle-income countries is frequently hampered by financial constraints, limited laboratory capacity, and inadequate staff knowledge and training in key areas such as hand hygiene, sterilization procedures, and isolation precautions.[2-4]

So, there is an urgent need for a systematic approach to detect deficiencies in infection control practices and to implement effective, affordable solutions. There are various assessment tools like Infection Control Assessment Tools

(ICAT) and Systems for Improved Access to Pharmaceuticals and Services (SIAPS) Program that provide an effective approach that can be used by hospital staff to identify and solve the problems economically.[5]

INTERACTIVE TOOLS FOR CONTINUOUS LEARNING AND INFECTION CONTROL

An "interactive and self-assessment tool for infection control" may be a digital platform or questionnaire that independently evaluates healthcare workers' current infection control practices knowledge, identifies their areas for improvement, and tracks the progress over time. It functions by recording the answers given by HCWs to questions about procedures, protocols, and resource availability related to preventing the spread of infections in ICUs or any other healthcare setting.[6,7] It is often based on established guidelines from the WHO or CDC. It includes scoring systems, feedback mechanisms, action plan generators, etc., to guide improvements.

The critical care nurses' infection prevention and control (IPC) practices can be crucial in reducing ventilator-associated pneumonia (VAP) and central line-associated bloodstream infection (CLABSI). Implementing IPC practices has been shown to reduce the incidence of HAIs in the ICUs. However, ICUs being a complex environment, there exist multiple barriers to IPC practice compliance. Some of the barriers to the successful implementation of IPC practices include the absence of local guidelines, inadequate knowledge and training, high workload, urgent patient needs, difficulty in integrating IPC practices in the workflow, and the lack of resources.[8-10] These barriers must be overcome to reduce HAIs successfully. Nowadays, social media platforms like Facebook, YouTube, Instagram, Twitter, WhatsApp, and Telegram have the advantage of connecting millions of users at the touch of a button. These can be utilized to share education and training materials, including videos and pictorial presentations, to create awareness among communities and healthcare professionals (HCP) on important topics like IPC practices, HAIs, and antimicrobial resistance. Some modes of dissemination being used widely are downloadable infographics, interactive blogs by experts, small video clips to promote knowledge and awareness, case studies, posts with thought-provoking questions, etc.

Bijarania et al. in a participatory study showed that implementing a multimedia tool in cardiac surgical ICU, improved compliance with IPC practices related to VAP and central-line-associated bloodstream infection (CLABSI), such as chlorhexidine baths, oral care, cuff pressure maintenance, hypertonic saline nebulization, endotracheal suctioning, scrubbing the hub for central line access, and assessment of the central line for removal.[11] Similarly, implementation of a computer-assisted learning package for IPC practices, particularly for the night-duty and weekend staff, leads to utilization of continuously available online tools.[12] Education tools on IPC involving self-study modules and pre- and postquestions are also beneficial in improving patient outcomes. Simulations and virtual reality are attractive teaching modalities capable of improving the knowledge of healthcare workers in infection control practices by offering real clinical care situations. Simulation-based training in the prevention of HAIs reduces the costs and complications.

Mobile apps can support widespread dissemination of evidence to reduce HAIs. Mobile apps can be utilized to reduce HAIs by providing easy access to guidelines, supporting hand hygiene monitoring, listing step-by-step procedures to reduce infections at the point of clinical care, or providing specific healthcare facility layout instructions to minimize HAIs. American Association of Critical-Care Nurses (AACN) Bedside Guideline Central, Infection Control Pocketbook, Infection Prevention, and Handwash Counter are some of examples of mobile applications providing guidelines for multiple HAI and complications. There are sections on core areas of infection control practices such as (1) prevention of catheter-associated urinary tract infection (CAUTI), CLABSI, SSI, VAP; (2) guidelines for multiple infections (including infection prevention); (3) diseases and conditions in healthcare facilities; (4) guidelines for infection control and prevention for healthcare providers; (5) list of precautions associated with preventing numerous infections; (6) track handwashing instances to promote infection prevention; (7) better hand hygiene; etc.

Self-assessment Tool for Intensive Care Unit Staff

Self-assessment tool helps to monitor the behavior of ICU staff against the National Standards for the Prevention and Control of Healthcare-Associated Infections. This tool comprises a series of specific questions in relation to:

- The hospital infection prevention and control program
- Training and implementation of related policies and protocols
- Systems to detect, prevent, and respond to healthcare-associated infections and multidrug-resistant organisms.

Self-assessment Tool for Hand Hygiene Practices

- In which of the following situations you should wash your hands with soap and water or an alcohol-based hand antiseptic?
    - Before contact with patients
    - After contact with individual patients or their immediate environment
    - Before manipulating medical devices such as intravenous catheters, or before handling wound dressing
    - After touching potentially contaminated objects or surfaces
    - After removing gloves
    - After using the bathroom, toilet, or latrine

- Is there a policy on keeping fingernails short and/or not using artificial nails or nail extenders? No/Yes
- Is it usual practice to wear gloves instead of washing hands for contact with patients or potentially contaminated environmental surfaces? No/Yes
- Is hand lotion (emollient) available for staff to use at the end of the working day? No/Yes (hand lotion in disposable containers)
- Is there a written policy or guide on hand hygiene in the ICU?
  - No written policy or guide
  - Policy/procedures communicated verbally only
  - Written policy/guide in a manual and also posted on walls in the ICU
- Does the ICU have a poster on hand washing? No/Yes
- What is the usual source of water for hand washing?
  - No water is usually available
  - Water is scooped from a basin and poured over hands
  - Water is usually poured over hands from a basin
  - Water is usually available from a cistern or container with gravity flow
  - Running water from the sink
- How frequently is running water available?
  - Never
  - Sometimes
  - Usually
  - Always
- What type of soap is most frequently available for hand washing?
  - No soap is available
  - Plain bar soap stored in a receptacle that does not allow water to drain
  - Plain bar soap stored in a receptacle that allows water to drain
  - Plain liquid soap
  - Liquid soap with an antimicrobial agent
- What types of dispensers are used in the facility for liquid soap?
  - Liquid soaps are not used
  - Handheld pour bottle dispenser
  - Hand-operated pump dispenser
  - Foot pump dispenser
- What method is usually available for drying hands after hand washing?
  - None (air dry)
  - Multiple-use cloth towel
  - Single-use cloth towel
  - Paper towels
  - Hot air dryer

Isolation Policies and Precautions

- Does the ICU have isolation for the following patients? Yes/No (TB, measles, cholera, *Clostridioides difficile*, influenza, *Staphylococcus aureus*, burn, transplant recipients, patients with neutropenia)
- Does the isolation precaution guidelines include instructions about the following?
  - Handling of linen
  - Handling of equipment and supplies
  - Disposal of waste and corpses
  - Cleaning
  - All of the above
- Does the isolation precaution guidelines include instructions about the following?
  - Patient placement in specific rooms according to their disease or mode of transmission
  - Transport of isolated patients to other locations in the facility

Environmental and Patient Equipment Cleaning

Table 1 shows environmental and patient equipment cleaning.

Prevention of Intravascular Catheter-related Bloodstream Infection

Table 2 shows the prevention of intravascular catheter-related bloodstream infection.

TABLE 1: Environmental and patient equipment cleaning.

There is a designated person with delegated responsibility for the management of environmental and patient equipment hygiene in the hospital	Yes	No
Training is provided to personnel prior to being allowed to perform environmental and equipment cleaning	Yes	No
Training is provided when new equipment or protocols are introduced for environmental and equipment cleaning	Yes	No
The hospital has protocols to ensure that healthcare personnel can readily identify equipment that has been cleaned and disinfected and is ready for patient use (e.g., tagging system, placement in a dedicated clean area)	Yes	No
The hospital regularly audits (monitors and documents) adherence to cleaning and disinfection procedures, including use of products in accordance with manufacturers' instructions (e.g., dilution, storage, shelf-life, and contact time)	Yes	No

TABLE 2: Prevention of intravascular catheter-related bloodstream infection.

The hospital has an up-to-date policy detailing measures to prevent intravascular catheter-related bloodstream infection that includes care bundle elements	Yes	No
The hospital has a competency-based training program for all clinical personnel who insert intravascular catheters	Yes	No
Training is provided to all personnel who are given responsibility for the insertion of intravascular catheters	Yes	No
The hospital regularly audits (monitors and documents) adherence to recommended practices for insertion of intravascular catheters	Yes	No
Evidence-based intravascular catheter care bundles are followed each time, including the insertion bundle, daily catheter care	Yes	No
Regular audit (monitors and documents) regarding adherence to evidence-based intravascular catheter care bundles	Yes	No
The hospital infection control committee monitors intravascular catheter-related infection and uses this information to take preventive measures	Yes	No

TABLE 3: Prevention of ventilator-associated pneumonia.

The ICU has an up-to-date policy detailing measures to prevent ventilator-associated pneumonia that includes care bundle elements	Yes	No
Regular training is provided to relevant clinical personnel in relation to the prevention of ventilator-associated pneumonia	Yes	No
Evidence-based ventilator-associated pneumonia care bundles have been implemented in clinical areas accommodating ventilated patients	Yes	No
The head end of the ICU bed is kept elevated	Yes	No
Stress ulcer prophylaxis is followed	Yes	No
Oral hygiene is maintained using chlorhexidine	Yes	No
DVT prophylaxis is administered	Yes	No
The hospital regularly audits (monitors and documents) ventilator-associated pneumonia care bundle compliance	Yes	No
The hospital provides feedback from audits to personnel regarding their compliance with ventilator-associated pneumonia care bundles	Yes	No
The hospital infection control committee performs ventilator-associated pneumonia infection surveillance and uses this information to direct prevention activities	Yes	No

(DVT: deep vein thrombosis; ICU: intensive care unit)

Prevention of Ventilator-associated Pneumonia

Table 3 shows the prevention of ventilator-associated pneumonia.

Prevention of *Clostridium difficile* Infection

Table 4 shows the prevention of *Clostridium difficile* infection.

TABLE 4: Prevention of *Clostridium difficile* infection (CDI).

The hospital performs CDI surveillance and uses the information gathered to direct prevention activities	Yes	No
The hospital has an up-to-date policy detailing measures to manage patients with CDI that includes care bundle elements	Yes	No
The hospital has specific antimicrobial stewardship strategies in place to reduce the incidence of CDI	Yes	No
At a minimum, systems analysis is performed for each episode of severe CDI and all cases of CDI associated with a cluster or an outbreak of infection	Yes	No
The hospital formally reviews management of CDI outbreaks/clusters in order to identify precipitating factors and necessary control measures	Yes	No
It is hospital policy that patients with potentially infectious diarrhea are promptly isolated in a single ensuite room until an infectious cause is ruled out	Yes	No

CONCLUSION

Interactive and self-assessment tools in infection control typically include questionnaires or checklists that healthcare workers can use or should be encouraged to use for evaluation of their current practices against established infection control standards, covering areas like hand hygiene, personal protective equipment use, environmental cleaning, patient placement, waste disposal, etc. It will allow them to identify areas for improvement and implement corrective measures through feedback mechanisms. All HCWs should be actively involved in and utilize this important endeavor, and can contribute towards achieving high-quality health care by practicing standard infection control practices, and help in the prevention of HAIs.

REFERENCES

1. Kubde D, Badge AK, Ugemuge S, Shahu S. Importance of Hospital Infection Control. Cureus. 2023;15(12):e50931.
2. Sengupta S, Barman P, Lo J. Opportunities to overcome implementation challenges of infection prevention and control in low-middle income countries. Curr Treat Options Infect Dis. 2019;11:267-80.
3. Ider B-E, Adams J, Morton A, Whitby M, Clements A. Perceptions of healthcare professionals regarding the main challenges and barriers to effective hospital infection control in Mongolia: a qualitative study. BMC Infect Dis. 2012;12:170.
4. Vilar-Compte D, Camacho-Ortiz A, Ponce-De-León S. Infection control in limited resources countries: challenges and priorities. Curr Infect Dis Rep. 2017;19(5):20.
5. SIAPS. 2013. Infection Control Self-Assessment Tool for Primary Health Care Facilities. [Online] Available from https://nest360-wp.newborntoolkit.org/wp-content/uploads/2021/11/USAID-SIAPS-Infection-Control-Assessment-Tool-for-Primary-Health-Care-Facilities.pdf [Last accessed August, 2025].

6. World Health Organization. (2016). WHO Guidelines on core components of IPC programmes at the national and acute health care facility level. [Online] Available from http://www.who.int/infection-prevention/publications/core-components/en/ [Last accessed August, 2025].
7. Improving infection prevention and control at the health facility level. Interim practical manual supporting implementation of the WHO guidelines on core components of infection prevention and control programmes. (http://www.who.int/infection-prevention/tools/core-components/en/, [Last accessed May, 2018].
8. Rehmani AI, Au A, Montgomery C, Papathanassoglou E. Use of nursing care bundles for the prevention of ventilator-associated pneumonia in low-middle income countries: a scoping review. Nurs Crit Care. 2024;29(6):1511e34.
9. Houghton C, Meskell P, Delaney H, Smalle M, Glenton C, Booth A, et al. Barriers and facilitators to healthcare workers' adherence with infection prevention and control (IPC) guidelines for respiratory infectious diseases: a rapid qualitative evidence synthesis. Cochrane Database Syst Rev. 2020;4(4):CD013582.
10. Croft K, Dallal-York J, Miller S, Anderson A, Donohue C, Jeng E, et al. Provision of oral care in the cardiothoracic intensive care unit: survey of nursing staff training, confidence, methods, attitudes, and perceived barriers. J Cont Educ Nurs. 2023;54(7):313e21.
11. Bijarania SK, Kaur R, Biswal M, Maheshwar S, Ganesan R, Puri GD, et al. A multimedia tool for infection prevention and control practices in the intensive care unit: a participatory interventional before-after study. Infect Prev Pract. 2024;7(1):100423.
12. Desai N, Philpott-Howard J, Wade J, Casewell M. Infection control training: evaluation of a computer-assisted learning package. J Hosp Infect. 2000;44(3):193-9.

24

CHAPTER

Key Tools for Practice

Vrunda Vijay Agre

LEARNING OBJECTIVES

- Prevent the spread of infection by using correct techniques and tools.
- Protect yourself and those you serve by understanding the chain of infection.
- Continuous surveillance of infection for early detection for which appropriate control measure is undertaken.
- Follow the intensive care unit (ICU) care bundles and antimicrobial stewardship policies.
- Control expenditure by reducing the need for intensive management in late stages of illness.

INTRODUCTION

In the intensive care unit (ICU), critically ill patients are vulnerable and are at high risk for hospital-acquired infection it's a significant challenge to patient's care, leading to increase mortality in ICU if we don't follow our protocols. The risk of infection in the ICU is very high due to the use of medical devices and the patient's critical condition, including comorbid condition. Despite adequate infection prevention and control (IPC) measures such as hand hygiene, environmental cleaning, and management of invasive lines, healthcare-associated infections remain high in ICUs worldwide.

This chapter aims to address the current recommendations for IPC in the ICU and improve patient outcomes by enhancing awareness and understanding of IPC.

INTENSIVE CARE UNIT BUNDLES

Ventilator-associated Pneumonia

Ventilator-associated pneumonia (VAP) is defined as a pneumonia that develops 48 hours after a patient has been placed on a mechanical ventilator. Ventilator-associated pneumonia should be suspected when a patient is on a mechanical ventilator and demonstrates progressive in filters on chest X-ray.[1]

Clinical Pulmonary Infection Score

Diagnosing VAP requires a high clinical suspicion combined with bedside examination. *Clinical Pulmonary Infection Score (CPIS)*—a scoring system

TABLE 1: Clinical pulmonary infection score (CPIS) points of different tests.

CPIS points	*0*	*1*	*2*
Tracheal secretions	Rare	Abundant	Abundant + Purulent
Chest X-ray infiltrates	No infiltrate	Diffused	Localized
Temperature (°C)	≥36.5 and ≤38.4	≥38.5 and ≤38.9	≥39 or ≤36
Leukocyte count (per mm^3)	≥4,000 and ≤11,000	<4,000 or >11,000	<4,000 or >11,000 + band forms ≥500
PaO_2/FiO_2 (mm Hg)	>240 or ARDS		≤240 and no evidence of ARDS
Microbiology	Negative		Positive

Note: The total score ranges from 0 to 10, with a score below 6 indicating the absence of VAP and a score of 6 or higher suggesting the presence of VAP.

(ARDS: acute respiratory distress syndrome; FiO_2: fraction of inspired oxygen; PaO_2: partial pressure of arterial oxygen)

that combines clinical, radiographic, and microbiological data to assess the likelihood of VAP, can be used **(Table 1)**.

Ventilator-associated Pneumonia Care Bundles

- Head-up tilt 30–45°
- Gastric ulcers prophylaxis—proton pump inhibitor (PPI)
- Chest X-ray, physiotherapy, suction endotracheal tube (ET), mouth, oropharynx
- Documentation 4 hourly
- Indication of VAP compliance
- Turn patient to side to back to side every 2 hourly
- Deep vein thrombosis (DVT) pump
- Daily assessment of readiness to be extubated
- Daily sedation vacations
- Keep ventilator tubing below the level of patient
- Moisturize mouth and lips
- Rinse Yankauer and suction tubing

Treatment

- Appropriate antibiotics as per hospital policy
- Follow VAP care bundles.

Central Line-associated Bloodstream Infection

As per the Centers for Disease Control and Prevention (CDC) definition, central line-associated bloodstream infection (CLABSI) is a surveillance definition used by the CDC and defined as the recovery of a pathogen from a blood culture (a single blood culture for an organism not commonly present on the skin and two or more blood cultures for an organism commonly present on the skin) in a patient who had a central line at the time of infection or within 48 hours before the development of infection. The infection cannot be related to any other infection the patient might have and must not have been present or incubating when the patient was admitted to the facility.[2]

Central line-associated bloodstream infection should be suspected when the patient has:

- A fever above 100.4°F (38°C) and chills
- Encephalopathy
- Shock
- Redness, pain, swelling, or drainage around the place where your central venous catheter (CVC) goes into your body

Exit site infection: Signs of inflammation confined to an area (typically <2 cm) surrounding the catheter exit site and the presence of exudate that proves to be culture-positive

Tunnel infection: Inflammation extending beyond 2 cm from the exit site (along with the track or cephalad toward the vein entry site or extending beyond the cuff), typically associated with pain and tenderness along the subcutaneous track and culture-positive exudate at the exit site that may not be seen unless expressed by palpation

Central Line-associated Bloodstream Infection Care Bundles

- Perform hand hygiene.
- Minimal barrier precautions
- Clean parts with 70% alcohol/chlorhexidine before use.
- Change wet insertion site dressing promptly.
- Semipermeable transparent dressing changes every 5–7 days
- Sterile gauze dressing changes every 24 hours
- Choosing proper central line insertion site (jugular, subclavian, and femoral); femoral line faces the highest risk for developing CLABSI
- Remove unnecessary central lines.

Post Insertion Care Maintenance

- Protective disk with chlorhexidine gluconate (CHG) is a polyurethane foam disk should be around the catheter making 360° contact proved to reduce local infections, catheter-related blood stream infections with skin to skin with blue side up.
- Dressing changed every 7 days
- Caps should be used at each lumen single use only
- Scrub the hub with chlorhexidine wipes for 15 seconds.

Catheter-associated Urinary Tract Infection

Catheter-associated urinary tract infection is defined as a urinary tract infection (UTI) where an indwelling urinary catheter (IUC) was in place for more than 2 consecutive days in an inpatient location on the date of event or the day before, with the day of device placement being day 1. If an IUC was in place for more than 2 consecutive days in an inpatient location and then removed, the date of event for the UTI must be the day of device discontinuation or the next day for the UTI to be catheter-associated.

Catheter-associated urinary tract infection should be suspected when a patient has any signs of infection post IUC insertion.

Catheter-associated Urinary Tract Infection Bundles[3]

- Perform hand hygiene and standard precaution.
- Insertion using sterile technique
- Proper care of perineal area
- Insert catheter only for appropriate indications.
- Maintain a closed drainage system.
- Secure drainage bag below bladder.
- Remove as soon as it is no longer needed.

Post Insertion Care and Maintenance

Catheter-associated urinary tract infections can lead to complications such as prostatitis, epididymitis, orchitis, cystitis, pyelonephritis, and gram-negative bacteremia.

Drug Infusion Pump Care

Indication: Infusion pumps are used in the ICU to deliver fluids, medications, and nutrients to a patient in controlled amounts.[4,5]

Cleaning of infusion pumps should be done as follows:

- *Gather necessary supplies:* Disinfectant wipes or solution, soft and lint-free cloths, isopropyl alcohol, water for rinsing, and gloves and protective gear
- *Power off and disconnect:* Turn off the infusion pump and disconnect it from the power source to avoid any electrical hazards during the cleaning process.
- *Disassemble (if applicable):* Some infusion pumps may have detachable components. Follow the manufacturer's instructions to safely disassemble the pump for thorough cleaning.
- *Clean infusion set connections:* Inspect the infusion set connections for any debris or residue. Clean the connections using a cloth dampened with isopropyl alcohol or a manufacturer-recommended disinfectant to ensure proper functioning and prevent contamination.

- *Wipe exterior surfaces:* Gently wipe down the exterior surfaces of the infusion pump, including buttons, screens, and casing. Take care not to allow moisture to seep into any openings. Allow the infusion pump to air-dry completely before reassembly or use.
- *Cleaning:* Clean with alcohol and allow it to dry.
- *Reassemble and test:* If you have disassembled any components, carefully reassemble the infusion pump according to the manufacturer's instructions. Perform a functional test to ensure that the pump operates correctly after cleaning and before using it for the next patient.

DONNING OF PERSONAL PROTECTIVE EQUIPMENT

The donning of personal protective equipment (PPE) is shown in **Figure 1**.

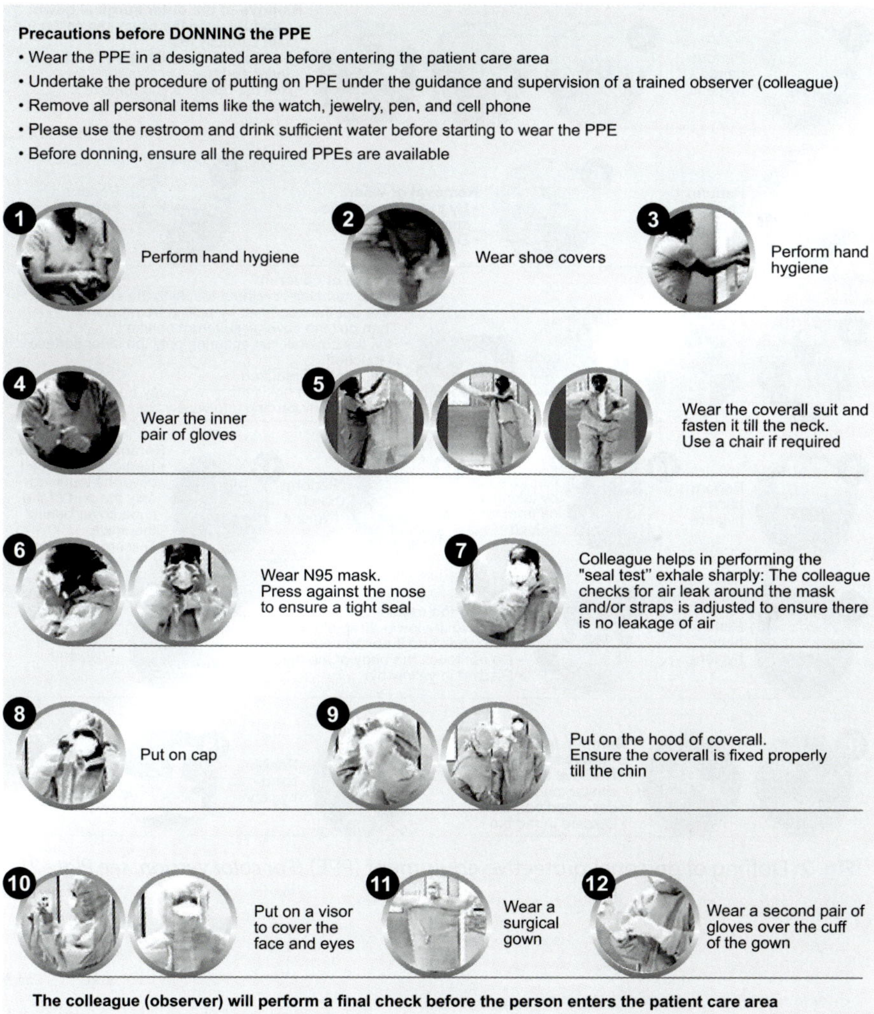

Fig. 1: Donning of personal protective equipment (PPE) *(For color version, see Plate 1)*.

DOFFING OF PERSONAL PROTECTIVE EQUIPMENT

The doffing of PPE is shown in **Figure 2**.

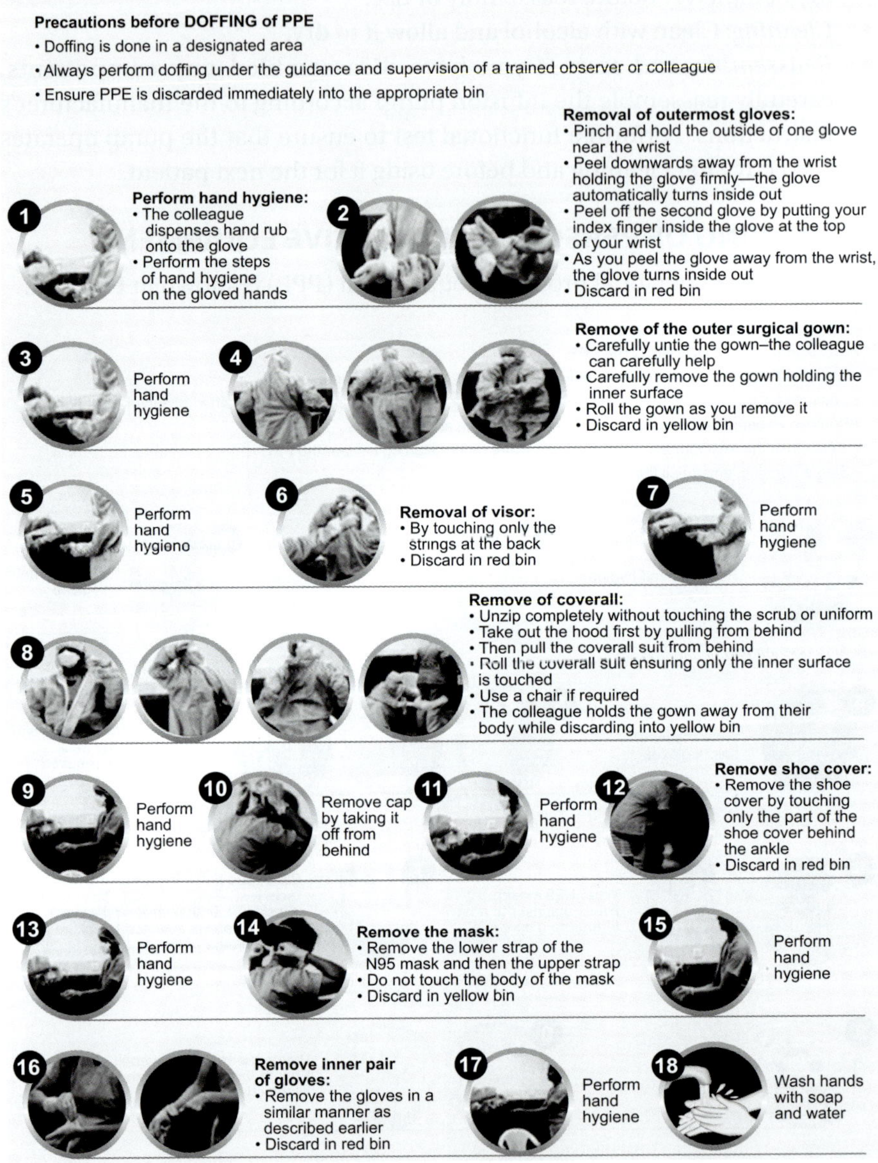

Fig. 2: Doffing of personal protective equipment (PPE) *(For color version, see Plate 2)*.

INFECTION CONTROL PROTOCOLS TO FOLLOW ON EXTRACORPOREAL MEMBRANE OXYGENATION

Patients on extracorporeal membrane oxygenation (ECMO) for prolonged duration are at high chances for nosocomial infection; hence, we have to follow the infection control protocols from day 1 of ECMO.[6,7]

- Follow strict aseptic precautions and bundles as per the hospital policy while cannulation of ECMO.
- Maintain sterility by following postinsertion care bundles.
- Do check complete blood count (CBC), C-reactive protein (CRP), procalcitonin (PCT), and blood cultures as and when required.

Bundles:[8-10]

- Hand hygiene before procedure
- Skin antisepsis with chlorhexidine
- Use a sterile technique during the procedure.
- Cover the ultrasonography machine with a sterile camera cover.
- Cover peripheral cannulas with chlorhexidine-impregnated bandages.
- Hand hygiene before touching cannula, hub, and ECMO circuit
- Change the ECMO dressing under all aseptic precaution (AAP).
- Use of antibiotic as per the patient's clinical condition and risk factor
- Follow the hospital antibiotic stewardship.
- Find a definitive solution for the patient's condition.
- Remove the ECMO as early as possible.

CONCLUSION

A good team work and a multidisciplinary approach to prevent infection and to reduce hospital acquired infection plays an crucial role in critical ill patient. Making a protocol and implementation of it will definitely improve the patient's outcomes and will decrease mortality in ICU. We should increase the adaptability to follow protocols in day-to-day practice which eventually evolve the health care system for better outcome the continuous education and training for all health care workers should be continued on regular basis.

REFERENCES

1. Koenig SM, Truwit JD. Ventilator-associated pneumonia: diagnosis, treatment, and prevention. Clin Microbiol Rev. 2006;19(4):637-57.
2. Haddadin Y, Annamaraju P, Regunath H. Central Line–Associated Blood Stream Infections. In: StatPearls [Internet]. Treasure Island (FL): StatPearls Publishing; 2025.
3. National Healthcare Safety Network (NHSN). Surgical Site Infection (SSI) Events. [online] Available from https://www.cdc.gov/nhsn/psc/ssi/index.html
4. Keely Boyle K, Rachala S, Nodzo SR. Centers for Disease Control and Prevention 2017 Guidelines for Prevention of Surgical Site Infections: Review and Relevant Recommendations. Curr Rev Musculoskelet Med. 2018;11(3):357-69.

5. Garvey M. Medical Device-Associated Healthcare Infections: Sterilization and the Potential of Novel Biological Approaches to Ensure Patient Safety. Int J Mol Sci. 2023;25(1):201.
6. Fartoukh M, Maitre B, Honoré S, Cerf C, Zahar JR, Brun-Buisson C. Diagnosing pneumonia during mechanical ventilation: the clinical pulmonary infection score revisited. Am J Respir Crit Care Med. 2003;168(2):173-9.
7. Klompas M, Branson R, Cawcutt K, Crist M, Eichenwald EC, Greene LR, et al. Strategies to prevent ventilator-associated pneumonia, ventilator-associated events, and nonventilator hospital-acquired pneumonia in acute-care hospitals: 2022 Update. Infect Control Hosp Epidemiol. 2022;43(6):687-713.
8. Patel PK, Advani SD, Kofman AD, Lo E, Maragakis LL, Pegues DA, et al. Strategies to prevent catheter-associated urinary tract infections in acute-care hospitals: 2022 Update. Infect Control Hosp Epidemiol. 2023;44(8):1209-31.
9. Richard VS, Kanchi M. A Practical Guide to a Safe Sequence of Donning and Doffing of Personal Protective Equipment in Relation to COVID-19. Journal of Cardiac Critical Care TSS. 2020;4(1):61-3.
10. Vazquez-Colon Z, Marcus JE, Levy E, Shah A, MacLaren G, Peek G. Infectious diseases and infection control prevention strategies in adult and pediatric population on ECMO. Perfusion. 2025;40(1_suppl):6S-14S.

Index

Page numbers followed by *b* refer to box, *f* refer to figure, *fc* refer to flowchart, and *t* refer to table.

A

D

J

K

L